P9-BAT-468

FITNESS
the new wave

THIRD EDITION

Roberta Stokes
Alan C. Moore
Clancy Moore
Sandra L. Schultz

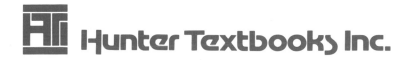

Hunter Textbooks Inc.

Copyright 1992 by Hunter Textbooks Inc.

ISBN 0-88725-170-6

All rights reserved. No part of this publication may be reproduced in any form or by any means including electronic, mechanical, photocopying, or recording without the prior permission of the publisher.

Inquiries should be addressed to the publisher:

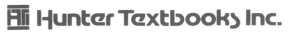 **Hunter Textbooks Inc.**

823 Reynolda Road
Winston-Salem, North Carolina 27104

Contents

1. Your Fitness 1

2. Analyzing Your Physical Fitness 11

3. Guidelines for Your Training Program 22

4. Selecting Your Fitness Program 35

5. Knowing Your Nutrition 75

6. Controlling Your Weight..110

7. Exercise and Your Cardiovascular System....................124

8. Your Respiratory System...144

9. Your Muscular System...156

10. Handling Stress 165

11. Special Concerns about Exercise and Fitness 175

12. Consumer Beware! 194

Glossary 199

Appendix A...207

Appendix B...229

Appendix C...249

Appendix D...261

Laboratory Exercises 267

Preface

Attainment of one's optimal level of health and physical fitness is truly the new wave sweeping across the United States. The average modern man or woman seems satisfied with reaching minimal standards rather than the highest or "optimal" level of health. Our error in the past has been in believing that a "normal" finding implied health. We now understand that these normal values or ranges are suspect because they have been based on studies of presumed healthy Americans, and the population has a high incidence of obesity, hypertension, smoking, a poor level of physical fitness, and a diet that leads to the development of cardiovascular heart disease. Therefore, only optimal standards can provide assurance of the highest level of health and establish goals for which individuals can aim.

The material presented in this book provides a scientific basis for the development and practice of lifetime exercise and a healthier lifestyle. The program is based on a rationale of testing and analysis and the concept that when students understand the values of exercise and the impact on their lifestyles, they will make wiser choices in planning a lifetime exercise program for a healthier life.

This new edition contains updated information about several topics: the latest nutrition research; charts on diet plans, fat and sugar substitutes; new exercise programs such as step aerobics; and additional stress reduction ideas. A new chapter on special concerns includes information about HIV/AIDS, osteoporosis, steroids, cancer, and low back exercises.

Throughout the text, new photographs and diagrams, as well as chapter objectives and key words, will help the reader gain understanding about the concepts presented. A glossary and new labs have also been added.

The authors believe that the information in this text can assist students in their quest for optimal health and fitness.

Acknowledgments

The authors of this book gratefully acknowledge the many suggestions and insights rendered by their colleagues. Special credit is given to the Health Analysis and Improvement instructors at Miami-Dade Community College and the staff of the University of Florida for their contributions to various portions of the text. Suggestions received from students and instructors using the text have also proved extremely valuable to us in maintaining a top-notch publication.

To the Reader:
The Decision is Yours

Maintaining personal health is largely a matter of individual initiative. In the United States we do not yet have a comprehensive system of truly preventive health care. Yet many of the health problems we develop result, to a large degree, from things which are under our own control—things we can do something about. The evidence is becoming clear that how we live determines to a great extent how long we live and how well we live. The decision to be healthy and fit is within our grasp. We must establish a lifestyle which enables us to achieve our highest potential for well being.

If we are to achieve optimal health, we cannot continue to maintain the attitude that we can abuse and neglect our bodies and then prescribe medicine to correct the damage. We don't want to watch our weight, find time for exercise, give up smoking, or limit our drinking. We want good health but only on our terms.

It is also difficult to persuade individuals to make these lifestyle changes when they are currently feeling "okay"—when the real benefits are long-term and not immediately noticeable. The human body is able to absorb large amounts of abuse and neglect without any overt signs of harm for many years, and this misleads people into thinking that what they are doing is all right. Most people seem to think there is time enough tomorrow to make these changes. Unfortunately, by the time tomorrow arrives it may be too late.

The evidence now indicates that the vast majority of deaths due to cardiovascular disease are "premature" since they occur in relatively young individuals. These deaths are clearly connected to negative lifestyles and habits related to exercise, diet, smoking, and stress. Many have called these the diseases of choice because they relate to the way we choose to live our lives. We each make personal choices that contribute to these early diseases and death. This lifestyle not only shortens life but, more importantly, it deprives each of us of maximum daily enjoyment and productivity.

Our goal is to help you achieve your optimal health. What is important is the quality of each day of your life. The goal is to feel the best you have ever felt in your life *now,* not just the distant future. It will take action and sacrifice on your part to improve your lifestyle. We can't guarantee you will live one day longer, but we can guarantee you a healthier, happier, and more productive life.

How important is health to you? Is your lifestyle worth dying for? The choice is yours!

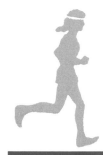

Your Fitness

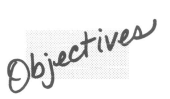

Objectives

- Describe the elements of health, wellness, and fitness
- Describe the benefits of physical exercise
- Describe the importance of lifestyle to health and fitness
- Describe the factors influencing fitness
- Define and describe health-related fitness
- Define and describe skill-related fitness
- Describe the health risk factors
- Describe the role of heredity, environment, and behavior in achieving fitness

Key Words

- Agility
- Balance
- Behavior
- Body composition
- Cardiovascular fitness
- Coordination
- Environment
- Flexibility
- Health-related fitness
- Heredity
- Muscular endurance
- Muscular strength
- Power
- Reaction time
- Risk factors
- Skill-related fitness
- Speed
- Wellness

Life is definitely a matter of balance, a matter of choice. The key to attaining an optimal level of health and fitness is a change in lifestyle. Our modern lifestyle contributes to our unfitness, but we can make choices in regard to exercise, smoking, diet, drugs, alcohol, and control of stress.

It is important that such changes in lifestyle be adopted and initiated as early in life as possible. Evidence shows that we can affect our chances of a longer life at almost any time in our lives, but the earlier we start, the better the chances of cutting our risks.

How Healthy Are You?

Most people when asked this question respond on the basis of whether or not they are sick—in other words, whether they have an illness or disease. However, true health should be evaluated in terms of a dynamic state of overall well-being—**a state of wellness.** For wellness refers to a lifestyle that enables you to live life to its fullest—to achieve full potential in all areas of your life. Wellness, therefore, includes all aspects of what has been previously referred to as total fitness—the physiological, the psychological, and the sociological well-being of an individual.

Achieving a state of wellness means taking responsibility for your own health and well being. It means:

- *learning* what it takes to achieve a high level of health.
- *taking control* of your health by practicing good health habits and avoiding harmful ones.

- reacting to the *warning signals* before problems become serious.

Those who are dedicated to a life of "wellness" are typically those who:

- Exercise regularly.
- Eat nutritional meals and maintain proper weight.
- Do not smoke, use drugs, or use alcohol to cope with life.
- Manage the stresses of life.
- Get adequate rest and sleep.
- Participate in some sort of recreational activity.
- Maintain a positive, optimistic outlook on life.
- Have identified personal goals.

These individuals are the ones you meet who seem to have endless energy; have fulfilling, constructive relationships; who handle stress well; who have a high resistance to illness; and who seem to get more enjoyment from all aspects of their lives (home, family, work, etc.).

Wellness consists of three major components: physical, social, and psychological. Each of these areas needs to be at an optimal level if a high level of wellness is to be achieved. Each is interrelated and dependent on the others. Actually wellness (and fitness and health) are part of a continuum—each of us has some degree of wellness. For instance, some of us may have a high level of physical fitness but do not have satisfactory interpersonal relationships. Individuals need to work for higher health levels in all the components for complete wellness.

The Wellness Continuum

Life Threatening Illness	Health Breakdown	No Obvious Illness	High Level Wellness
Bedridden or Unable to Function	Temporarily Incapacitated	Sporadic Efforts Toward Better Health	Committed to a Program of Healthy Living

TOTAL FITNESS OR WELLNESS

Total fitness has been defined by numerous authors in various ways. However, the expression "being able to live most and serve best" seems to express the concept as well as any.

Factors Influencing Your Fitness

You should assess the changes you are required to make in order to achieve the level of fitness you desire. In identifying your goals it is important to realize that three factors influence not only your current level of fitness but the potential level you can achieve: heredity, environment, and behavior.

Heredity. Each of us is born with certain strengths and certain weaknesses which determine to some extent our size, intelligence, personality, and many other things which make us what we are. It may be said that **heredity sets limits on our potential.**

Environment. Numerous group studies have graphically reflected the tremendous effect of one's environment on the potential and total well-being of an individual. Recent legislation which attempts to equalize educational and economical opportunities has done much to neutralize this powerful force. Even so, it still must be said that **environment limits the opportunities which may be available.**

Behavior. In the last analysis, total fitness will probably be determined by one's behavior. It is certain that some people might have everything going for them (i.e., good hereditary factors, the best environment) and yet, because of unwise behavior, place in jeopardy the future well-being of

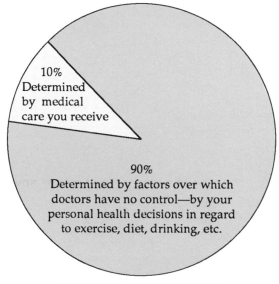

FACTORS DETERMINING YOUR HEALTH

themselves and their children. One example might be the effect of smoking or alcohol abuse on the unborn fetus by an expectant mother.

It is fairly clear that while each aspect of total fitness plays a unique role in well-being, it is equally true that **each aspect influences the others and they are interrelated in very complex ways.** In summary, then, of the factors influencing your total fitness, behavior is the only one totally within your control.

In the following chapters you will find information to guide you in making key lifestyle changes which will assist you in achieving total fitness or wellness. While the emphasis in this text is on the health-related concepts of fitness, nutrition, weight control, and stress management, we hope you realize the importance of setting wellness goals in the other areas:

- job satisfaction.
- relationships: family/social.
- recreational activities.
- emotional, psychological, spiritual life.

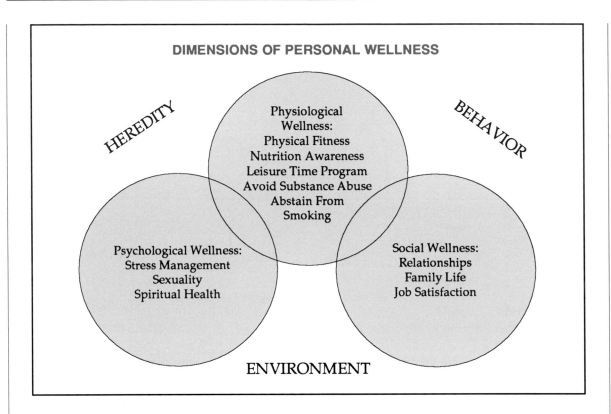

DIMENSIONS OF PERSONAL WELLNESS

HEREDITY

BEHAVIOR

Physiological
Wellness:
Physical Fitness
Nutrition Awareness
Leisure Time Program
Avoid Substance Abuse
Abstain From
Smoking

Psychological Wellness:
Stress Management
Sexuality
Spiritual Health

Social Wellness:
Relationships
Family Life
Job Satisfaction

ENVIRONMENT

HEALTH RISK FACTORS

In addition to striving to reach the optimal standards of health and fitness, you can significantly influence your future health and life expectancy by controlling the primary risk factors associated with disease, disability or premature death. The removal or reduction of even one personal risk factor can generally reduce the threat of several diseases. The most commonly identified risk factors are **heredity, inactivity, obesity, high blood pressure, smoking, stress, high levels of cholesterol, diabetes,** and **gender.**

In determining one's probability for developing a disease or developing a health problem, it is common to refer to one's "risk" and specific "risk factors." In the case of coronary heart disease, many of the risk factors are related to lifestyle health habits.

The primary and secondary risk factors most commonly identified for coronary heart disease are:

Primary Risk Factors
Cigarette smoking
Hypertension
Elevated blood cholesterol

Secondary Risk Factors
Obesity
Pulmonary function abnormalities
Diabetes
High uric acid levels
Sedentary lifestyle
Family history (heredity)
High stress lifestyle
Age
Sex
Race

Lab 2 (in the back of the book) will help you assess your overall risk and consider lifestyle changes you should pursue.

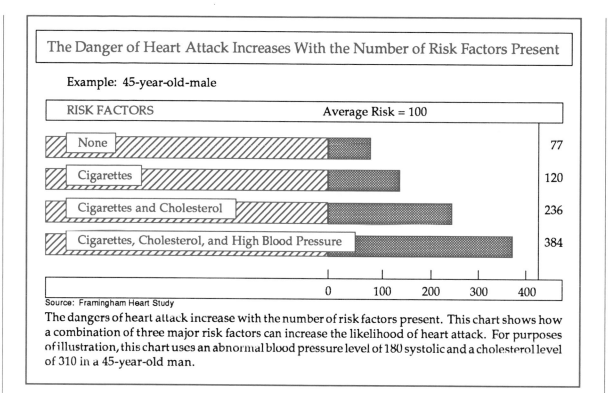

The Danger of Heart Attack Increases With the Number of Risk Factors Present

Example: 45-year-old-male

RISK FACTORS	Average Risk = 100	
None		77
Cigarettes		120
Cigarettes and Cholesterol		236
Cigarettes, Cholesterol, and High Blood Pressure		384

0   100   200   300   400

Source: Framingham Heart Study

The dangers of heart attack increase with the number of risk factors present. This chart shows how a combination of three major risk factors can increase the likelihood of heart attack. For purposes of illustration, this chart uses an abnormal blood pressure level of 180 systolic and a cholesterol level of 310 in a 45-year-old man.

THE CASE FOR EXERCISE

A significant study published November 1989 in the *Journal of the American Medical Association* reported that even a minimal amount of exercise—a brisk half-hour walk once a day— is enough to provide significant protection not only from cardiovascular disease and cancers but also against a number of other diseases. In short, the study states that people who exercise just a little bit tend to live longer. The study, which involved 13,344 men and women, was conducted at the Institute for Aerobics Research in Dallas and evaluated participants for an average of eight years.

There is now clear evidence to support the important role of exercise in the development of a lifestyle of wellness. Although research indicates significant gains in the reduction of the mortality rates attributed to cardiovascular heart disease, heart attacks continue to be the number one cause of death in the United States with over 550,000 fatalities each year. Each year about 1,500,000 people have heart attacks. Also, according to data from the Framingham, Massachusetts Heart Epidemiology Study, which evaluated 2,282 middle-aged men over a ten-year period, approximately 45% of all male heart attack victims were less than 65 years of age and about 5% were under 40 years of age.

It is estimated that more than 95% of all movement used to produce goods is now mechanical rather than human. It is little wonder that this drastic change in lifestyle has produced a nation of people who are experiencing a wide assortment of physiological and psychological problems. Many of these problems are directly related to body image and lack of self-concept brought on by limited movement and physical deterioration.

Premature death costs American industry billions of dollars each year. This cost and the fact that health care costs have increased more than twice the rate of inflation have caused American businesses and industries to reassess practices and to organize Employee Fitness/Wellness programs. Some of their results have been impressive.

Obesity has long been a major American health problem. It is estimated that nearly half of the American public is obese as defined by the Metropolitan Life Insurance Company, which has been gathering this type of data for more than fifty years. (2)

From a psychological viewpoint, W. C. Meninger, Director of the famous Meninger Clinic, has stated, "There is a direct correlation between good mental health and the capacity and willingness to play." (1)

Increased pressures brought about by density in population and the complexities of our modern civilization are exacting a tremendous toll from the American people. As one example of the inability of people to adjust, we have doctors reporting that approximately seventy percent of the pseudo-physical ailments which they see are really illnesses that are psychosomatic in origin. (5) *Among college students, suicide ranks second (after accidents) as the leading cause of death.*

Most physical educators and sociologist believe that exercise and play offer valuable resources for the cultivation and retention of good mental health. It is certain that basic psychological needs such as status, security, affection and independence can be fostered through wise choice of activities. Physical fitness and exercise also contribute to psychological well-being by providing a mental and emotional release of tension and frustration brought on by life's daily problems.

Harry Truman, one of our more colorful presidents, had a small wooden sign on his desk which read, "The Buck Stops Here." In a like manner, the ultimate decision as to whether you achieve and maintain a state of physical fitness rests with you.

It is the purpose of this book to provide factual information and to challenge you so that you are able to make intelligent decisions concerning the role of exercise in your daily lives. In this case "The Buck Stops With You." What are you going to do?

WHAT IS PHYSICAL FITNESS?

Physical fitness means different things to different people. Obviously there is a vast degree of difference in the level and kinds of fitness required by the highly trained athlete as compared to the average person in our society. However, physical fitness is not only one of the most important keys to a healthy body, it is the basis of dynamic and creative intellectual activity. The relationship between the soundness of the body and activities of the mind is subtle and complex. Much is not yet understood, but we do know what the Greeks knew, that intelligence and skill can only function at the peak of their capacity when the body is healthy and strong. As President John F. Kennedy once said, "Hardy spirits and tough minds usually inhabit sound bodies."

Physical fitness, then, is one aspect of total fitness, which includes the social, mental and emotional makeup of each individual. Since physical fitness is composed of several elements, we must develop a fitness profile utilizing various test batteries to accurately measure this elusive component. The components of physical fitness are generally classified into two groups: health-related and skill-related.

The following information is presented to assist you in developing your personal concept of physical fitness, and to aid you in understanding the various parameters of physical fitness.

Health-related Components

Health-related components are those qualities which are more important to a person's health, as contrasted to the ability to perform specific motor tasks. Achievement of an optimal level of health-related physical fitness indicates the ability to perform daily activities with vigor and capacities that are associated with low risk of premature development of diseases associated with physical inactivity (hypokinetic disease).

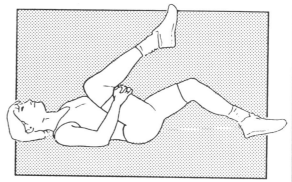

Flexibility: The functional capacity of a joint to move through a normal range of motion. The muscular system is also involved.

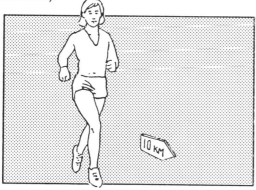

Cardiovascular Endurance: The ability of the body to persist in strenuous tasks over a prolonged period of time.

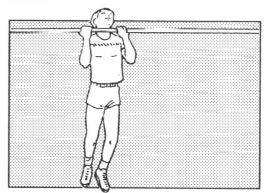

Muscular Endurance: The ability to continue selected muscle group movements for prolonged periods of time.

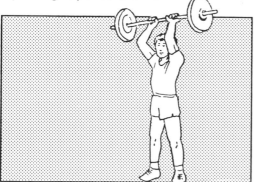

Muscular Strength: The ability of a muscle group to contract against a resistance.

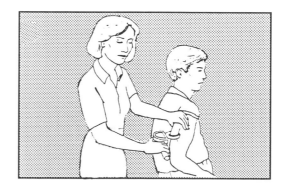

Body Composition: One of the newer attributes to be included as a component of physical fitness, this term refers to the relative distribution of lean and fat body tissue.

Skill-related Components

Skill-related components are those qualities which enable a person to perform motor tasks.

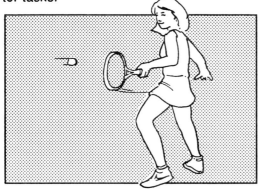

Coordination: The ability to integrate the senses with the muscles so as to produce accurate, smooth, and harmonious body movement.

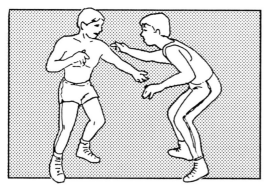

Agility: The capacity to change direction of the body quickly and effectively.

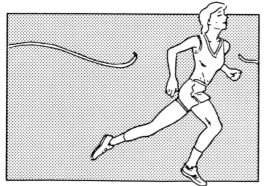

Speed: The ability to move one's body from one point to another.

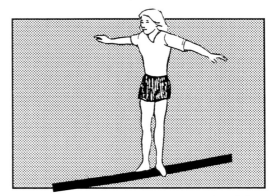

Balance: A kind of coordination involving vision, reflexes, and the skeletal muscular system which provides the maintenance of equilibrium.

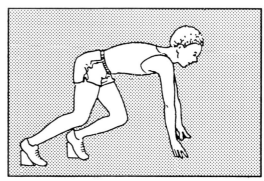

Reaction Time: The time required to respond or initiate a movement as a result of a given stimulus.

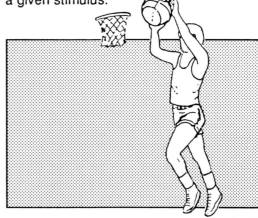

Power: Power is sometimes confused with strength; however, speed of contraction is the basic ingredient which, when combined with strength, provides an explosive type of movement.

QUESTIONS AND ANSWERS

Is there a point in life when it is too late to begin an exercise program?

Mrs. Eula Weaver didn't think so. At age 65, she was treated for angina (a heart disease); at age 75, she was hospitalized with a severe attack of angina; and at age 81, she experienced congestive heart failure and suffered from hypertension and arthritis.

When she began her exercise plan of diet and walking at age 81, her condition was so poor she was able to walk only 100 feet without rest, and the circulation in her hands was so impaired that she had to wear gloves to keep them warm even in the summer. A year after beginning her program, Mrs. Weaver was asymptomatic and no longer required medication.

At age 85, after four years of training, Mrs. Weaver won two gold medals in the Senior Olympics. Her events—the half-mile and the mile! A year and a half later, she duplicated the effort. Mrs. Weaver's daily routine involved running one mile and riding a stationary bicycle 10-15 miles. (3)

Approximately 42% of the runners who finished the 1989 New York Marathon were over the age of 40 and 56 of the finishing runners were over age 70. The oldest finisher of the 26 mile race was 91 years old. His time? A mere six hours and forty-three minutes.

Does exercise slow the aging process?

It is now recognized that many problems long attributed to aging are, in fact, infirmities that could be avoided if people would only be more active.

The list of infirmities includes reduced muscle strength, shortness of breath, slowed reflexes, soft bones, stiffness, se-nility and a double chin. We now know one can limit these "symptoms of aging" by one of the most natural of activities—walking. Exercise makes us breathe and thus increases the oxygenation process at the molecular level. After age 20, we process an average of one percent less oxygen every year. The result of this cutback is a commensurate decline in cellular activity. In reality, our bodies begin to suffocate. Studies have shown that people who remain active as they grow older can maintain breathing capacities equal to people 40 years their junior.

The human body responds to physical stress by adapting and growing stronger. Heart and lungs don't get tired as we get older; they get lazy. Bones respond to environmental stress (exercise) accordingly. As bones are stressed by muscular contraction and compressional impacts of exercise, they respond by taking on more calcium and phosphorus—getting thicker, denser, and stronger as a result.

The skin becomes thicker, stronger, and more elastic as a result of good oxygen uptake capacity. Skin reflects an adaptation to habitual endurance training by increasing its mass and strengthening its structure.

Exercise seems to strengthen nerve tissue in about the same manner as it does muscles. The increased enzyme activity and abundant blood flow caused by exercise appear to safeguard the overall health of the central nervous system—the brain included.

Can exercise increase the body's defense against disease?

A lot of people think so. Let's look at what happens when an infectious agent enters the human system. White blood cells are soon triggered which surround and destroy the bacteria; however, something else also happens. The cells release protein which travels in the blood to the brain triggering an increase in body temperature (fever). This creates an environment in which bacteria cannot reproduce. Also, the blood level of iron is decreased, and bacteria must have iron to thrive.

Many studies have indicated that aerobic exercise increases the number of white blood cells in the body, and secondary exercise elevates the body temperature for a period of time.

Dr. Kenneth Cooper, noted aerobics authority, tends to think that regular exercise may produce a "pasteurizing effect" on the blood. (2) Before you go off full-tilt, however, remember that *excessive* exercise leading to chronic fatigue may make you more prone to infectious disease. So remember Socrates' proverb, "Moderacy in all things."

Does education contribute to improved physical fitness?

Most people think so, and that is the reason for this course. For instance, research has indicated the following:

1. In the late 1960s, doctors were dis-covering and controlling only 10-15% of high blood pressure cases. By the 1990s, this percentage has increased to more than 50%.

2. In the 1960s, middle-aged men had average cholesterol levels of 245-250. By the 1990s, this level had dropped to 210-215.

3. In the early 1960s, about 24% of adults were exercising regularly. Recent studies indicate that now two-thirds of all adults exercise regularly.

4. And finally, in 1964 more than 50% of Americans smoked cigarettes. That figure is now less than 33%.

In summary, education does make a difference, and the earlier you start the better chance you have of living a healthy, productive life.

Unfortunately, education is not an "instant" process—it does take time—so "hang in there" as you go through the course. You will come out of the experience knowing more about what you need to do to maintain a lifetime of fitness; you will be more physically fit; and more important, you will feel better about yourself. Good luck in your search for the "good life."

REFERENCES
1. AAHPERD, "Quotes and Facts Supporting Comprehensive Programs of HPER." Washington, D.C.
2. *Aerobics.* The Aerobics Center. Dallas, Texas. May/June 1983.
3. Allsen, P. et al., *Fitness for Life,* Dubuque: William C. Brown Co., 1989.
4. Armstrong, L. H. "Is Fluid Intake Important in the Control of Body Temperature?" *National Strength and Conditioning Journal,* Vol. 13, Number 1, 1991.
5. *Military Medicine,* Vol. 152, June 1987.

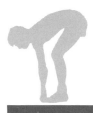

Analyzing Your Physical Fitness

Objectives

- Discuss who should have a medical exam before beginning an exercise program
- Describe the elements of physical fitness: cardiovascular endurance, body composition, flexibility, muscular fitness
- Discuss the tests for cardiovascular endurance: 1 mile walking test, bicycle ergometer test, 12 minute run/1.5 mile test, Harvard Step test, 1 minute step test, resting heart rate, lung capacity, and blood pressure
- Explain tests to evaluate body composition
- List and explain tests to evaluate flexibility
- Explain tests to evaluate muscular fitness

Key Words

- Bicycle ergometer
- Blood pressure
- Body mass index
- Cardiovascular endurance
- Cholesterol
- Diastolic
- Electrical impedance
- Flexibility
- Hypertension
- Maximal oxygen uptake
- Muscular endurance
- Muscular fitness
- Resting heart rate
- Skinfold caliper
- Sphygmomanometer
- Spirometer
- Strength
- Systolic
- Vital lung capacity

11

The Medical Examination

The best way to determine your physical condition is a thorough medical examination. The medical examination by a physician can identify areas requiring special attention as well as provide guidance in establishing a fitness program.

Before attempting to establish an individual physical fitness program, you should have some idea of your current level of fitness. By measuring your initial status of fitness, you can determine your needs accurately and design a sound and safe plan for achieving them. The evaluation of key components of fitness can provide you with important information as to your current physical condition and also serve as a basis for setting personal goals. Such an evaluation will prove extremely beneficial as a basis for measuring improvement and determining the effectiveness of your training program.

Following are several tests and activities which provide valuable information to help you analyze your physical fitness profile.

According to the American College of Sports Medicine, **apparently healthy** individuals can begin **moderate** exercise programs such as walking or increasing normal daily activities without the need for exercise testing or a medical examination. The exercise should proceed gradually and should be within the individual's capacity so that he/she can sustain it for a prolonged period (up to 60 minutes).

Individuals at or **above age 40 in men or age 50 in women**, should have a medical examination and a maximal exercise test before beginning a **vigorous** exercise program. A vigorous exercise is intense enough to present a substantial challenge and result in significant increases in heart rate and respiration. Usually this type of exercise cannot be sustained by untrained individuals for more than 15-20 minutes. However, a medical exam is not necessary if the person begins with a moderate intensity exercise program and gradually builds on it.

A medical examination before beginning an exercise program is indicated for **anyone** who has two or more of the major **coronary risk** factors:

- Diagnosed hypertension or systolic **blood pressure** greater than **160** or diastolic blood pressure greater than **90** on at least two separate occasions or someone on **antihypertensive** medication
- Serum **cholesterol** greater than **240**
- Cigarette **smoking**
- **Diabetes** mellitus
- **Family history** of coronary or other atherosclerotic disease in parents or siblings prior to age 55

The Pre-Participation Health Questionnaire and Consent Form

Participants may be asked to complete a self-evaluation of their current health status and a review of family history before taking part in an organized activity program. This evaluation will assist the exercise leader in identifying and excluding individuals with medical contraindications to exercise and those who may have special needs for safe exercise (i.e., the elderly and pregnant women). A sample health questionnaire is included in this book on page 269. All participants may also be asked to complete a consent form before participating in activities. This form indicates an awareness of the activities being planned and verification that to one's knowledge he or she is capable of safely participating in them.

SUGGESTED HEALTH SCREENING TESTS

Blood Pressure

If you have had a complete physical examination, your blood pressure was checked. The procedure involves wrapping an inflatable cuff on your arm and pumping enough air into the cuff to temporarily cut off circulation with a device called a **sphygmomanometer.** Then the pressure is slowly released so that the blood begins to flow. Your blood pressure is recorded in two numbers and is measured in millimeters of mercury. The first number recorded is called the **systolic** pressure and is your blood pressure at the moment blood is ejected from the heart. The second number is the **diastolic** pressure and represents the blood pressure between beats when the heart is relaxed. The acceptable range for your blood pressure is stated as 120-140 for systolic and 70-90 for diastolic. Generally blood pressure will rise with either an increase in cardiac output or with an increase in resistance to blood flow.

Of course, physical activity requires your heart to pump more blood. If you are not in good physical condition, there may be a sharp rise in both systolic and diastolic pressure. As your physical fitness improves there will be a smaller rise in the blood pressure. As a matter of fact, highly trained endurance athletes may have no significant increase in diastolic pressure or it may be a little lower during sustained vigorous exercise than at rest.

Even though the blood pressure may go up and down within a limited range during exercise, if it starts high and stays high during rest, it is called **hypertension**. Many people with moderately elevated blood pressure can significantly lower this pressure by altering their lifestyle. In any case,

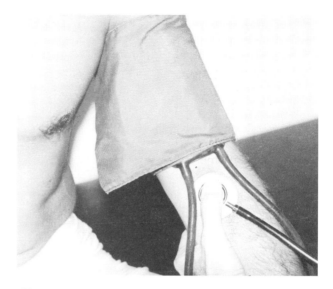

Blood pressure is taken with a sphygmomanometer.

you should definitely know what your blood pressure level is, the factors affecting it, and what you can do to control it. See Appendix A-9 concerning specific directions for measurement and Appendix B-1 for classification levels for blood pressure. Additional information on blood pressure can be found in Chapter 7.

Resting Heart Rate

Each time the heart beats a wave is initiated that travels throughout the arterial system. This is commonly referred to as the pulse or heart rate. This pulse can be felt wherever a large artery lies near the surface of the skin. One's pulse rate changes throughout the day. It is lowest after one sleeps for six or more hours. When one awakens, the heart rate generally increases 5-10 beats and then increases another 5-10 beats during the day.

How high the heart rate is when you are at rest is one other indication of your heart's condition. The best measure of resting heart rate is determined by taking the pulse for one minute just after waking in the morning and while in a sitting position.

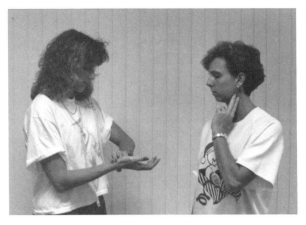

The pulse can be felt wherever a large artery lies near the surface of the skin.

The American Heart Association identifies the normal range for resting heart rate as between 50-100. However, a resting heart rate above 80 beats per minute puts a person in a higher risk category for heart attack. Such a high rate indicates a potential underlying problem. A high rate may be the result of cigarette smoking, too much coffee, anxiety, an overactive thyroid, or more commonly, a poor level of general physical fitness. In addition, we know that those who develop high levels of cardiovascular endurance often have resting heart rates below 50 beats per minute.

The resting pulse rate will go down gradually in response to a program of regular endurance activities. By keeping a record of your resting heart rate, you can follow the progress being achieved through your fitness training program. See Appendix B-1 for classification levels for resting heart rate.

The Blood Cholesterol Test

(Note: See Chapter 7 for a complete explanation of cholesterol.)

Cholesterol is one of the fat-like substances transported in the blood. When there is too much cholesterol in your bloodstream, it can become trapped in the walls of your coronary arteries and increase your chances of getting heart disease. A high cholesterol level may put you at greater risk for participating in an exercise program and therefore it is important you understand the test and consider whether you need to be tested.

If you are over 20 years of age and you have never had a blood cholesterol test you should have one. Those with a family history of heart disease or high blood fats should discuss with their doctor the need for a test earlier than age 20.

The cholesterol blood test will measure several factors:

- Total cholesterol—all the cholesterol that is in your blood. It is reported in milligrams of cholesterol per deciliter of blood—about 1/10 of a quart.
- LDL Cholesterol Level (low-density lipoprotein cholesterol)—the amount of cholesterol being transported in the blood that promotes the formation of plaque on the walls of the arteries.
- HDL Cholesterol Level (high-density lipoprotein cholesterol)—the amount of cholesterol being transported in the blood that protects against plaque formation.
- Total Cholesterol/HDL Ratio—the amount of total cholesterol divided by the HDL amount.
- Total Triglycerides—the amount of blood fats (indicates how much fat is being formed in the liver from the fats you eat or from the body's synthesis of internal fat).

In order to have your blood cholesterol measured, a simple blood analysis is done by a reputable lab. Due to the variations found in some blood test results, it is recommended you use a lab certified by the College of American Pathologists or one that uses standards established by the Lipid Research Clinics. A simple screening test which is being used in some situations is the "finger-stick" test. This test can provide a fairly accurate measure of one's total cholesterol if conducted accurately by trained personnel. Its primary use is as a preliminary screening test to encourage those with high levels to seek a full blood test by a lab.

Once you have the results of a blood test, the tables below will help you evaluate your risk and need for further testing, dietary changes, or additional medical advice.

Total Blood Cholesterol

Age	Recommended	Borderline-High Risk	High Risk
Less than 20	Less than 180 mg/dl		
20 or above	Under 200 mg/dl	200-239	240 or above

LDL Cholesterol Level*

Below 130	Desirable
130-159	Borderline High
160 or greater	High risk

*From the National Cholesterol Education Program

HDL Cholesterol Level*

	Men**	Women
Very low risk (1/2 aver.)	over 65	over 75
Low risk	55	65
Average risk	45	55
Moderate risk (2 times aver.)	25	40
High risk (3+ times aver.)	under 25	under 40

*From the Framingham Study
**Male sex hormones tend to decrease HDL, while female hormones have the opposite effect. After menopause, however, a woman's HDL cholesterol does generally begin to fall.

Total Cholesterol/HDL Cholesterol Ratio

Risk	Men	Women
Very low (1/2 aver.)	under 3.4	under 3.3
Low risk	4.0	3.8
Average risk	5.0	4.5
Moderate risk (2 times aver.)	9.5	7.0
High risk (3+ times aver.)	over 23	over 11

*From the Framingham Study

Triglycerides Level

Risk	Level
Low	less than 100
Average	120
High risk	200 or more

Lung Capacity

Vital lung capacity is a measurement of the maximum amount of air that can be expired after a maximum inspiration. This test can serve as an excellent screening device for determining the condition of the lungs and whether any airway obstruction is present. The test is performed by having the subject inhale as deeply as possible and then exhale forcefully and completely into a device called a spirometer. See Appendix A-5 for methods of calculating normal vital capacity and Appendix B-1 for standards to compare results.

HEALTH-RELATED FITNESS TESTS

Cardiovascular Endurance

Cardiovascular endurance is a measure of ability of the heart to pump blood, of the lungs to breathe volumes of air, and of the muscles to utilize oxygen. No matter how fit one might look, if the cardiovascular and respiratory systems cannot meet the demands of sustained activity one has a low level of fitness. Tests designed to measure cardiovascular endurance involve vigorous physical activity that make high demands on the heart and lungs. One's level of cardiovascular endurance is generally considered the most important single measure of his or her overall level of fitness because it reflects the condition of the heart, blood vessels, and lungs as well as the general condition of the muscles.

In attempting to measure your cardiovascular endurance or working capacity, the best and most accurate measure is the maximum amount of oxygen your body can utilize. The maximum oxygen consumption that you can attain measures the effective functioning of the heart, lungs, and vascular system in the delivery of oxygen during periods of heavy work. The higher the maximum oxygen consumption, the more effective the system. The following tests are excellent measures of one's cardiovascular endurance.

One-Mile Walking Test

A simple, safe test which can be used to identify a general level of fitness is a one-mile walking test. This test involves finding an area which measures one mile and walking it as quickly as possible. The time it takes to complete the walk indicates the general fitness category.

The Rockport Walking Institute has identified a complete analysis of fitness category based on time and heart rate and a suggested fitness program. See Appendix A-1 for these charts.

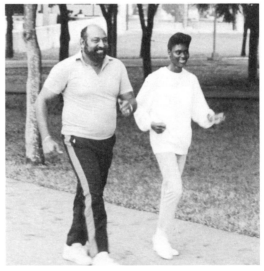

A one-mile walking test can help you determine your level of fitness.

One-Mile Run Test

Another test of cardiovascular endurance which can be used when a group includes individuals who are at the walking level as

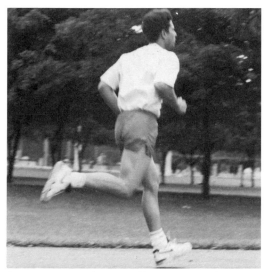

Joggers can use the one-mile run test to determine levels of fitness.

well as joggers is the one mile run test. Both groups can be timed with walkers using the Rockport Walking Institute scale to evaluate results (see Appendix B-2) and the runners using the one-mile run test scale. (See Appendix B-2.)

Bicycle Ergometer Test

An excellent estimate of work capacity is provided by the submaximal bicycle ergometer test. This test is performed on a special stationary bicycle which has an adjustable and precise pedaling speed and work load. The changes in heart rate are recorded each minute during a period of at least six minutes. After approximately five to six minutes, your heart rate will begin to stabilize—reach a steady state or level off. If the difference between heart rates for the fifth and sixth minutes is within five beats, then the test is completed. The average for the last two measured heart rates represents your exercise heart rate for that particular work load. Your maximal oxygen uptake (VO_2 maximum) is predicted or estimated from the exercise heart rate obtained. The higher your level of fitness, the lower your heart rate for a given work load.

Appendix A-2 contains more complete information and specific methods of predicting maximal oxygen uptake through bicycle ergometer testing. See Appendix B-2 for norms of maximum oxygen uptake.

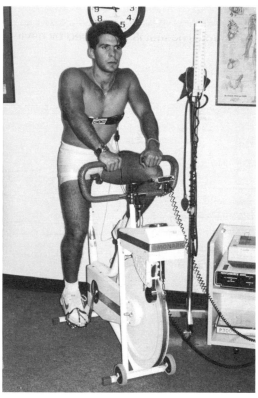

The bicycle ergometer test is an excellent way to determine fitness levels.

12 Minute Run/1.5 Mile Test

A simple test of working capacity which correlates well with laboratory measurements such as the bicycle ergometer is the 12 minute run-walk test developed by Dr. Kenneth Cooper. The test involves measuring the distance covered by running, or running and walking, for a time of 12 minutes. By evaluating the distance covered, one can be rated in terms of maximum oxygen consumption. See Appendix B-2 for prediction of maximum oxygen uptake (VO_2 Max) based on test results.

An alternate method of field testing which correlates well with maximum oxygen consumption determined from laboratory results is the 1.5 mile run test. The time it takes the individual to walk-run a distance of 1.5 miles is recorded to the nearest hundredth of a second. See Appendix B-2 for prediction of maximum oxygen uptake based on the 1.5 mile run.

Harvard Step Test

The Harvard Step Test was developed at the Harvard University Fatigue Laboratories as a relatively simple, easily administered measure of cardiovascular endurance. The test is based upon the premise that for a given work task, the person with a higher level of cardiovascular fitness will have a smaller increase in heart rate, and that following the task, heart rate will return to normal much faster than for a person who has a lower level of cardiovascular fitness. The test consists of stepping up and down on a bench or box (20 inches high for men, 16 inches for women) for five minutes at the rate of 30 times per minute or until unable to continue the exercise at the prescribed rate. The test is scored by counting the recovery pulse rate after one minute, two minutes, and three minutes of rest. Each time the pulse is counted for 30 seconds. The sum of these three pulse rates is used in calculating test results. See Appendix A-3 for specific scoring procedures and evaluation of results.

One Minute Step Test

Another method of evaluating cardiovascular fitness is by measuring heart rate recovery after a one-minute step test. Although the test is conducted in a manner similar to the Harvard Step Test, because it is shorter in duration more individuals will be able to maintain the correct cadence for the entire test. In addition, the results are based on relationship to the starting heart rate rather than an absolute norm. See Appendix A-4 for specific testing procedures and Appendix B-2 for evaluation for results.

Body Composition

A complete fitness evaluation should include various body measurements including height and weight and selected skinfold fat measurements. An accurate estimation of one's desirable body proportions and body weight can be made after such an evaluation. From the standpoint of your fitness level, the key aspect of body weight is the proportion of fat. There is a clear relationship between excess amounts of fat and low levels of physical fitness and a higher risk of cardiovascular disease.

The chief limitation of the evaluation of body weight measurement is that most tables describing "normal" weight for a particular age, height, frame size, and sex are based on "averages" taken from the general population that is not necessarily "optimal." Also, the tables are based on frame size which currently cannot be accurately determined by any reliable measure. Another major limitation of the tables is the lack of close correlation between body weight and percentage of body fat. The key factor which must be evaluated is the proportion of lean body mass to body fat.

Unfortunately, the most accurate method of measuring body fat is underwater weighing, a complicated process which requires special equipment that may not be available.

A slightly less accurate, but practical, method is the use of **skinfold caliper** measurements. By measuring the thickness of skinfolds at specific body sites (the

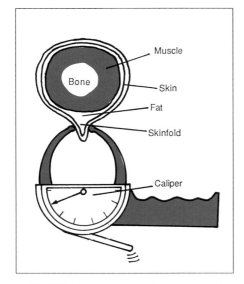

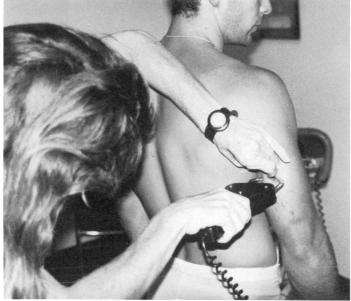

A skinfold caliper measures the amount of fat between two layers of skin.

hips, triceps, abdominals, subscapular, etc.), it is relatively easy to obtain an estimate of body fat percentage.

A new technique being used to measure body fat is an **electrical impedance** unit. These units measure the electrical resistance of the body by detecting changes in electrolyte levels. They work on the principle that lean tissue has a far greater electrolyte content than fat; therefore, the less electrical resistance measured, the more lean tissue a person has and, by inference, the less fat.

According to some authorities, water and bone content vary tremendously from person to person and affect body density independently from fat. It is also apparent that exercise (sweating), dehydration, eating, and drinking affect impedance. The readings can be totally off when the body's water compartments are high or low. Dr. Michael Pollock, a noted exercise physiologist, states that he is not certain that electrical impedance will ever match its commercial "hype" because "it overestimates lean individuals and underestimates fat people."

Electrical impedance can also be distorted by inherent differences in skin resistance. In addition, day-to-day fluctuations do not pose problems for skinfold testing as they do for electrical impedance. The standard error for electrical impedance testing thus far has been much too high. Therefore, at present, only skinfold calipers and underwater weight results are considered reproducible (and therefore scientifically valid).

The optimal range of body fat for men is between 10% and 15% and for women between 15% and 20%. Directions for measuring body fat using skinfold calipers and tables showing the percentage of body fat based on the specific measurements may be found in Appendix A-6. See Appendix B-3 for body fat evaluation.

Body Mass Index

Another valuable measure of body composition that can be done without special equipment is the Body Mass Index. Use the measure of your weight in kilograms divided by your height in meters squared (wt/ht^2). If this value is above 27.8 kg/m^2 for men or 27.3 kg/m^2 for women one is considered at an increased risk of disease or death.

Note: To calculate weight in kilograms:
Divide weight in pounds by 2.2
To calculate height in meters:
Multiply height in inches by 2.54, divide by 100

It is also important to consider where one's weight is distributed on the body. If the fat is located in the abdominal area (apple shape) rather than the extremities (pear shape), one is at greater risk. The "apple" type of fat distribution tends to be from the inside out being stored within the abdominal cavity. However, those with a "pear" shape have fat as subcutaneous fat just under the skin.

A simple measure to check this is the waist/hip ratio (measure the circumference of the waist and divide it by the circumference of the hips). A ratio over .95 for men and .85 for women significantly increases the individuals risk of disease or death.

Muscular Fitness

The term muscular fitness is used to refer to the interrelationship of strength, endurance, and flexibility in the muscles. Maintaining an optimal level of muscular fitness is particularly important in order to perform the essential daily tasks, to improve posture, and to prevent or reduce low back pain.

Muscular Strength

Strength is the ability to exert force against resistance. Although many people seem to think that strength is needed only by athletes, this is not true. The average indi-vidual would benefit greatly and be better prepared to meet the demands of everyday living if he or she had a higher level of strength.

Stronger muscles better protect the joints they cross and thus the individual is less likely to suffer strains, sprains, and pulls that sometimes occur when participating in physical activity. In addition, stronger trunk muscles aid in preventing postural problems such as round shoulders and low back pain. Persons who possess optimum levels of strength are likely to derive more satisfaction from participating in recreational sports and are less likely to experience fatigue.

An optimal level of strength is especially important in the abdominals, arm and shoulders, and hand (grip).

Measures of static strength are specific to the muscle group used and the joint angle involved during the test. These tests have limited ability to predict overall muscular strength. Other tests which can be included involve the performance of one-repetition maximum using weights (i.e., the maximum amount one can lift in one bench press, one leg press, etc.). These tests should be performed carefully following a warmup and using a gradual increase in weights.

Muscular Endurance

Muscular endurance is the ability of a muscle group to perform repeated contractions over a period of time. Tests of muscular endurance generally require the muscle contraction to be performed continually without rest until the muscle is fatigued or until time expires (sit-ups, push-ups, dips, chins). Appendix A-8 describes specific tests for muscular endurance and Appendix B-4 provides standards for comparison.

Flexibility

Flexibility is the ability of an individual to move the various body joints through a maximum range of motion. It is an important aspect of physical fitness and the lack of flexibility can lead to numerous physical disorders and problems. Generally, the loss of the ability to bend, twist, and stretch is due to the lack of muscle use. Those with sedentary lifestyles involving long periods of sitting or standing are particularly prone to a lack of flexibility.

No single test can measure flexibility since it is specific to each joint. However, the following tests provide an indication of flexibility in various parts of the body: the shoulder lift test, the trunk extension test, and the sit and reach test. Appendix A-7 contains instructions for the tests and Appendix B-4 contains tables for evaluation of the results.

SUMMARY

The objective of this chapter has been to assist you in gaining a better understanding of your physical strengths and weaknesses. By using various measures of physical fitness, you can obtain the information needed to develop an individualized physical improvement program.

In evaluating the results of each test, you should establish a goal of "optimal" physical fitness. The optimal level refers to the highest obtainable level—to the achievement of your maximum potential. Each individual should strive for his or her personal best rather than settle for "normal" or "average" standards. These optimal levels can be reached if you are willing to work for them and willing to make the essential changes in living habits and lifestyle.

REFERENCES
1. Cooper, Kenneth, *The Aerobics Way.* New York: M. Evans and Company, Inc. 1977.
2. Cooper, Kenneth. *Controlling Cholesterol.* New York: Bantam Books, 1988.
3. Elrick, H., J. Crakes and S. Clerk. *Living Longer and Better.* California: World Publications, 1978.
4. American College of Sports Medicine, *Guidelines for Exercise Testing & Prescription.* Philadelphia: Lea & Febiger, 1991.

SUGGESTED LABS

Beginning with this chapter, you will find suggested laboratory activities to supplement the information presented in each chapter. These labs begin on page 267.

Suggested labs: 1, 3, 4, 6, 7, 8, 9, 10, 11, 12, 26.

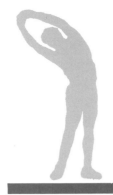

Guidelines for Your Training Program

Objectives

- Define a training program
- Describe the principles of training
- Describe training factors: progression, specificity, retrogression, use and disuse, muscle recruitment, skill, and individual rates of response
- Describe the method of determining the target heart rate
- Describe the components of the exercise session
- Describe the training guidelines
- Describe the process of setting up an exercise program

Key Words

- Frequency
- Intensity
- Muscle recruitment
- Overload
- Progression
- Recovery heart rate
- Retrogression
- Specificity
- Target heart rate
- Time
- Training
- Use and disuse

A sound exercise program is one developed on an individual basis, taking into consideration differences in abilities, capacities, likes and dislikes. Selection of activities within an individualized exercise program is based on results of the testing program and development of a physical fitness profile. Once the profile has been developed, specific exercises for the various areas of weakness can be suggested.

The following exercise program guidelines for cardiovascular endurance, strength, and flexibility should enable you to develop a program suited to your specific needs. Within each area you will find several effective training methods, and you are encouraged to select those toward which a real commitment can be made. Factors such as available equipment and facilities, as well as personal interests, must be taken into consideration.

Training is a term that applies to the procedure of systematically preparing a person in the most efficient manner to perform strenuous work and to recuperate from that work as quickly as possible. The process of conditioning is a deliberate one and, for the most efficient results, should follow specific guidelines for each exercise session and basic training principles.

THE EXERCISE SESSION

According to the American College of Sports Medicine, a complete exercise session should include the following phases and be conducted for the time specified for each level of exerciser:

The Warmup
Beginner:	8-10 minutes
Intermediate:	6-8 minutes
Advanced:	5-7 minutes

The Workout
Beginner:	10-20 minutes
Intermediate:	15-45 minutes
Advanced:	30-60 minutes

Cool Down I
Beginner:	3-5 minutes
Intermediate:	3-5 minutes
Advanced:	3-5 minutes

Muscle Toning
Beginner:	8-10 minutes
Intermediate:	10-12 minutes
Advanced:	12-15 minutes

Cool Down II
Beginner:	4-7 minutes
Intermediate:	4-7 minutes
Advanced:	4-7 minutes

Each of these phases is explained below. Included are recommendations for activities to include in that phase.

The Warmup

The purpose of the warmup phase is to prepare the body for the increased stress which will be placed upon it. If possible, the warmup activity should relate specifically to the exercise to be performed. There are three important benefits to the warmup session:

1. The heart rate is gradually increased from the resting pulse.
2. The temperature within the muscles is increased.
3. Chances of muscle soreness and injury are lessened.

Both static stretching and rhythmic movement should probably be included during the warmup. A combination of both performed smoothly at a moderate pace will provide a more complete warmup.

The Workout

The purpose of this phase is to elevate the heart rate and achieve aerobic fitness.

23

Activities which may be included in this phase include walking, jogging, running, swimming, bicycling, rope skipping, and aerobic dance. This phase should follow the principles of training in regard to frequency, intensity, and time. (A complete description of the principles of training follows this section.) Reaching the target heart rate and maintaining the intensity of the workout for the specified time are important guidelines for this phase.

Recently the American College of Sports Medicine modified its recommendations to encourage two or more sessions per week of moderate intensity strength training. The workout should include 8-10 exercises involving the major muscle groups. The reason for this change is to encourage a more well-rounded exercise program and emphasize the need for upper body fitness.

Cool Down I

The purpose of this phase is to slowly decelerate the heart rate. The body should be kept moving during this time and either walking or slow rhythmic movements along with static stretches are particularly good activities. The participant should remain in the standing position and avoid bouncing or sharp moves.

Muscle Toning

The purpose of this phase is to work on muscular strength and endurance. Isolated exercises for various muscle groups should be performed: legs, hips, buttocks, arms, and abdominals. The muscle groups used can be alternated on different days. Try doing sets moving from side to side and stretch out the muscles before moving to the next group.

Cool Down II

The purpose of this phase is to improve flexibility and to relax. Static stretching exercises should be included. Avoid bouncing and tensing movements. A final pulse check is also done during this phase. The recovery heart rate (120 or less after five minutes and below 100 after ten minutes) should be reached.

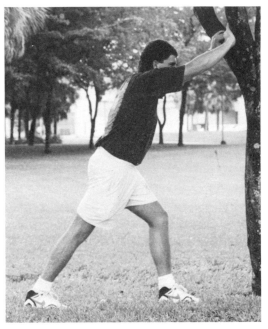

The Achilles tendon stretch should be performed in the Cool Down II phase.

PRINCIPLES OF TRAINING

Three basic principles will determine the effectiveness of any training program. Understanding and applying these principles is essential to developing a program which will produce improvement. In addition, following these principles will enable you to engage safely in a progressive training program. These three principles are **overload, progression,** and **specificity.**

Overload

Overload occurs when increased demands are made upon the body. This increased stress causes the body to adapt and, consequently, an improvement in physical condition will result. Overload can be accomplished in three general ways:

1. **Frequency.** By increasing how often one exercises; the number of times per day and/or week that an activity is performed.

2. **Intensity.** By increasing the difficulty of an exercise such as increasing the speed of a run, amount of weight lifted, or distance stretched.

3. **Time (or duration).** By increasing the length of each training session.

Each of these overload factors can and should be applied to the specific training: cardiovascular, strength and endurance, or flexibility.

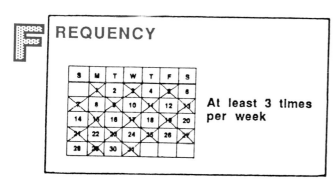

REQUENCY

At least 3 times per week

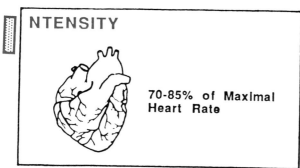

NTENSITY

70-85% of Maximal Heart Rate

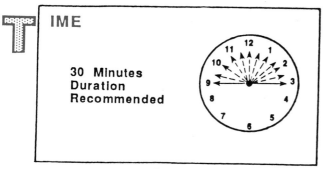

IME

30 Minutes Duration Recommended

Figure 3.1.

*Note: Some individuals may need to start as low as 50% and build up to the 70% level.

Progression

Progression is a combination of adaptation and overload. Adaptation refers to the body's ability to adapt to stress. This means that as you force your body to work harder, it will eventually adjust so as to work more efficiently.

Since the body adjusts to stress, the amount of work must be periodically increased in order for improvement to occur. For example, if you began an exercise program that involves running one mile a day in eight minutes, you would probably find the workout stressful. You would, therefore, improve your cardiovascular function for the next several weeks if you continued the eight-minute rate. But if you continued to perform at that level (i.e., run the same distance in the same time), cardiovascular improvement would stop and adaptation would occur. To continue improving, you would have to increase your stress on your cardiovascular system; and, therefore, the overload principle would go into effect again. In a few weeks or months, additional overload would again have to be added.

Specificity

The specificity principle implies that the improvements made in training are specific to the type of training undertaken. For example, a strength program will develop strength, but not an appreciable amount of cardiovascular endurance. Another illustration is the person who has trained adequately for a sport such as swimming, but when that person participates in basketball or some other sport, he or she quickly becomes fatigued during play and muscle-sore later. Each activity requires specific demands, and doing the event is the best way to train for the event.

Training is specific to the:
- fitness component
- muscle group
- range of motion
- joint angle

Additional Training Factors

Retrogression. During a training program, you may find that at certain levels in the program you reach a plateau or seem to slightly decrease in performance. Try as you may, it seems you are unable to regain or surpass your previous level. Then suddenly, for no apparent reason, you may surge ahead surpassing all previous performance levels. The reasons for such retrogression are not clear except that the body may be making adjustments to meet the demands of the overload. When the adjustments are effected, then progress or improvement is made.

Use and Disuse. Use and disuse, simply stated, means that if you train, there will be improvement. If not, physical performance will decline. Use stimulates the function of the organism, and disuse results in a deterioration.

Muscle Recruitment. The ability of the body to call upon additional muscle units depends on an individual's level of training. Thus, if the load or task is slight, a few units

are stimulated; if the load is heavy, many units are stimulated or "recruited."

Skill. Improvement in muscle usage facilitates improvement in skill, which in turn improves physical performance and results in improved coordination.

Individual Rates of Response. Each person will have his or her own level of response to a training program. Many people who train or participate on athletic teams seem to arrive at a high level of condition long before others. The reason is probably dependent upon many factors, some of which are emotional and some of which are hereditary. A few of the variables may be (1) present physical condition; (2) age; (3) body type; (4) weight; (5) rest, sleep and relaxation; (6) nutrition; (7) freedom from disease; (8) proneness to injury; (9) motivation; and (10) ability to learn new skills readily.

DETERMINING TARGET HEART RATE

Target heart rate refers to the optimal rate at which the heart should be beating during exercise to achieve a cardiovascular training effect. Actually, the "target" is within a range of minimum and maximum heart rates so that one is also exercising within a generally safe upper limit. The procedure for determining your target heart rate is relatively simple and should be done before engaging in a cardiovascular workout.

To begin with, it is important to know your resting heart rate. Refer to Chapter 2 for the correct procedure for obtaining your resting heart rate. Next, calculate your predicted maximum heart rate which is 220 minus your age. The basis for this formula is that as you age, the maximum heart rate declines. (See Fig. 3.2.) The next step is to subtract the resting rate from the predicted maximum heart rate. Your resting heart

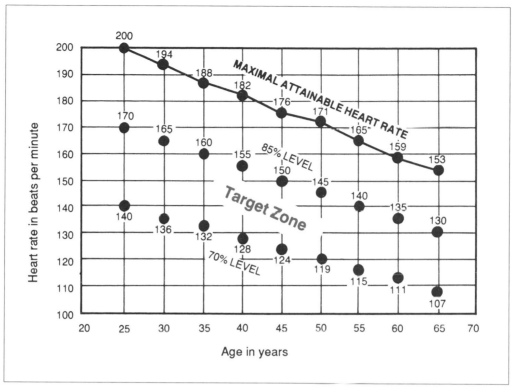

Figure 3.2.: Summary of changes to maximal heart rate resulting from age and target zones for each age group. Note: Some individuals may need to start at the 50% level for the target heart rate.

rate should be taken into consideration because it is a fairly reliable guide to your cardiovascular condition, and it reflects your starting point before exercise. For instance, the target heart rate zone of an 18-year-old with a resting heart rate of 74 is 163-182 beats per minute. See Lab 5 for a step-by-step procedure for calculating the target heart rate zone.

A model cardiovascular training pattern is illustrated in Figure 3.3. It demonstrates how the heart rate should be increased gradually to the target zone, level off for the training session, and then gradually be brought down to the starting level.

If a person has not exercised for some time or is extremely overweight, he or she should not go to the full overload of intensity and duration, but rather should begin at a lighter load (i.e., a 50% working rate) and gradually progress to a full overload at 80-85%. The cardiovascular system will adapt to the overload placed upon it, although an excessive amount of overload could be harmful to your physical health. On the other hand, a person in superior physical condition may desire to train at a level above 85%.

The progression may increase safely depending on recovery heart rate. The guiding principle is that 5-6 minutes after the workout, your heart rate should return to about 120 beats per minute; and after 10 minutes, it should drop to less than 100 beats per minute. **NOTE:** It is extremely important that you frequently monitor your recovery heart rate after engaging in a cardiovascular fitness program.

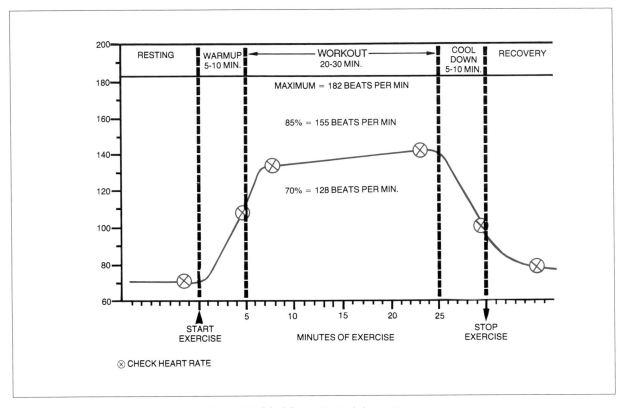

Figure 3.3: Model exercise training pattern.

The heart rate can be monitored at several points throughout an exercise session:

- before exercise begins (resting heart rate)
- after the warmup phase
- every 4-5 minutes during the aerobic phase at natural breaks (training heart rate)
- during the cool-down phase
- after relaxation techniques or at the conclusion of class

The Recovery Heart Rate

One final check on the quality of any exercise session can be made by checking the recovery heart rate. If the intensity and duration of your workout were appropriate, your heart rate five minutes after the exercise should be below 120 beats per minute. A heart rate higher than this indicates that perhaps the intensity of the program should be lowered and/or that the duration should be less. Remember your goal is to have an effective program but one that is not greatly uncomfortable—one that you can enjoy!

TRAINING PROGRAM GUIDELINES

The following chart describes how the training guidelines can be applied to exercise programs for each of the health-related fitness components.

Cardiovascular Endurance

Frequency	3-5 days per week
Intensity	60-90% of Maximum Heart Rate
Time (Duration)	20-60 minutes
Mode	Large muscle movement (walking, cycling, jogging, swimming, aerobic exercise to music)

Flexibility

Frequency	At least 3 times per week
Intensity	Slow, sustained stretch for 3 repetitions
Time (Duration)	Easy stretch 5-10 seconds; developmental stretch 10-20 seconds
Mode	Stretching

Muscular Strength

Frequency	Every other day (3 days per week)
Intensity	High resistance-low repetitions
Time (Duration)	3 sets
Mode	Isometrics, isotonic, isokinetic

Muscular Endurance

Frequency	Every other day (3 days per week)
Intensity	Low resistance-high repetitions
Time (Duration)	3 sets
Mode	Isometrics, isotonic, isokinetic

Body Composition

Frequency	3-5 days (daily is best)
Intensity	Expend 300 calories per session
Time (Duration)	20 minutes at least
Mode	Large muscle movement (walking, cycling, jogging, swimming, aerobic exercise to music)

TRAINING GUIDELINES

The basic purpose of any exercise program is to cause the body to improve—to adapt and adjust to the increased stress placed upon it. The body is a remarkable structure which is capable of adapting to stress and continually improving its efficiency. An improvement in physical condition results when exercise is increased in intensity and when an overload is presented to the body. One can overload the body by increasing the resistance or work being done, by increasing the speed of the repetitions, or by increasing the number of repetitions. Once the body adapts to this stress, the amount of work must be periodically increased in order for improvement to continue to occur. The progression should be gradual to prevent strain and soreness.

And finally, it must be realized that no two people are alike. Everyone does not progress or improve at the same rate. Each person will respond to the training program in his or her own unique way and unique rate. Concentrate on the changes you are achieving and do not compare your progress with that of others. If you are observing the principles and guidelines described in this chapter, you will eventually achieve your optimal level of fitness. Keep working but be patient!

DESIGNING YOUR PROGRAM

There are many different activities which can be included in your program. As you design a program you may find it helpful to refer to the suggested training programs for the activities listed in Chapter 4. If you decide to include a sport or recreational activity in your plan, be certain you monitor whether the guidelines for training are met for the particular fitness component you are trying to develop. While following your exercise program, keep the following questions in mind:

- Which activities do you most enjoy?
- Do you prefer to select one activity and stick with it, or do you prefer a variety of activities?
- Do you need special equipment for the activity? If so, is it easily available to you?
- How far must you travel to do the activity? Will transportation be a potential problem?
- Which days of the week and which time of day are best for you? Will you need to make changes in your schedule from week to week? Are you a morning or an evening person?
- Is your time schedule realistic? Will you be so rushed that you are tempted to skip the workout?
- Do you need to have someone to exercise with you, or do you prefer to do it alone? If you need others, do you have a partner or will you join a group?
- What potential obstacles could interfere with your plan—illness, weather, injuries, school, job, or other activities? How can you overcome them?
- Do you need motivation to get you going? If so, how can you get assistance?
- Do you need assistance in "staying with it?" If so, do you have someone to rely on?

The next step is to put your plan in writing. Use the sample on the next page to help you complete Lab 13 in the back of the book.

SAMPLE

DESIGNING YOUR EXERCISE PROGRAM

NAME _Judy Miller_ WEIGHT _124_ RESTING HEART RATE _73_

Fitness Area	Current Level	Activity or Activities	Specific Exercises	Place	No. Days	Time of Day	How Long	Alone or With Others	Cost
Cardiovascular	Very Good	Cycling	Stationary Cycling	Local health club	3	4:00 PM	1 Hr.	Group	$20 per mo.
		Aerobic Dance	Jumping Twisting	"	2	"	"	"	
Flexibility	Very Good	Stretching	Suggested by health club	"	5	"	15 min.	"	
Muscular Strength & Endurance	Poor	Weights	Exercises for Strength	"	2	"	30 min.	"	

List below any sports or recreational activities which you plan to include in your exercise program. Be certain to include any intramural, varsity, or recreational sports in which you participate.

Sport or Recreational Activity	Your Skill Level	How Often	How Long	Fitness Benefits of Activity
Racquetball	Good	2 - 3 days per week	2 Hrs.	Cardiovascular Flexibility

Selecting An Activity

Factors to consider:
1. age
2. health status
3. present level of fitness
4. previous activity and training experience
5. psychological factors and motivation
6. goals

Setting Up An Exercise Program

1. Set realistic goals. In establishing goals for your exercise program, keep in mind that changes will not happen overnight. The following chart indicates the average time needed for significant changes to occur.

Cardiovascular endurance	12 weeks
Muscular strength	8 weeks
Muscular endurance	8 weeks
Flexibility	8 weeks
Body Composition	12-16 weeks

2. Keep a record of workouts (time, distance, heart rate, etc.).
3. Plan for obstacles (weather, time, soreness, etc.).
4. Use appropriate training techniques to maximize the effect.
5. A lower level of intensity is suggested for those with a lower initial level of fitness.
6. The less fit and middle-aged and older participants should take more time to warm up.
7. The initial level of exercise should be maintained for a longer period of time for the unfit participant (2-4 weeks). After this time a steady progression can be utilized.
8. The maximum increase in total work should not exceed 10% per week.
9. Initially it is best to increase duration and/or frequency of training rather than intensity.
10. Participants should monitor their bodies and feelings during exercise and use this information to provide input on the rate of progression.
11. The intensity of effort needed to reach a minimum threshold for improvement and rate of progression will vary from individual to individual. These differences must be taken into account.
12. Avoid competing with others or pushing yourself unrealistically.
13. If the individual stops completely, all improvements are lost within 3-8 months. A significant loss in fitness occurs in just 1-2 weeks.
14. Fitness must be maintained on a regular basis—it cannot be stored!
15. It takes more effort to gain fitness than it does to maintain it.

Evaluating Your Plan. After you have followed the plan for at least six weeks, take time to evaluate it. Consider the following questions about your program:

- Were you able to complete the program as planned? If not, what obstacles prevented you from doing so?
- Did you really enjoy the activities? If not, which ones would you change?
- Have you noticed any changes in your health and fitness level? If so, what are they? If not, why do you think that is so?
- What changes would you make to improve your plan?

QUESTIONS AND ANSWERS

What causes muscle soreness?

Most muscle soreness occurs between 24-48 hours after the exercise. Although the specific cause is not known, it appears to be due to small tears in the muscle or connective tissue around the muscle. Previous theories linked the soreness to a buildup of lactic acid in the muscle during sustained activity. In any case, you can help prevent the pain and stiffness by proper warming up and cooling down, by gradually getting into your exercise program, by progressing slowly, and by avoiding ballistic or bouncing-type stretching exercises.

What exactly is "second wind?"

During the first phase of a workout, energy comes from the stored fuel in the muscles. The breakdown of this fuel occurs without the benefit of oxygen and is called anaerobic energy consumption. In this phase, lactic acid builds up which causes muscle ache and tiredness. After you have been exercising a while, you pass over the anaerobic threshold and depend more on the oxygen breathed to help produce fuel. This is aerobic energy or the second wind. With this energy there isn't the lactic acid buildup so you do not feel as tired.

How will I know if I have exceeded the safe limits for exercise?

There are several warning signs which indicate you are over-exercising and should reduce the intensity of your workout: excessive heart rate, labored breathing, pale skin, flushness, and a prolonged heart rate recovery time after exercising.

Any of the following signs indicate that exercise should be stopped immediately because the participant may be in danger: difficulty in breathing (not just deep breathing), loss of coordination, dizziness, or tightness in the chest.

If the participant exhibits any of these danger signs, medical advice should be sought before continuing with the exercise program.

What do we know about the effects of physical activity and sport on women?

It is generally recognized that strength in women is approximately fifty to sixty percent that of men. The male advantage is due to several factors including anatomical and hormonal factors, greater size, and less fatty tissue.

Endurance studies have shown that males have ten to twelve percent more hemoglobin per milligram of blood and approximately eight percent more red blood cells per cubic centimeter. Men have larger hearts and lungs, have slower heart rates and ventilate less frequently during exercise. Females generally have ten to fifteen percent more body fat, which provides more load on the cardiovascular system and offers more of a thermal barrier to the dissipation of body heat.

This evidence does not indicate that women should not be allowed to participate in endurance type activities, only that males have a functional advantage necessitating separate competition for some competitive activities.

Why do I sweat more after I stop exercising than during exercise?

Since the body has a limited amount of blood with which to nourish the great demand by the skeletal muscles, it shunts blood from the skin of the muscles, thereby causing a buildup of body heat. After you stop exercising, the body sends an overabundance of blood to the skin for cooling and you sweat more to dissipate the excess heat. Also, in jogging, movement causes your sweat to evaporate more quickly than when standing still.

Does it really matter which exercises I choose to do?

All exercises are not the same. Not only do some exercises burn more calories per minute, exercises provide benefits which are specific to the type of exercise. For instance, stretching exercises will only contribute to a gain in flexibility—not to strength or endurance. The exercises requiring continuous activity and involving large muscle groups will provide the greatest caloric expenditure. Therefore, you must select exercises which meet your needs — whether for a specific fitness component or for weight control.

Does missing a few sessions cause me to lose my fitness?

All the gains of an exercise program are not lost by missing a few days. However, when you begin exercising again you should start at a lower level. Depending on the number of days you missed and how you feel while exercising, it is suggested you begin at half to two-thirds your usual exercise level. Once you have missed the days, don't worry about them — just get back on schedule and work toward achieving your goal.

Some people say exercise is good for everything and anything! Is this true?

Exercise does have many benefits, but it is not a cure-all. Combined with caloric intake, it helps to reduce and control weight, but will not change the structure of the body. Exercise does not guarantee good posture, but it does help in acquiring and maintaining it.

Are there any easy ways to exercise?

None that are beneficial. All require time and effort. However, it is possible to select activities that are enjoyable.

What are the effects of training on the cardiovascular system?

1. Longer resting phase of heart cycle which enables the heart to have a more complete filling of the chambers, resulting in the myocardium receiving proper nutrients and expediting removal of waste products.
2. Hypertrophy of the heart muscle which ultimately results in a stronger heart.
3. Increased contractility of the heart muscle.
4. Stroke volume is increased enabling more blood to be pumped with each stroke. This improves the ability to more rapidly transport life-sustaining oxygen from the lungs, the heart and ultimately to all parts of the body.
5. Cardiac output is increased (minute volume).
6. There is an increase in blood volume—a temporary anemia may occur as a result of this change and a fragmentation of red blood cells during heavy training.
7. Venous return is increased due to "muscle pump."
8. Increase in red blood cells.
9. Increase in hemoglobin.
10. Lactic acid formation is lower due to increased oxygen supply.
11. Increase in white cells following muscular work.
12. Increase in blood pressure during exercise is less in the trained individual.
13. Increase in buffering capacity of the blood.
14. Blood pressure is lowered.
15. Increase in high density lipoprotein ratio.

SUGGESTED LABS: 5, 13.

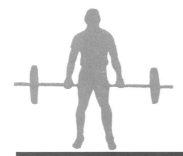

Selecting Your Fitness Program

Objectives

- Describe cardiovascular fitness programs: walking, jogging, interval training, cycling, aerobic dancing, rope jumping, aqua dynamics
- Describe muscular strength programs: isotonics, isokinetics, isometrics
- Describe a flexibility program
- Describe guidelines for selecting and designing a fitness program
- Describe exercises to be avoided

Key Words

- Aerobics
- Cross Training
- Interval Training
- Isokinetic Training
- Isometric Training
- Isotonic Training
- PNF Stretch
- Step Aerobics

Since no two people are alike, exercise programs should be tailored according to ability, preference, and capacity to fit individual needs. The foundation of your program will be based on the results of your lab tests and the resulting fitness profile.

The following guidelines for strength building, flexibility, and the development of cardiovascular fitness should enable you to make wise choices as you develop a program suited to your needs. Because of factors such as available equipment, facilities, and diverse interests, several effective training methods are presented for each fitness area. The rest will be up to you.

Whichever training program is selected, each workout should consist of three essential phases: (1) the warmup, (2) the training session, (3) the cool-down. All three phases are important for a sound program which will safely provide maximum results. See Chapter 3 for specific suggestions.

CARDIOVASCULAR FITNESS PROGRAMS

The main objective of all cardiovascular programs is to increase the body's ability to utilize oxygen within a controlled time span and specifically to develop cardiovascular endurance.

The word **aerobics** means *with oxygen* and involves those activities that can be performed for at least fifteen minutes without developing an oxygen deficit. Oxygen deficiency occurs when the oxygen consumption is below that required. Supplying the body with sufficient oxygen is vital if the body is to produce the energy necessary for the completion of the activity. While this is a complex procedure, cardiovascular fitness is dependent upon the interaction of the heart, lungs, blood, and blood vessels.

Your heart rate is the key to cardiovascular fitness. In order to actually improve this aspect of fitness, the target heart rate must be maintained for a minimum of fifteen minutes. For optimal results, a period of at least thirty minutes is required. A frequency of three days is necessary for minimal results, with four days required for optimal achievement. Remember that the intensity, duration, and frequency need to be progressive.

The following principles govern whether an exercise program is considered aerobic:

1. The exercise must involve large muscle groups.
2. The exercise must elevate your heart rate to the target heart rate zone.
3. The exercise must sustain the target heart rate at least fifteen minutes.
4. The exercise must be performed at least three times per week (on alternate days).

Tables 4-1 through 4-5 represent a basic training progression for use in several aerobic activities—walking, cycling, jogging, interval training, jumping rope, aqua dynamics and swimming.

Walking—Technique

- Remember that walking for fitness is not the same as pleasure walking. No shuffling, strolling, or sauntering is allowed!
- Concentrate on really using your muscles (and contracting them), the feet, thighs, calves, buttocks, diaphragm, etc.
- Make certain you are in an upright position and that your entire foot is placed on the ground—heel first, then toes.
- Arms should be at a 90° angle; one arm swings forward as the opposite foot moves forward.
- Wear good walking shoes. Follow these

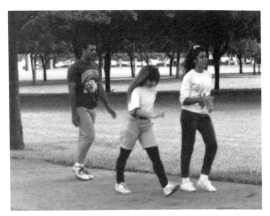

Walking is an excellent aerobic activity.

helpful tips from the American Podiatrists Association for obtaining a suitable pair:

— Arch supports that are wide and comfortable.
— Sturdy uppers of mesh fabric or leather.
— Heavy but *flexible* soles that are cushioned. Crepe or rubber soles work well.
— A slightly elevated heel.
— A firm heel counter to prevent sliding and blistering.
— A good shoe fit, about one-fourth inch between your longest toes and the end of the shoe, and a wide enough shoe to allow for foot expansion.

Procedure

• Start slowly and use the first three to five minutes as a warmup. Increase your pace gradually.
• Try to get rhythm with a natural, effortless motion.
• Use a stride that is natural for you but lengthen your stride gradually to increase the speed of your walking.
• As you quicken your pace, thrust harder with your legs, increase your arm swing, and breathe naturally.

Jogging

Jogging is a form of exercise that involves alternate walking and running at a slow-to-moderate pace or running at a slow, even pace. Jogging is advantageous to the person watching his or her weight. It is good for the legs, helps to firm the abdominal region and trim flab. This method of exercise is the basis of the aerobics program since it is one of the best for developing the cardiovascular system.

A physical examination before initiating a jogging program is recommended if you have been inactive for a period of time, or if your medical history indicates heart, blood vessel, or lung problems.

Clothing for jogging should be loose and comfortable. Choose shoes having a good arch support and a firm sole. Avoid wearing rubberized clothing since this material does not allow sweat to evaporate, thereby

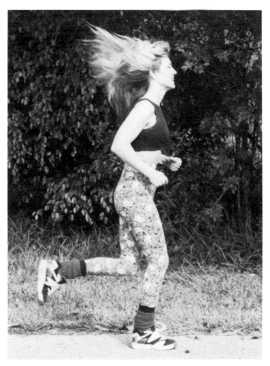

Jogging is one of the best activities for developing the cardiovascular system.

causing excessive heat buildup and dehydration which may result in heat stroke.

The beginning jogger should run on a track or a grass or dirt path and not on a hard surface. A park or golf course should also be considered for a change in scenery. In the initial stage of your jogging program, jog every other day until your body adjusts, then plan a daily jog.

The following procedures outline basic jogging technique:

- A warmup, consisting of a brief walk and stretching exercises should precede your jog.
- The back should be kept as straight as is comfortable with the head up, looking toward the horizon with the jaw loose. Avoid a forward lean; keep the pelvis tucked under.
- The head and shoulders should be relaxed.
- The elbows are bent at a 90° angle and held slightly away from the body. The arm swing should be forward to the mid-line of the body.
- The best way for your feet to hit the ground is to land first on the heel and then rock forward on the ball of the foot. Avoid landing on the ball of the foot, as this puts excessive strain on the calf muscles.
- Breathing should be regular and deep, through the mouth and nose, with maximum exhalations.
- At the end of a jogging session, taper off with a walk.

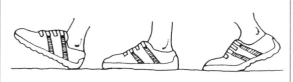

Correct jogging technique: land on the heel, then rock forward on the ball of the foot. Avoid landing on the ball of the foot.

Interval Training

While most people agree that running or jogging long, slow distances is an excellent means of improving cardiovascular endurance, another method called interval training has also gained widespread acceptance.

The chief differences between the two systems are the length of work periods and the degree of intensity. A common interval workout usually consists of three to seven work periods of three to five minutes duration, and at about 80% maximum capacity. These periods of work are broken by short rest periods of walking or jogging to partially recover for the next work period. The length of the rest or recovery period is usually based on a heart rate recovery plan, with 120 beats per minute classified as minimal. That is, if your heart rate reaches 160 during the exercise bout, you must jog or walk until your heart rate drops to 120 beats per minute. As your system becomes more efficient, your recovery rate time will decrease.

The advantages of interval training over continuous training appear to be the following:

1. More work can be accomplished in less time.
2. Greater flexibility in the work program reduces boredom.
3. Because of the short work periods, the intensity of the work can be greater.

Designing Your Interval Program

The requirements of an effective interval program are the following:

1. The length of the rest period should be no greater than 1:3, and should be 1:2 or 1:1. (This means that if the work period is 30 seconds, the rest period

should be 60 seconds or 30 seconds.)

2. If aerobic power is the objective, then the length of each work period must be at least 3-5 minutes.

3. The heart rate intensity should be 70-80% of maximum.

Overload for this system or training can be achieved or increased by:

1. Reducing the length of the recovery period.

2. Increasing the intensity of the work period.

3. Increasing the number of work periods.

4. Increasing the length of the period.

5. Any combination of the above.

Cycling—Technique

• Make certain the seat height is correct for you. Comfortable padding on the seat is a must for long rides!

• Adjust the handlebars to a position which is comfortable for your riding style.

• Pedaling must be vigorous and sustained to achieve real benefits.

• Try to relax and enjoy the sights!

Procedure

• Start with a moderate pace so your leg muscles can adjust gradually to the increased activity.

• Remember, it takes skill to safely handle a bike in traffic, on narrow roadways, and in tight situations. Learn how to handle your bicycle effectively before you attempt difficult situations such as heavy traffic or steep, winding roads. Be alert to holes or debris on the road.

• Generally, you need to cycle twice as fast as you would jog to achieve your target heart rate. But, in the beginning, strive for a sustained ride and gradually increase your time or distance.

Aerobic Exercise to Music

Aerobic exercise to music incorporates a variety of movements—high hopping, stepping, jumping, twisting, stretching, swinging, and skipping—set to almost any type of music. The reason for its popularity is that the benefits of exercise are achieved by utilizing the appeal of music and dance.

Most people seem to feel that aerobic exercise to music makes exercising and training more enjoyable. Once you have learned the basics you can combine dozens of movements into routines, or you can use one of the many prepared records or tapes to guide you. There are also regularly scheduled aerobic

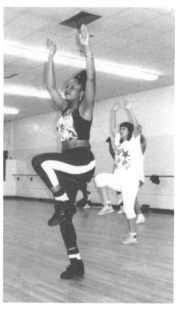

For a fun workout, try aerobic exercise to music.

workouts appearing on several television stations. When selecting an aerobic exercise workout whether on tape, film or in an exercise facility, it is important to know that the leader is qualified and will follow the training principles and guidelines described in the previous chapters.

Low Impact Aerobics

Low impact aerobics refer to those programs in which the stress and shock to the participant's joints are minimized. An example is low-impact aerobic dance in which the activities and movements always leave one foot on the floor.

Step Aerobics

A relatively new type of exercise being included in many aerobics classes is referred to as step aerobics, bench stepping, or step training. The participant steps on and off a bench while working to music and attempts to maintain a rate of 80-120 steps per minute. Not only does a pumping action of the arms contribute to the workout, but light (1 pound) weights can add to the calorie expenditure.

Beginners should use a 4 inch step and gradually increase to 8-12 inches. To avoid the risk of knee strain and injury, the knee should not flex (bend) beyond 90° as you step up. The knee should be slightly bent and the entire foot (not just the toes or ball of the foot) should be placed flat on the center of the step. The landing on the floor should be with the ball of the foot first and then the heel with the knee bending to

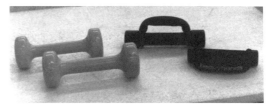

Using light weights during step aerobics will increase calorie expenditure.

absorb the impact. Wearing the proper shoes is important for safety—those made for aerobics or cross training are recommended. Running shoes and those with extensive treading may cause problems. Good posture should be maintained—lean forward slightly at the hips (not the waist). Keep the chest up and hips tucked under.

The bench can also be used during the workout for stretches (hamstring and calves) by dropping the heels toward the floor and for exercises such as push-ups (place hands on the step) or sit-ups (place feet on the step).

Some commercial step benches are 42 inches long and 14 inches wide with an adjustable height. Get those with non-skid top surfaces. One word of caution: Be certain you avoid overuse injuries by cross training and limiting step workouts to no more than three per week.

Rope Jumping

Rope jumping is a form of endurance training in which various rhythmical jumping, hopping and gymnastic dance steps are performed over a steadily rotating or swinging rope held in the hand of the individual. The length of the rope should be such that it will reach the armpits when held to the ground beneath the feet.

When running and rope skipping are compared at equal levels of exercise intensity and duration, running creates a larger

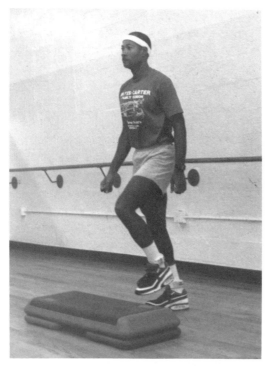

Beginners should use a four-inch step for step aerobics.

oxygen demand and burns a greater number of calories than rope skipping. Studies indicate that the energy expenditure for jumping 125, 135, and 145 skips per minute averages 14-16 calories per minute (equivalent to jogging 7.5 minutes per mile). Rope jumping does have an advantage in regard to improving footwork, agility and coordination.

You should first practice the footwork without twirling the rope. Don't jump too high—about one-half inch above the floor is sufficient. Now combine footwork with the rope twirling; one jump for each rotation of the rope. The rope should hit the floor to the side of you as you are in the air.

Finally, practice the complete skill. Start with the rope behind you, one end in each hand forming a loop; jump over the rope as it is rotated over your head and beneath your feet. Avoid large arm circling in twirling the rope; emphasize wrist action. When an error or "miss" occurs, continue footwork while you recover rope action. Other activities such as walking briskly can be alternated with periods of rope jumping.

To achieve the aerobic training effect, you should determine if the activity produced your target heart rate. If this level was not reached immediately after jumping, then you must increase the load by jumping faster or for longer time intervals. After the appropriate jumping pattern has been found and the pattern is followed for a period of time, the amount should be increased.

Aqua Dynamics

An aqua dynamics program is a series of water exercises and/or lap swimming designed for use in achieving cardiovascular fitness. Water exercises can be performed by most people—swimmers and non-swimmers—regardless of age and physical condition.

Technique

- Use the activities beginning on page 45 to improve not only cardiovascular fitness but to increase muscle tone, flexibility, calorie burn-up, and tension release.
- The exercises are for the swimmer and/or the non-swimmer.
- If possible, stay in water that is shoulder-level—the resistance of the water increases the strenuousness of your workout.

Procedure

- Swimmers can add lap swimming to their programs. Choose a variety of strokes and make your workout continuous. Alternate strokes when you need a change. See the suggested starter program (Table 4-6).
- Select a variety of exercises and perform them in a sequence that will keep your heart rate in the target zone.
- Consider having music available and combining aerobic dance steps with the usual water exercises.

Cross Training

A popular method of training being used by many exercisers today is cross training: using one or more activities to train for another. Alternating the type of sport or exercise you do is an excellent way of providing good overall conditioning, reducing the risk of injury and avoiding boredom.

These workouts allow you to exercise more muscle groups—especially those involving complementary muscles (i.e. the hamstring muscles strengthened by running and the quadriceps strengthened by cycling). Achieving better muscle balance is important in avoiding injury.

Cross training also helps reduce the risk

of injury caused by overtraining the same set of muscles and joints over a period of time. Giving muscle groups a day of rest while working others is a wise training guideline.

The concept behind muscle balance is the fact that muscles work in groups. Every time you move, a muscle shortens as it initiates motion and an opposing muscle lengthens as it stabilizes and balances the joint. The muscle which is considered the prime mover becomes developed while the opposite muscle which controls the motion's intensity stays largely undeveloped. Cross training enables you to correct these muscle imbalances and assures the proper working of all muscle groups.

The chart below identifies the major muscle groups and indicates the opposing muscles which should be well-balanced.

Achieving Muscle Balance

Training for muscle balance should involve strengthening the weaker muscles and stretching the stronger ones to increase flexibility.

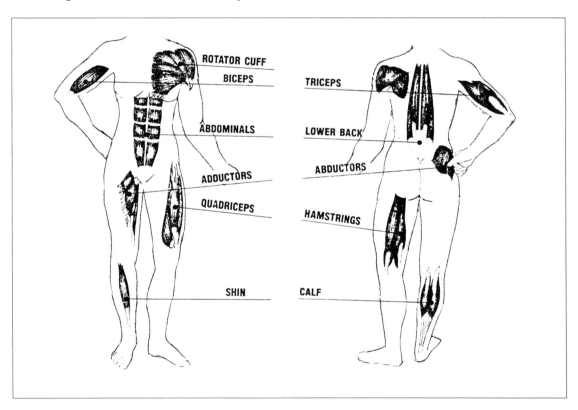

TABLE 4-1
WALKING EXERCISE PROGRAM

Week	Distance (miles)	Time Goal (minutes)	Frequency (per week)
1	1.0	18:00	4
2	1.5	26:00	4
3	2.0	35:00	3
4	2.0	32:00	4
5	2.0	30:00	5
6	2.5	38:00	5
7	2.5	37:00	5
8	2.5	36:00	5
9	3.0	44:00	5
10	3.0	43:00	5
11	3.0	42:00	5
12	3.0	41:00	4

TABLE 4-2
RUNNING/JOGGING EXERCISE PROGRAM
(Start by walking, then walk and run, or run as necessary)

Week	Distance (miles)	Time Goal (minutes)	Frequency (per week)
1	1.5	20:00	3
2	1.5	18:00	3
3	1.5	15:00	4
4	2.0	32:00	3
5	2.0	32:00	4
6	2.0	30:00	4
7	2.0	28:00	4
8	2.0	26:00	4
9	2.0	24:00	4
10	2.0	22:00	4
11	2.0	20:00	4
12	2.5	25:00	4
13	2.5	25:00	4
14	3.0	30:00	4

TABLE 4-3
INTERVAL TRAINING — SAMPLE PROGRAM

Session	Activity	Time	Session	Activity	Time
1	Walk	3 minutes	5	Walk	2 minutes
	Jog	1 minute		Jog	5 minutes
	Walk	3 minutes		Walk	2 minutes
	Jog	2 minutes		Jog	4 minutes
2	Walk	3 minutes	6	Walk	2 minutes
	Jog	3 minutes		Jog	5 minutes
	Walk	2 minutes		Walk	2 minutes
	Jog	3 minutes		Jog	4 minutes
3	Walk	2 minutes	7	Walk	2 minutes
	Jog	3 minutes		Jog	6 minutes
	Walk	2 minutes		Walk	2 minutes
	Jog	4 minutes		Jog	5 minutes
4	Walk	2 minutes	8	Walk	2 minutes
	Jog	4 minutes		Jog	6 minutes
	Walk	2 minutes		Walk	2 minutes
	Jog	4 minutes		Jog	6 minutes

TABLE 4-4
CYCLING EXERCISE PROGRAM

Week	Distance (miles)	Time Goal (minutes)	Frequency (per week)
1	3.0	18:00	4
2	3.0	15:00	5
3	4.0	18:00	4
4	4.0	15:00	4
5	4.5	20:00	4
6	5.0	18:30	4
7	5.0	18:00	5
8	6.0	24:00	4
9	6.0	22:00	4
10	7.0	28:30	4
11	7.0	27:00	4
12	8.0	35:00	4
13	8.0	34:00	4
14	8.0	32:00	4

During the first six weeks, warm up by cycling slowly for three minutes before attempting the specified distance and time. Cool down by cycling slowly for three minutes at the conclusion of exercise.

TABLE 4-5
SUGGESTED ROPE JUMPING PROGRAM

Week	Activity
1	Jump five 2-minute series. (Stretch between each series.)
2	Jump five 3-minute series. (Stretch between each series.)
3	Jump three 5-minute series. (Stretch between each series.)
4	Jump two 7-minute series. (Stretch between each series.)
5	Jump ten minutes, stretch, then jump five minutes.
6	Jump fifteen minutes and stretch.

Aqua Dynamics

Alternate Toe Touch

Standing in waist-to-chest-deep water:

1. Raise left leg, bringing right hand toward left foot, looking back and left hand extended rearward.
2. Recover to starting position.
   Repeat.
   Reverse.

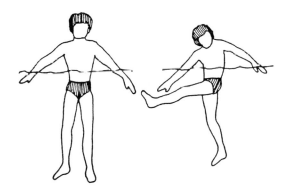

Side Straddle Hop

Standing in waist-to-chest-deep water with hands on hips:

1. Jump sideward to position with feet approximately two feet apart.
2. Recover.

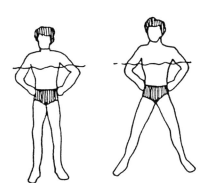

Stride Hop

Standing in waist-to-chest-deep water with hands on hips:

1. Jump, with left leg forward and right leg back.
2. Jump, changing to right leg forward and left leg back.
   Repeat.

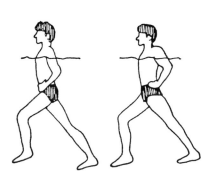

45

Walking Twists

With fingers laced behind neck:

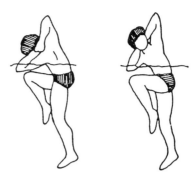

1. Walk forward, bringing up alternate legs, twisting body to touch knee with opposite elbow.
   Repeat.

Leg Out

Standing at side of pool with back against wall:

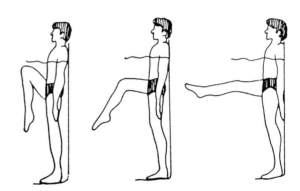

1. Raise left knee to chest.
2. Extend left leg straight out.
3. Stretch leg.
4. Drop leg to starting position.
   Repeat.
   Reverse one leg.

Gutter-Holding Drills

Pool-side Knees Up

Supine, holding on to pool gutter with hands, legs extended:

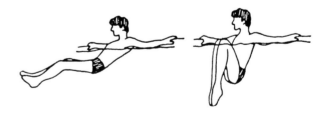

1. Bring knees to chin.
2. Recover to starting position.
   Repeat.

Knees Up Twisting

Supine. holding on to pool gutter with knees drawn up to chest:

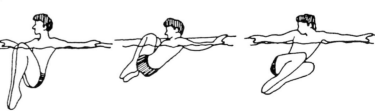

1. Twist slowly to left.
2. Recover.
3. Twist slowly to right.
4. Recover.
   Repeat.

Leg Crosses

Supine, holding on to pool gutter with legs extended:

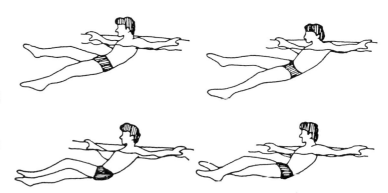

1. Swing legs far apart.
2. Bring legs together crossing left leg over right.
3. Swing legs far apart.
4. Bring legs together crossing right leg over left.
   Repeat.

Alternate Raised Knee Crossovers

Standing, holding on to pool gutter with hands, back to wall:

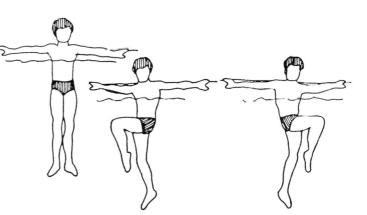

1. Lift left knee and cross it over. Twist to the right.
2. Recover.
3. Lift right knee and cross it over, twisting to the left.
4. Recover.

Legs Together on Back

Supine, holding on to pool gutter with hands, legs together and extended with feet about 6 inches under water:

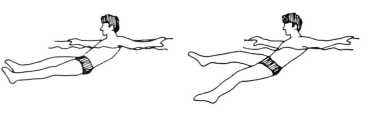

1. Spread legs apart as far as possible.
2. Pull feet and legs vigorously together.
   Repeat.

Legs Together on Front

Prone, holding on to pool gutter with one hand flat on wall to push legs out, with feet together:

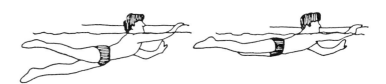

1. Spread legs apart as far as possible.
2. Pull feet and legs vigorously together.
   Repeat.

Leg Swing Outward

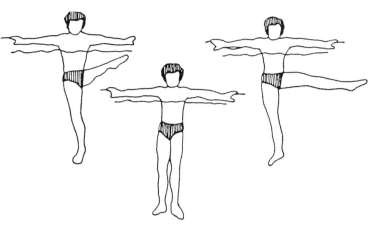

Standing with back against pool side and hands sideward, holding gutter:

1. Raise left foot as high as possible with leg straight.
2. Swing foot and leg to left side.
3. Recover to starting position by pulling left leg vigorously to right.
   Repeat.
   Reverse to right leg.
   Repeat.

Back Flutter Kicking

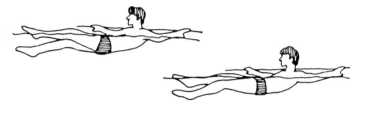

Lying in a supine position and holding on to side of pool with hand(s):

1. Flutter kick.

Left Side Flutter Kicking

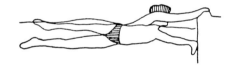

Lying on left side position holding on to side of pool with right hand, with left hand braced on pool wall:

1. Flutter kick.

Right Side Flutter Kicking

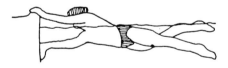

Lying on right side position holding on to side of pool with left hand, with right hand braced on pool wall:

1. Flutter kick.

Front Flutter Kicking

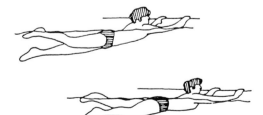

Lying in a prone position holding on to side of pool with hand(s):

1. Kick flutter style in which toes are pointed back, ankles are flexible, knee joint is loose but straight, and the whole leg acts as a whip.

Climbing

Hands in pool gutter, facing pool side and feet flat against side and approximately 16 inches apart:

1. Walk up side approximately six short steps.
2. Walk down side to starting position. Repeat.

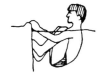 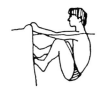

With Kickboards

1. Flutter kick
2. Side stroke

With Balls

1. Hold under water
2. Basketball or keep-away

Arm Exercises:

Shoulders in water
Palm up and down
Breast stroke
Circling

DEVELOPING YOUR MUSCULAR STRENGTH AND ENDURANCE PROGRAM

Training for muscular strength and endurance involves using the overload principle by using weights, immovable bars or objects, pulleys, straps, or springs. The muscle responds to the intensity of the overload, not the actual method of the overload, and in general the muscular overload is increased by:
— either increasing the "load" or the "resistance" to be lifted;
— increasing the number of times or "repetitions" the exercise is done;
— increasing the "speed" of muscular contractions; or
— by a combination of these.

The key to the development of muscular strength is regular participation in a systematic training program.

There are three different methods for developing strength, and it is possible to use any one or a combination of them to achieve results: isotonic, isometric, and isokinetic.

Isotonics

Isotonic training involves lifting a constant resistance through the range of motion. Lifting weights such as barbells or using equipment such as the Universal Gym are examples of isotonic training. It should be noted that when lifting a constant resistance the muscle will not be exercised to the same extent as it goes through the range of motion. The reason for this is that the strength of a muscle varies at different angles through the range of motion.

Several isotonic strength training principles, if followed, will allow you to get the most out of your workouts. (1)

1. **Strength training should be progressive.** A constant attempt should be made to increase resistance or repetitions in every workout.
2. **The higher the intensity, the better the muscles are stimulated, the more strength is built.**
   • Muscle fibers operate on the "all or nothing" basis; i.e., only the number of muscles actually required to move a weight are involved in any movement.

49

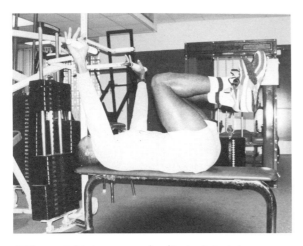

Lifting weights is an example of isotonic training.

- If a set is ended before the point of failure then the maximum number of muscle fibers available have not been used.
- If effort is decreased even slightly, the result will be out of proportion to the effort.
- It is not possible to measure less than 100% effort.
- To increase muscular strength, the intensity of the lift should be 80% of the maximum one can lift and the duration should be 8-12 repetitions. Occasional multiple sets may be performed.
- To increase muscular endurance, the intensity of the lift should be 30-50% of the maximum one can lift and the duration should be 12-20 repetitions. Three sets are recommended.

3. **Repetitions should be performed slowly, with a great range of movement, and after pre-stretching the muscles involved.**
   - Movement should not be too fast or too slow.
   - Avoid jerky or uneven movements.
   - Each repetition should include as great a range of movement as possible.
   - Each repetition should start from a pre-stretched position.

4. **For best results, select exercises that involve the greatest range of movement in the major muscle groups.**
   - Usually, the greater the muscle mass involved, the better the value of the exercise.
   - Include supplementary activities such as running, aerobic sports, calisthenics and gymnastic activities.

5. **Begin your workout by using the largest muscle groups, proceeding gradually to the smallest.**
   - Overall strength will be greater if the largest muscular structures of the body are exercised first.
   - If muscle growth is proportionate it will occur at a faster rate.

6. **Strength is best developed by brief and infrequent muscle training.**
   - Since it is not possible to have high intensity exercise and a large amount of exercise, high intensity training must be of short duration.
   - High intensity workouts should allow 48-72 hours of rest between sessions.
   - A "good" strength training workout should not exceed 30 minutes.
   - Advanced lifters do not require more exercise than beginners; they usually need less exercise, but of a more intense nature.

Women are frequently concerned that they will acquire large, bulky muscles by participating in weight training. Actually, the opposite occurs. A trim, firm, well-contoured figure is usually found among women who participate in regular exercise of this kind.

Females have the same muscle properties as males; however, they do not have the same potential for developing muscular bulk and body size because of a male hormone called testosterone, which is produced at a higher level in males. Conversely, males lack the hormone estrogen, which is produced at a much higher level in women. Men or women having an unusual amount of the opposite hormone in their bodies will tend to display characteristics of the opposite sex. It is not the weight training that does it. It should be noted that most weight training programs for women rely more upon increasing the number of repetitions than increasing the weight.

Safety Precautions for Weight Training

- Warm up properly before beginning the training program.
- Barbell plates should be properly secured to prevent slipping.
- Keep hands dry by using carbonate of magnesia.
- Use the overhand grip for overhead lifts.
- Avoid stiff leg positions when lifting weights from the floor (lower back injuries are frequently the result of this lifting position).
- Avoid the full squat position, "deep knee bend" (one-half knee bends achieve good results with less chance of knee injury).
- Avoid holding breath while lifting - breathe naturally. Holding the breath while lifting or jerking heavy weights is a common practice. However, this procedure closes the glottis (opening of the breathing tube), causing pressure which delays blood

flow into the left ventricular, lowering the blood pressure and causing blackout.

- Unless spotters are present, do not perform the "bench press" or other lifts in which you may be "pinned" if control is lost.
- Avoid informal, all-out effort, lifting contests.
- The stooped or squat position is used in a number of weight-training exercises and is the first phase of the "clean and jerk" lift. This position restricts the blood flow in the legs and, if combined with one or both of the other factors, can cause blackout by reducing the cerebral blood flow.
- To avoid blackouts, breathe normally before lifts. Do not hold your breath during lifts. Slowly exhale or inhale through all moving phases of a lift and return to normal breathing in the stationary phases of the lift. Be brief in the squatting position.

Isokinetics

Isokinetic exercises are muscle contractions in which the muscle contracts maximally at a constant speed over a full range of movement with variable resistance.

In an isokinetic contraction the tension developed by the muscle as it shortens is kept at maximum through the full range of motion by the use of special equipment with which the weight or resistance can be decreased or increased as the muscle moves through the range of motion. Therefore, strength is developed through the total range of motion. You must have special equipment such as Cybex, Orthotron, Biodex or minigym devices to apply the principle of isokinetics, and many health spas, colleges, YMCAs, etc. make use of this equipment in their conditioning program.

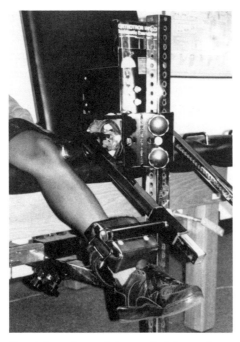

Special equipment is needed to perform isokinetic exercises.

Isometrics

Another method of developing muscular strength is by isometric training. Isometric is a derivation of the Greek preface *iso* (equal) plus *metron* (measure), i.e., *equal measure.* It is a form of strength-building exercise in which short bouts of maximum effort are applied to immovable resistance so that, in effect, the degree of resistance is equal to the force applied to it.

The exercises involve static contraction of a muscle group. As tension is increased, however, the muscle length and joint angle remain constant.

Basic Principles

1. The duration of the contraction should last for ten seconds. The first four seconds are used to obtain maximum contraction. Maximum contraction is then maintained for six seconds.
2. One maximum contraction per day will produce only very limited effect. Several repetitions, adjusted to individual requirements and desired results, are recommended.
3. Strength gain is specific to the angle of contraction. Therefore, contractions should be performed at various joint angles.
4. As with isotonic exercises, you should not hold your breath while performing these contractions. Normal breathing is essential.

Any program of isometric exercise should be considered only as an adjunct or complement to a balanced and comprehensive strength program which includes isotonic and or isokinetic exercise.

Advantages of Isometrics

The following are valid considerations favoring isometric exercises as a part of your total fitness program:
1. Noticeable and excellent results can quickly be obtained.
2. Exercise routine can be accomplished in a short length of time.
3. Can be accomplished indoors in a small space without elaborate and expensive facilities and equipment. For example, your bedroom has all the necessary immovable objects, such as chairs, desks, doorways, towels, and of course, one's own body parts, to contract against.
4. Special attire is not required.

Disadvantages and Limitations of Isometrics

Although there are some specific advantages of isometric exercise, a few limitations should be considered. They are:
1. Accomplishes only one fitness objective, i.e., strength. Muscular and

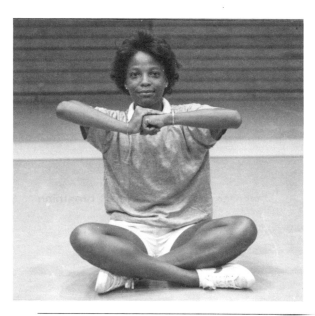

cardiovascular endurance are not improved, nor is flexibility.

2. Difficult to judge when maximum effort is reached without expensive electronic apparatus.
3. Accompanying rise in blood pressure may be harmful to some persons.
4. Feeling of accomplishment may be lacking; therefore, motivation is more difficult.
5. Muscles and joints are not moved through a full range of motion.

Isometric exercises can be performed without expensive and elaborate equipment.

Comparing Muscle Resistance Methods

Method	Potential Value	Advantages	Cautions
Light weights— 1 or 2 lbs. that wrap or buckle around wrists, ankles, etc. or tiny hand weights	Very little strength— mainly toning.	Can increase calorie burning when used with aerobics or with exercisers to increase tone.	Never use these as ankle weights while aerobic dancing. Can be effective for floor exercises.
Elastic bands or surgical tubing	Can add strength and toning—especially wide bands (4")	Inexpensive, portable	Use those bands made for exercise that will not snap if they break.
Hand weights— dumbbells	Many possible strength exercises— can help develop specific body spots	Progressively heavier weights can be used—adds to proper posture by using large muscle groups for stability while lifting.	Start with a weight easy to use and increase gradually.
Weight machines— Universal, Nautilus, etc.	Excellent for overall strength development—one can lift heavier weights.	Safer than the free weights and do not require spotters.	Make certain you know how to use the equipment before beginning—some machines may be too heavy for women to start with.

53

MUSCLES OF THE BODY

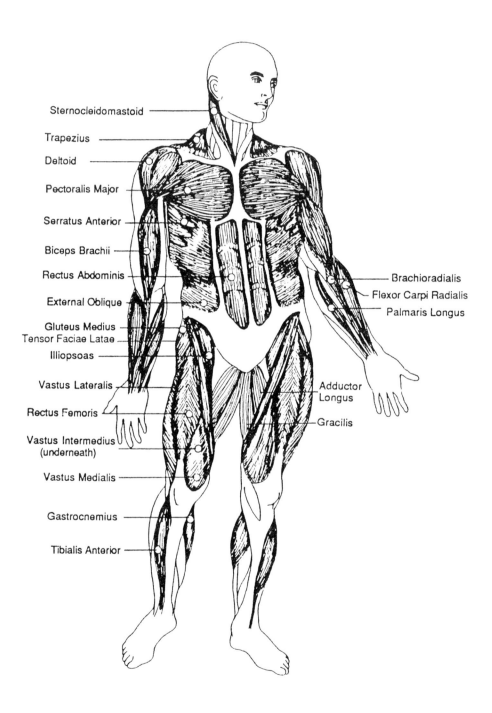

Sternocleidomastoid

Trapezius

Deltoid

Pectoralis Major

Serratus Anterior

Biceps Brachii

Rectus Abdominis

External Oblique

Gluteus Medius
Tensor Faciae Latae

Illiopsoas

Vastus Lateralis

Rectus Femoris

Vastus Intermedius
(underneath)

Vastus Medialis

Gastrocnemius

Tibialis Anterior

Brachioradialis

Flexor Carpi Radialis

Palmaris Longus

Adductor
Longus

Gracilis

MUSCLES OF THE BODY

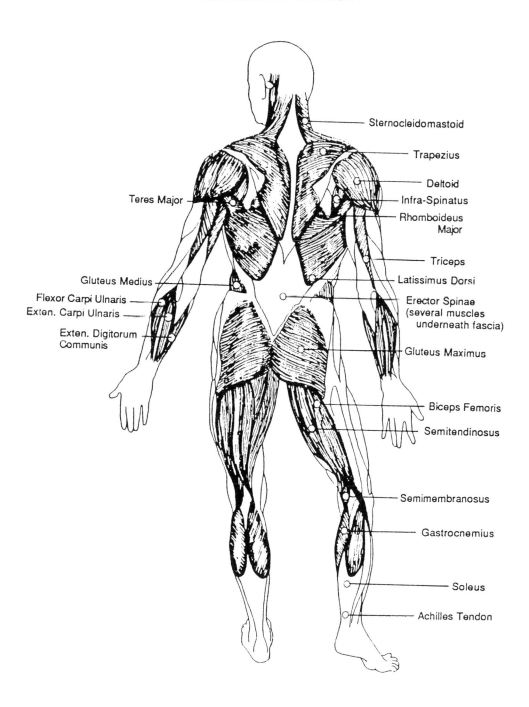

Sternocleidomastoid

Trapezius

Deltoid

Infra-Spinatus

Rhomboideus Major

Teres Major

Triceps

Latissimus Dorsi

Gluteus Medius

Erector Spinae (several muscles underneath fascia)

Flexor Carpi Ulnaris

Exten. Carpi Ulnaris

Gluteus Maximus

Exten. Digitorum Communis

Biceps Femoris

Semitendinosus

Semimembranosus

Gastrocnemius

Soleus

Achilles Tendon

EXERCISES FOR THE MAJOR MUSCLE GROUPS

Muscle Group	Weights	Calisthenics	Partner Exercises
UPPER ARM & SHOULDER			
Biceps	Arm curls Pull downs Upright rowing	Pull ups	One arm curl
Deltoids	Military press Upright rowing Bent arm pull overs	Pull ups	Seated military press
Latissimus Dorsi	Bent arm pullover Rowing Pull downs	Pull ups	Seated Rowing
Pectoralis major	Chest press Bench press Pull overs	Push ups	Push ups
Rhomboids	Rowing	Pull ups	Seated row
Trapezius	Military press	Pull ups	Shrugs
Triceps	Bench Press Tricep extension French curl	Dips Push ups	Push ups
TRUNK			
Obliques Rectus Abdominus	Twisting crunches Sit-up Crunch	Twisting crunches Sit-up Crunch	Abdominal curl Abdominal curl
LOWER EXTREMITY			
Gastrocnemius Gluteus maximus	Heel raise Squat Leg press	Calf raise Knee bends	Calf raise Single leg press
Hamstrings	Squat	Towel curl	Leg curl
Quadriceps	Leg extension Leg press Squat	Knee bends Sit-ups	Single leg press

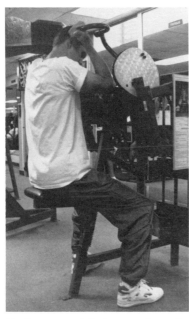

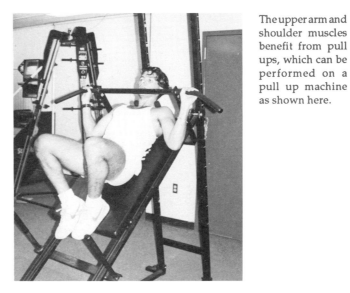

The upper arm and shoulder muscles benefit from pull ups, which can be performed on a pull up machine as shown here.

Curls are one of the best workouts for the biceps.

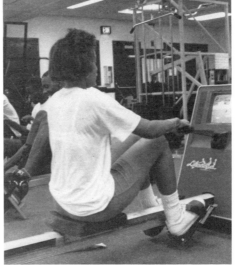

Rowing is an excellent exercise for the latissimus dorsi muscles.

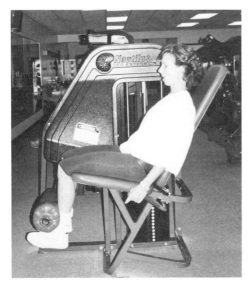

Leg extensions are a popular exercise for the quadriceps.

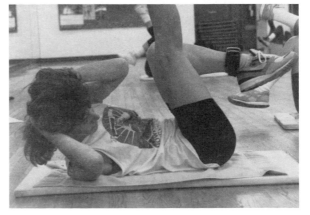

Twisting crunches are great for the obliques.

57

Home Exercise Program

The following exercises can be done at home without weights to improve muscular strength and endurance.

Abdominal Muscular Strength and Endurance

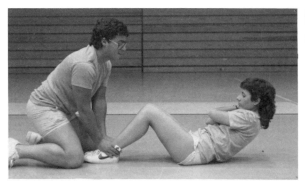

Curl Up—Arms Crossed

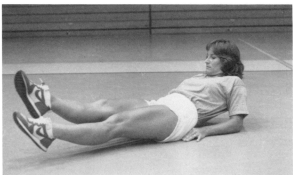

Lower Abdominals

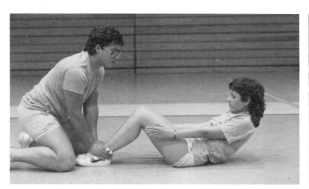

Curl Up—Arms Extended

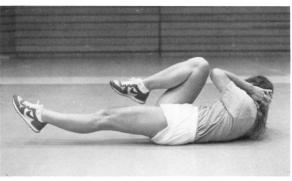

Advanced Lower Abdominal Crossovers

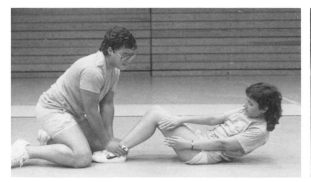

Obliques—Both Arms Reaching to Side

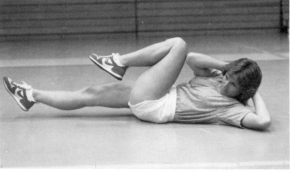

Advanced Lower Abdominal Crossovers

Abdominal Muscular Strength and Endurance, continued

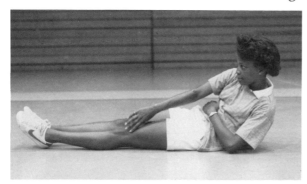

Obliques

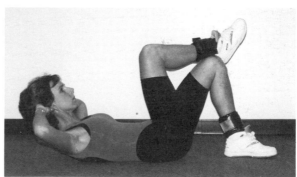

Crunches With Weights

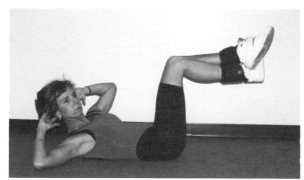

Obliques With Crossed Legs Bent

Abdominals With One Leg Extended

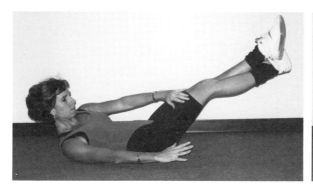

Obliques With Straight Crossed Legs

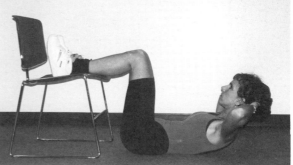

Abdominals With Legs Elevated

Triceps

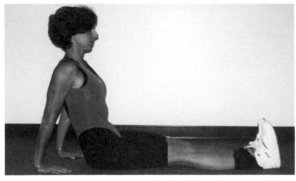

Floor Dips—Position 1

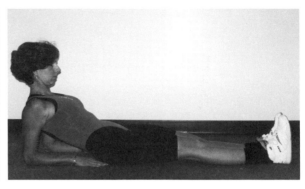

Floor Dips—Position 2

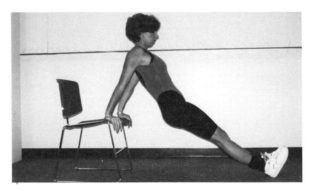

Chair Dips

Strength and Endurance for the Back Muscles

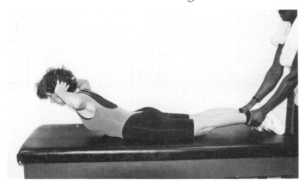

Upper Body Lift

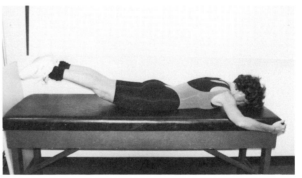

Table Leg Lift

Strength and Endurance for the Back Muscles, continued

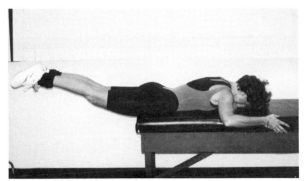

Advanced Table Leg Lift

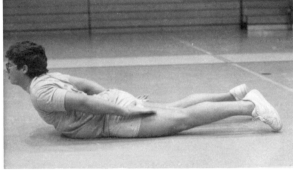

Floor Upper Body Lift

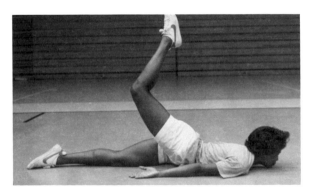

Floor Leg Lift

Thigh Muscle Exercises

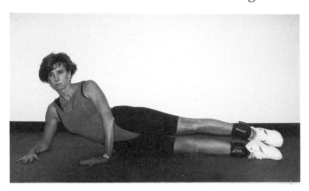

Outer Thigh Lift—Starting Position

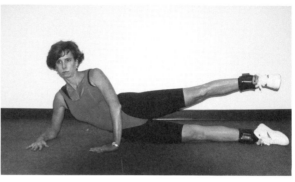

Outer Thigh Lift

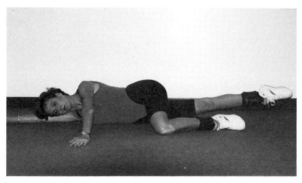

Beginner Inner Thigh Lift

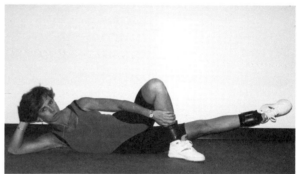

Inner Thigh Lift

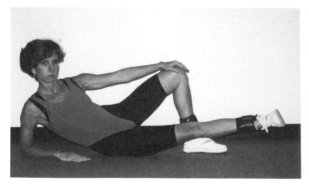

Advanced Inner Thigh Lift

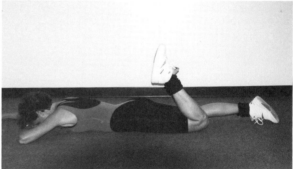

Hamstrings and Buttocks

DEVELOPING YOUR FLEXIBILITY PROGRAM

Flexibility is a very important part of physical fitness and is all too frequently overlooked when programs are being planned.

Flexibility is important for the average person because of its relationship to health and a person's working capacity. Short muscles can become sore muscles when exposed to physical exertion. In addition, inflexible joints and muscles can limit working efficiency and cause problems such as those associated with the lower back.

Flexibility is the ability of a person to move body joints through a maximum range of motion without undue strain. It is not a general factor, but is specific to given joints, sports, and physical activities. It is more dependent upon the soft tissues, tendons, ligaments and muscles of a joint than upon the bony structure of the joint. The bony structures of certain joints place certain limitations of flexibility; an extension of the knee illustrates this limitation graphically. Also, overextension of the spinal column is limited by the shape and position of the spinous processes in the column.

Flexibility is related to activity, body size, age, and sex. Active people tend to be more flexible than inactive people; as the soft tissues or joints tend to shrink they lose extensibility when the muscles are maintained in a shortened position.

Physical activity with wide ranges of movement will help prevent the loss of extensibility. An increase in body fat usually decreases flexibility and girls are generally more flexible than boys of the same age. Also, as a person grows older there is a gradual decrease in flexibility as the soft tissues lose their extensibility.

Flexibility development and training techniques are progressive and to improve your range of motion you will need to relax so that you can proceed to a more intense level of stretch.

Experts generally agree that soft tissues and muscles are most affected by the slow, sustained (static) stretch which involves holding a muscle at a greater than resting length in a stationary position for a period of time, usually 20-30 seconds. The **ballistic stretch** (dynamic stretch) involves putting a muscle in a longer than resting position and bobbing or bouncing against the muscle in an attempt to increase the length of the muscle. The use of a fast, forceful or bobbing type of stretching is less effective and dangerous; it may cause the body to bring into play the stretch reflex, which is the automatic contraction of a muscle in response to the muscle's being suddenly stretched beyond its normal length and this causes considerable pain and muscle soreness.

The developmental phases of flexibility training are:
1. Easy stretch, held for about 5-10 seconds as you relax and let gravity and/or a body part do the work.
2. Developmental stretch allows the muscle fibers to stretch out slowly and to stay stretched for a period of 10-20 seconds.

The PNF Stretch

Proprioceptive Neuromuscular Facilitation (PNF) is a group of stretching techniques which involve alternating contractions and relaxations of the opposing muscle groups. Several techniques can be used:
1. slow—reversal—hold—relax
2. contract—relax
3. hold—relax techniques

Each technique involves the assistance of a partner in alternating a contraction and relaxation of the muscles involved (i.e., a ten-second pushing phase followed by a ten-second relaxing phase). Following are three more specific examples.

1. The muscle is stretched until there is slight discomfort, then you push against your partner who applies resistance for 10 seconds while your partner uses passive pressure to stretch the original muscle group. This sequence is repeated at least three times.
2. The muscle is isotonically contracted so that it actually moves away during the push phase.
3. The hold—relax method involves an isometric contraction during the push phase and during the relaxation phase both muscle groups (original and opposing) are passively stretched.

Six Guidelines for a Flexibility Program

1. Brief cardiorespiratory warmup (2-5 minutes), such as easy jogging, running in place, rope skipping, or inverted bicycling, and preliminary movements of the skeletal structure, such as arm circles and joint swings, should be done. This warmup is necessary to increase circulation and body heat for the tissues, ligaments, and joints, thus increasing flexibility of the muscle and skeletal systems.
2. Exercises must be performed for each muscle group or joint in which flexibility is desired.
3. The stretching should be gradual and progressive. It should be done with full extension and flexion being placed on the joint for a period of 20-30 seconds.
4. Stretching should be distributed rather than massed; thus exercises should be performed at least several times a day and four to five days a week.
5. Stretching should be gentle and gradual so as not to cause overstretching, since the stretch reflex may come into play, thus causing soreness and possible damage to the soft muscle tissues, ligaments, or tendons.
6. Breathing should be slow, rhythmical and relaxed.

Suggested Flexibility Exercises

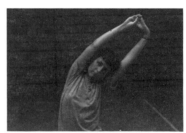

Sidewinder

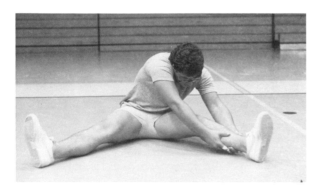

Saddle Stretch

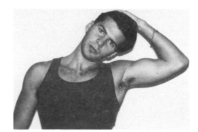

Neck Stretch

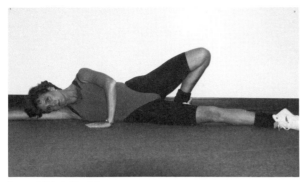

Inner Thigh Stretch

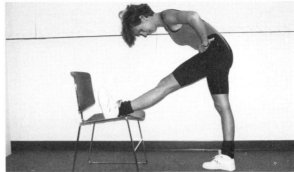

Hamstring Stretch

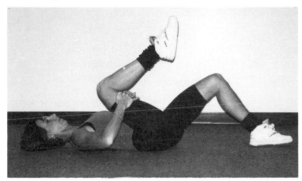

Hip Flexor

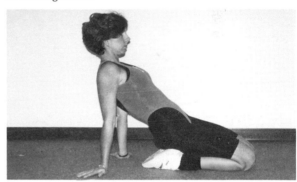

Quadriceps Stretch

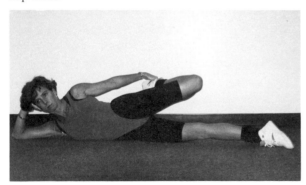

Quadriceps Stretch

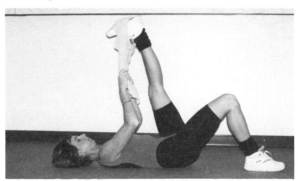

Hamstring Stretch

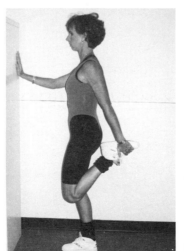

Quadriceps Stretch

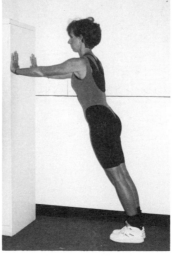

Gastrocnemius
and Achilles
Tendon Stretch

65

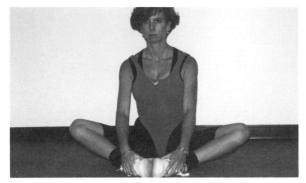

Hip Stretch

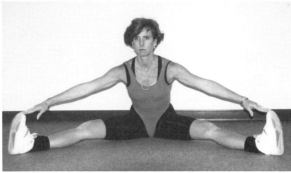

Hip Stretch

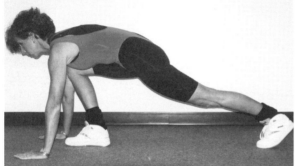

Low Lunge Stretch

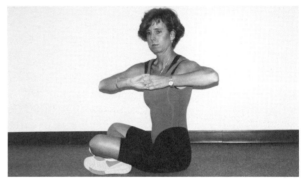

Back Stretch

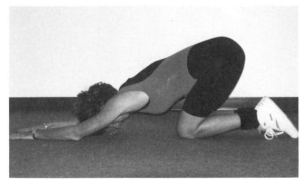

Back Stretch

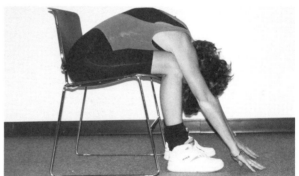

Back Stretch

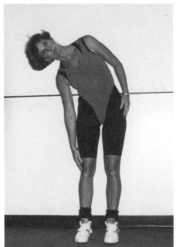

Back Stretch

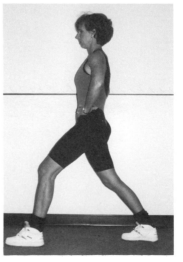

Hip and Calf Stretch

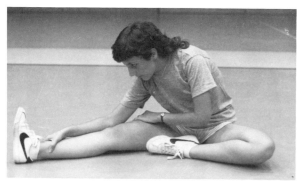

Forward Hurdle Stretch

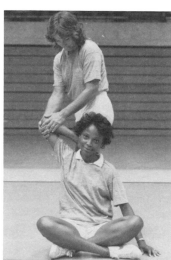

Upper Leg and Back Stretch

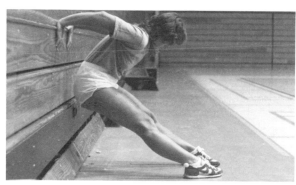

Shin Stretch

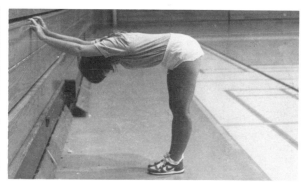

Back Stretch

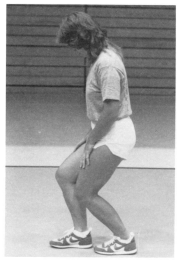

Quadriceps Stretch

Shoulder Stretch

Partner Resistance

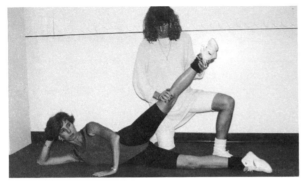

Outside of Thigh

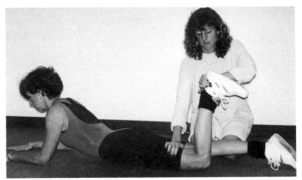

Lower Back

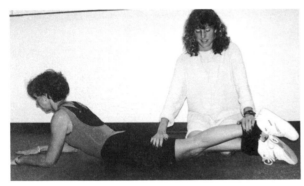

Hamstring Curl

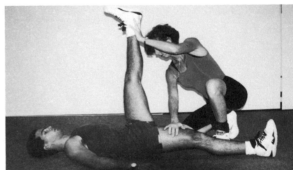

Hamstring Curl

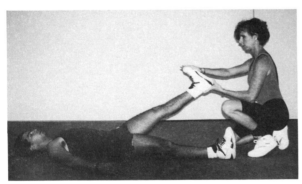

Calf and Achilles Tendon

Hamstrings

Potentially Harmful Exercises

Recently some reports have indicated that certain exercises may be harmful or dangerous and should be avoided. However, James Garrick, M.D., orthopedic surgeon and director of the Center for Sports Medicine at St. Francis Memorial Hospital in San Francisco, says: "There is very little evidence about whether specific exercises are good or bad. Most experts agree that exercise programs should be individually tailored to previous problems and to present goals." This means that there should be differences in the exercises utilized by the budding or accomplished young athlete as opposed to the sixty-year-old with osteoporosis or arthritis—just as there should be a difference between programs for the sixty- and thirty-year-old who enjoy good health, but who exercise for recreational reasons.

There does seem to be a group of exercises that have the potential to cause some people problems. They are usually classified under neck, back, or knee exercises.

Potentially Harmful Exercises — Neck

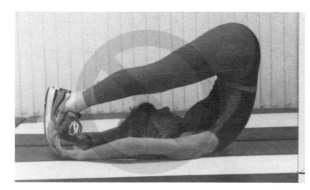

The Yoga Plough

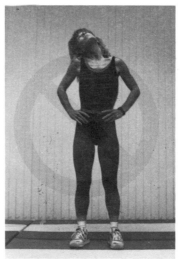

Full and Fast Neck Circles

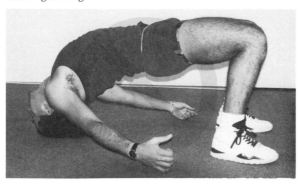

The Wrestler's Bridge

Potentially Harmful Exercises — Knee

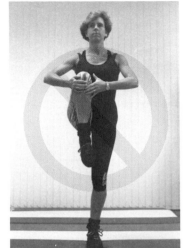

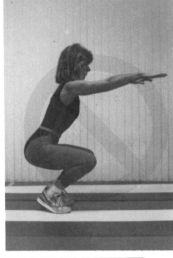

Knee Pull-Down (Correct method is to pull on the thigh instead of the knee.)

Full Squats or Duck Walk

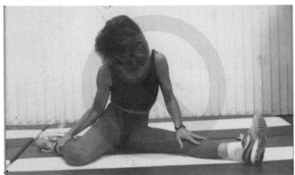

Hurdler's Stretch

Potentially Harmful Exercises — Back

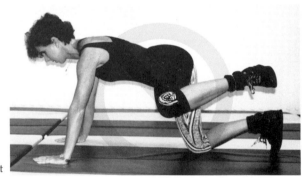

Donkey Kick or Fire Hydrant

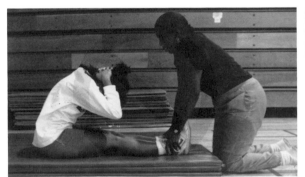

Straight Leg Sit-ups

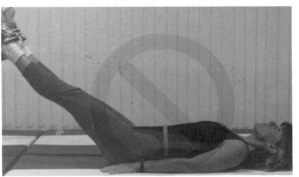

Double Leg Lifts

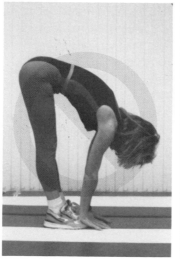

Standing Toe Touch with Locked Knees

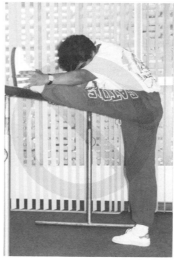

Ballistic (Bouncing) Bar Stretch

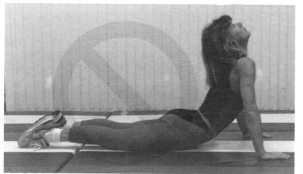

The Cobra

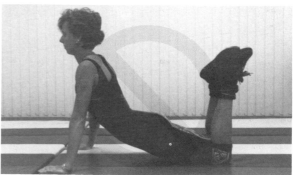

Arched Push-ups from the Knees

Getting Started

Many people procrastinate or hesitate when beginning their exercise program. The following suggestions may help you:

Start today—not tomorrow. Put your decision into action before you think of all the negatives or dwell on your doubts and fears. No matter how little you do the first day, *do something*—take a walk, jog in place, stretch, etc.

Start out easy. Pushing yourself too hard in the beginning may cause injury, sore-ness, and extreme fatigue. Follow the training guidelines to gradually increase your workload.

Set specific goals and reward yourself for reaching them. Promise yourself something special after successfully completing one week of your plan—a new outfit, a warmup suit, or something you have wanted to buy or do but, for some reason, have not.

Put exercise at the top of your "to do" list—make it a priority. Remind yourself that you want to exercise, therefore, you will

71

find a way to fit it into your schedule. Use cues and prompts to reinforce your decision—put your exercise clothes out the night before or before you leave for work; put your bicycle in a conspicuous place; leave your jogging shoes where you will see them as you come in the door.

Emphasize the positive. Give yourself a pep talk. Congratulate yourself for doing the workout. Feel good about sticking to your plan—for not letting yourself make excuses. If you miss a day, don't give up—realize you can recover the lost ground. Even if changes in your body are not noticeable right away, remind yourself that you have overcome the most difficult part—the beginning. Remind yourself of the benefits you are receiving every day.

Be flexible. If you always work out in the morning but have an early appointment and cannot, work it into your afternoon schedule. If you don't feel like jogging one day, try something different—a swim, aerobic dance, etc. You may find the change and variety very enjoyable.

QUESTIONS AND ANSWERS

I usually stop running to take my pulse. Does this prevent me from getting an accurate reading of my pulse when jogging?

If you can take it within 10 seconds after stopping, it should accurately reflect your true rate while exercising.

Since my heart rate increases during weight training, can weight training be considered an aerobic exercise?

No. In this case, an increased heart rate can be a misleading indication. Although the heart rate is elevated during weight training, the oxygen delivery system is not challenged or overloaded, which is an important phase of aerobic exercise. During powerful muscle contractions, the blood flow through the muscles is actually shut off. The blood flow rushes into the muscles after the contraction. During aerobic exercise, the blood flows continuously through the muscles, and oxygen consumption by the muscles is high.

Which type of exercise will help me burn up the most calories?

The basic rule is that the fuel you burn is governed by the amount of weight you move and the distance you move it. Therefore, the same exercises which contribute to cardiovascular fitness are those which burn the most calories. Select activities which involve total body activity, which are rhythmical and which can be maintained for a longer time. Aerobic dance is great!

Is an aerobic workout in water of any value or better than a dry-land workout?

Two recent studies have concluded that water exercise increased oxygen consumption according to the depths of the water. This was determined by walking subjects on a dry-land treadmill then on one submerged at ankle-level water, knee-level, mid thigh-level, and waist-level.

This study, conducted by the Nicolas Institute of Sports Medicine and Athletic Trauma of Lenox Hill Hospital in New York City, concluded that water depth significantly increased calories burned during walking.

Another study conducted by the Human Performance Lab at Adelphi University found that water walking used more than twice as many calories per minute as treadmill walking, and only 23% less than treadmill running.

Why should I do my weight program three or four times a week rather than every day?

Research indicates little difference in strength gains between a three- or four-day program as opposed to a seven-day program. Also, the body requires a certain amount of rest for rejuvenation and growth.

What is the difference between "negative" work and "positive" work?

These terms refer to whether a muscle contraction is eccentric or concentric. An eccentric muscle contraction is known as "negative" work and occurs when a muscle is lengthened while you are actually contracting it. An example is lowering yourself from a chinning bar as you resist the pull of gravity. A concentric muscle contraction is the shortening of a muscle as it works. Raising yourself up to a chinning bar is an example of a positive contraction. It is important to include both types of training in your conditioning program. By doing negative work, you also improve your ability to do the positive work since the negative work contributes to strength development.

How much should I increase my "weight load" from week to week?

Since many weight machines increase their weights in increments of 10-25 pounds, this can present a problem.
Remember that:
- Each person is different and does not respond to training in the same way.
- The entry level of strength will be different for each person.
- Maximum strength limits will be different.
- Initial gains will be greater for those who are farther from their limit.
- Less gains always occur as an individual approaches his or her maximum limits.

The wise person will increase weight by no more than five percent each week, and as the limit is reached, this may well drop to two and a half percent.

As a female, I am not interested in gaining great strength, but I would like to body build in a few spots. Any suggestions?

Assuming you are in good health, the following guidelines for training should be helpful:
- Remember to begin with light weights to practice the basic techniques.
- Do only one set of 10-12 reps per exercise.
- Work every other day for one or two weeks, then increase your workout to two sets.
- After one or two weeks increase your workout to three sets.
- The next step is to increase your weight and to drop back on reps and/or sets.
- Remember that calcium is important for bone strength and muscle contractions. About 1,000 mg per day are recommended for women under age 30.

After exercise, how long must I wait to fully regain my strength?

Laboratory experiments indicate that if a muscle is fully fatigued it will take approximately 45 minutes for partial recovery.

Under ideal conditions, a muscle will regain 70 percent of its initial strength within 30 seconds and will be able to perform with 80-90 percent normal strength within seven and a half minutes.

My grandparents are becoming pretty feeble. Would weight training be of any benefit to them?

Dr. Maria Fiatarone recently completed an interesting study at the Hebrew Rehabilitation Center for Aged in Boston. She experimented with 10 patients ranging in age from 86 to 96; all were inactive and frail, four had high blood pressure, six had heart disease, and seven had arthritis.

They performed weight training exercises for quadriceps muscles three times a week for eight weeks, and increased weight lifted from 15 to 43 pounds. At the conclusion of the study they had experienced an average strength gain of 174%. In addition, two no longer required canes to walk, and one of the three, who was wheel chair confined, was able to rise and stand without using his arms for assistance.

Weight training is not the only activity that seniors can engage in with success. For example, just recently, Gertrude Zint, age 67, swam the 100 yard individual medley in 1:46.6 during the Northern Illinois Senior Olympics in DeKalb. And Bryon Fike, at age 72, ran the mile in 6:40 during the Ohio Senior Olympics.

Once I acquire the strength I need, what do I have to do to keep it?

Strength can be maintained by exercising at least once weekly. However, all body parts must be exercised at a close to maximum repetition. It should be noted that this type of workout may cause muscle soreness.

Do jogging and walking use the same total energy?

No. Jogging utilizes more total calories and more fat calories. If loss of body weight and body fat are your objectives, stick with jogging.

Are there any risks in jogging?

Although jogging is an excellent aerobic exercise, it is not risk-free. The Center for Disease Control in Atlanta reports that 17% of all female runners and 13% of all male runners seek medical attention for running-related injuries each year.

If you have been inactive for a period of time, if you have old leg injuries, or if you are excessively overweight, you may develop problems. Inadequate shoes and hard surfaces also contribute to difficulties.

However, before you throw your running shoes away, consider that most of us end up each year visiting the doctor for the common cold, and that many running problems can be treated with the RICE formula—i.e., **R**est, **I**ce, **C**ompression, and **E**levation. At the appropriate time, heat is also a valuable aid in rehabilitation.

REFERENCES
1. Tuten, R., V. Knight and C. Moore. *Weight Training Everyone*. 3rd ed. Winston-Salem, NC: Hunter Textbooks, Inc., 1990.
2. Knopf, Fleck & Martin. *Water Workouts*. Winston-Salem, NC: Hunter Textbooks, Inc., 1988.
3. Floyd, P. and J. Parke. *Walk, Jog, Run for Wellness Everyone*. Winston-Salem, NC: Hunter Textbooks, Inc., l990.

SUGGESTED LABS: 13, 14, 15, 16, 17, 18, 19, 20.

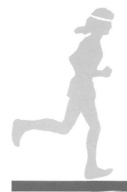

Knowing Your Nutrition

Objectives

- Describe the nutrients (carbohydrates, proteins, and fats) and their functions, sources, and recommended percentage in the diet
- Describe the reasons for limiting sugar intake
- Describe the important role of fiber in the diet
- Describe the importance of controlling cholesterol in the diet in lowering the risk of cardiovascular disease
- Describe the problem with fast foods and identify nutritional values of many fast foods
- Describe the role of vitamins and minerals in the diet as well as sources and functions
- Describe the potential problems with salt in the diet
- Describe the important role of water to the body
- Describe the Recommended Dietary Goals providing recommended food sources
- Describe how to compute daily target fat rate

Key Words

- Amino acids
- Carbohydrates
- Cholesterol
- Complete protein
- Disaccharides
- Electrolyte
- Fat soluble vitamin
- Fiber
- HDL
- Hydrogenated
- Incomplete protein
- Polysaccharides
- LDL
- Minerals
- Monosaccharides
- Monounsaturated fat
- Proteins
- RDA
- Saturated fat
- Triglycerides
- Unsaturated fat
- Vitamins
- Water soluble vitamin

Anyone interested in his or her level of fitness and health should learn the basic facts about good nutrition. Nutrition is the study of the food we eat and how the body uses it. The most important practical use of the science of nutrition is as a guide for selecting and eating foods that will provide the body what it needs to function effectively. The study of nutrition allows you to disregard the faddist, quacks and advertising experts who try to influence the uninformed individual. Unfortunately, most people seem to have very limited knowledge of such basic information as the nutritive value of foods and even less knowledge of applying this to meal planning.

Obviously we are creatures of what we eat, but we are also creatures of what we fail to eat. In order to maintain optimal health, we must supply our body with the right foods in sufficient amounts. Whether at work, in school, in sports or in leisure activities, we can perform only as well as our physical well being allows.

Through better nutrition you can improve the quality of all aspects of your life. Nutrition affects virtually every function of the body and good nutrition can act as preventive medicine. Since you control the types and amounts of food you eat, you alone are responsible for the nutritional state of your body. You cannot consistently deprive your body of the essential nutrients it needs, for effects of a diet deficiency or imbalance are slow and subtle, but inevitable.

As a consumer, it is also important to have a thorough knowledge of nutrition. A wise consumer knows that nutritionally good food need not cost any more than nutritionally inadequate food and may often cost less. With constantly rising food cost, it is important for you to get the best nutrition for your money. Once you have knowledge of the nutritional value of various foods, you can eat more economically by decreasing or eliminating foods that have little nutritional value.

U.S. DIETARY GOALS

In November of 1990 the U.S. Department of Health and Human Services released the updated Dietary Guidelines for Americans. These seven recommendations are designed to provide advice on the dietary pattern Americans should follow. These guidelines are briefly described below.

1. **Eat a variety of foods.**

A varied and balanced diet is described as one with these daily servings:
    3-5 servings of vegetables
    2-4 servings of fruit
    6-12 servings of grains (breads, cereals, rice, pasta)
    2-3 servings of milk, yogurt, and cheese
    2-3 servings of meat, poultry, fish, dry beans, peas, eggs, nuts

2. **Maintain healthy weight.**

A major change is a new table of suggested weights for adults which puts men and women together with the higher weights in the range applying to men. The report also emphasizes that one must evaluate a "healthy weight" in relationship to blood pressure and blood cholesterol levels. If one is at risk in these areas, then it may be necessary to lower one's weight. In addition, one's body shape has been found to be an important factor in relation to weight. Research indicates that excess fat in the abdomen (apple shape) presents a greater risk than excess fat in the hips or thighs (pear shape). (See the chapter on Weight Control for a method of determining your body shape.)

3. **Choose a diet low in fat, saturated fat, and cholesterol.**

The recommendation encourages individuals to limit fat in the diet to 30% or less of the total calories and no more than 10% from saturated fat. It also provides advice on how to reach these goals.

4. **Choose a diet with plenty of vegetables, fruits, and grain products.**

This recommendation specifically encourages the intake of foods with adequate fiber and starch.

5. **Use sugars only in moderation.**

In addition to recommending the limited use of sugars, the guidelines list some names for sugars that often appear on food labels (glucose, fructose, corn syrup, etc.) and sugar's role in tooth decay is described.

6. **Use salt and sodium only in moderation.**

The recommendation points out the relationship of salt and sodium use to high blood pressure and provides advice for selecting foods to control the intake (i.e., fresh vegetables rather than canned).

7. **If you drink alcoholic beverages, do so in moderation.**

The definition of moderate drinking is no more than one drink a day for women and no more than two drinks a day for men. One drink is considered to be one 12-ounce beer, 5 ounces of wine, or 1 1/2 ounces of distilled spirits.

These dietary guidelines should form the basis of the food selection and preparation for all Americans. However, to achieve a high level of wellness one must go beyond these basics to a more complete understanding of nutrition.

THE BASIC FOOD GROUPS

Nutritionists have long recognized four basic food groups as being the key to obtaining a well-balanced, nutritious diet. Essentially these food groups can still be used as a guideline for proper eating. However, in view of the information now available concerning the possible dangers of some foods, we need to carefully select those that are low in fat, saturated fat, and cholesterol. Although the groups are not new, the emphasis on which foods are given priority has changed. By selecting the correct number of servings from each of the food groups each day, one would have a balanced diet; however, this is only a quantitative measure of your diet. To ensure a quality diet, one should give careful consideration to the selection of foods from within each of the four food groups.

Described on the next page are the food groups, the recommended number of servings per day and suggestions for quality selections. Also noted are those high in fat and cholesterol.

THE NEW AMERICAN EATING GUIDE

Beans, Grains, and Nuts
(4 or more servings per day)

Anytime	In Moderation	Now and Then
Bread and rolls (whole grain)	Cornbread[8]	Croissant[4, 8]
Bulgur	Flour tortilla[8]	Doughnut[3 or 4, 5, 8]
Dried beans and peas	Granola cereals[1 or 2]	Presweetened cereals[5, 8]
Lentils	Hominy grits[8]	Sticky buns[1 or 2, 5, 8]
Oatmeal	Macaroni and cheese[1, (6), 8]	Stuffing (with butter)[4, (6), 8]
Pasta, whole-wheat	Matzoh[8]	
Rice, brown	Nuts[3]	
Sprouts	Pasta, refined[8]	
Whole-grain hot and cold cereals	Peanut butter[3]	
Whole-wheat matzoh	Pizza[6, 8]	
	Refined, unsweetened cereals[8]	
	Refried beans[1 or 2]	
	Seeds[3]	
	Soybeans[2]	
	Tofu[2]	
	Waffles or pancakes with syrup[5, (6), 8]	
	White bread and rolls[8]	
	White rice[8]	

Fruits and Vegetables
(4 or more servings per day)

Anytime	In Moderation	Now and Then
All fruits and vegetables except those at right	Avocado[3]	Coconut[4]
Applesauce (unsweetened)	Cole slaw[3]	Pickles[6]
Unsweetened fruit juices	Cranberry sauce[5]	
Unsalted vegetable juices	Dried fruit	
Potatoes, white or sweet	French fries[1 or 2]	
	Fried eggplant[2]	
	Fruits canned in syrup[5]	
	Gazpacho[2, (6)]	
	Guacamole[3]	
	Potatoes au gratin[1, (6)]	
	Salted vegetable juices[6]	
	Sweetened fruit juices[5]	
	Vegetables canned with salt[6]	

[1] Moderate fat, saturated.
[2] Moderate fat, unsaturated.
[3] High fat, unsaturated.

[4] High fat, saturated.
[5] High in added sugar.
[6] High in salt or sodium.

(6) May be high in salt or sodium.
[7] High in cholesterol.
[8] Refined grains.

THE NEW AMERICAN EATING GUIDE, continued

Poultry, Fish, Meat, and Eggs
(2 servings per day; vegetarians should eat added servings from other groups)

Anytime	*In Moderation*	*Now and Then*
Cod	Fried fish[1 or 2]	Fried chicken, commercial[4]
Flounder	Herring[3, 6]	Cheese omelet[4, 7]
Gefilte fish[(6)]	Mackerel, canned[2, (6)]	Whole egg or yolk (limit to 3 a
Haddock	Salmon, canned[2, (6)]	week)[3, 7]
Halibut	Sardines[2, (6)]	Bacon[4, (6)]
Perch	Shrimp[7]	Beef liver, fried[1, 7]
Pollock	Tuna, oil-packed[2, (6)]	Bologna[4, 6]
Rockfish	Chicken liver[7]	Corned beef[4, 6]
Shellfish, except shrimp	Fried chicken in vegetable oil	Ground beef[4]
Sole	(homemade)[3]	Ham, trimmed[1, 6]
Tuna, water-packed[(6)]	Chicken or turkey, boiled, baked	Hot dogs[4, 6]
Egg whites	or roasted (with skin)[2]	Liverwurst[4, 6]
Chicken or turkey, boiled, baked, or	Flank steak[1]	Pig's feet[4]
roasted (no skin)	Leg or loin of lamb[1]	Salami[4, 6]
	Pork shoulder or loin, lean[1]	Sausage[4, 6]
	Round steak or ground round[1]	Spareribs[4]
	Rump roast[1]	Red meats, untrimmed[4]
	Sirloin steak, lean[1]	
	Veal[1]	

Milk Products
(3 to 4 servings per day for children, 2 for adults)

Anytime	*In Moderation*	*Now and Then*
Buttermilk (from skim milk)	Cocoa with skim milk[5]	Cheesecake[4, 5]
Low-fat cottage cheese	Cottage cheese, regular[1]	Cheese fondue[4, (6)]
Low-fat milk (1%)	Frozen yogurt[5]	Cheese soufflé[4, (6), 7]
Low-fat yogurt	Ice milk[5]	Eggnog[1, 5, 7]
Nonfat dry milk	Low-fat milk (2%)[1]	Hard cheeses: blue, brick,
Skim-milk cheeses	Low-fat yogurt, sweetened[5]	Camembert, cheddar,
Skim milk	Mozzarella, part-skim[1, (6)]	muenster, Swiss[4, (6)]
Skim-milk and banana shake		Ice Cream[4, 5]
		Processed cheeses[4, 6]
		Whole milk[4]
		Whole-milk yogurt[4]

[1] Moderate fat, saturated.	[4] High fat, saturated.	[(6)] May be high in salt or sodium.
[2] Moderate fat, unsaturated.	[5] High in added sugar.	[7] High in cholesterol.
[3] High fat, unsaturated.	[6] High in salt or sodium.	[8] Refined grains.

Copyright 1986, 8th printing, CSPI. Reprinted from *New American Eating Guide* which is available from CSPI, 875 Connecticut Ave. N.W. #300, Washington, DC 20009 for $4.95.

THE MAJOR NUTRIENTS

Nutrients are chemical substances which are obtained from food. Nutrients are utilized by the body to build and maintain body cells, to regulate body processes, and to supply energy. There are about fifty known nutrients plus water (and possibly others not yet discovered) which have been chemically classified as proteins, carbohydrates, fats, vitamins, and minerals. In maintaining optimal health, it is important to include a variety of foods, because no single food—not even mother's milk—contains all the nutrients we need in the proper amounts we need.

Carbohydrates

Carbohydrates are the most important source of energy available to the body. Consisting of sugars and starches, they yield four calories of energy for each gram consumed. The confusion and concern about carbohydrates in our diet have developed because of the great variability between sugars and starches.

One group of carbohydrates is made up of the sugars that are quickly broken down and absorbed by our bodies. These simple carbohydrates include refined sugars and carbohydrates such as white bread, rolls, snack food, candy bars, jellies, and hot fudge sundaes. In addition, fructose, a simple carbohydrate found naturally in fruits, is more slowly digested and is packed with vitamins, minerals and fibers.

The complex carbohydrates are those identified as the starches which provide a more stable form of energy and have great supplies of other nutrients needed by the body. Generally, complex carbohydrates are found in the natural types of foods—vegetables, cereals, whole grains and beans.

Carbohydrates are the number one source of energy and are found primarily in plants. There are three main groups of carbohydrates according to the number of sugar units (saccharides) in the basic structure.

Monosaccharides are the simplest form of carbohydrate and consist of a single sugar. This group includes glucose, fructose, galactose, and mannose. The two most common monosaccharides or single sugars are glucose and fructose, which are found abundantly in fruits and vegetables. The amount of sugar in fruit depends somewhat on the degree of ripeness. As the fruit ripens, some of the starch changes to sugar. The single sugars require no digestion.

Function	Sources	Calories per gram	Recommended % in diet
Broken down into glucose, which is the major source of energy	Fruits	4	50-66%
Some is stored in liver and muscles in the form of glycogen	Vegetables		
Supply fiber	Grains Cereals		

They are quickly absorbed from the intestines into the bloodstream and are carried to the liver where they are converted into glycogen (stored glucose) or used immediately as energy needs. Glycogen stored in the liver can be converted to glucose later to meet the body's energy needs.

Disaccharides are a more complex form of carbohydrates and consist of two sugars or two monosaccharides. This group includes sucrose, lactose, and maltose. Sucrose is the common granulated table sugar, known also as beet or cane sugar. Sucrose is sugar—granulated, powdered, or brown. White sugar contains no vitamins, no minerals, no protein, no fat, no fiber, but has 770 calories per cup. Molasses, a by-product of sugar manufacturing, is also a form of sucrose. Lactose is the sugar present in milk and is the only common sugar not found in plants. It is less soluble and less sweet than sucrose.

Polysaccharides are the most complex carbohydrates and consist of many units of monosaccharides. This group includes cellulose, pectin, starch, and glycogen. Good sources of polysaccharides are potatoes, beans, peas, grains (wheat, oats, corn, and rice), flour, macaroni, spaghetti, noodles, grits, bread, and breakfast cereals.

The end product of the breakdown of carbohydrates is glucose (blood sugar), which is used by the cells to furnish energy for the body's activities. Carbohydrates differ in their nutritional value, though. For instance, potatoes and fruit supply essential vitamins and minerals but sugar provides nothing but calories.

Sugar

It is important to realize the potential problems related to refined carbohydrates. In addition to increased dental problems, dietary sugar causes a rapid elevation of blood sugar, elevation of blood triglycerides, and may stimulate the liver to produce more cholesterol. Because sugar is quickly converted to glucose and rapidly gets into the bloodstream, there may be a short feeling of quick energy. However, the pancreas releases insulin necessary for the utilization of the sugar in such large amounts that the blood sugar level is then driven lower than normal. As a result, you may experience the uncomfortable sign of hypoglycemia: light-headedness, weakness, depression, and even dizziness.

Part of the problem with the high intake of refined sugar is the "hidden" sugar in so many foods. Processed foods and beverages account for more than two-thirds of the refined sugar we consume. You may be surprised to read the label of many foods and find that sugar has been added. There is also confusion as to whether honey, brown sugar, and molasses are better substitutes for table sugar Honey is still straight sugar, brown sugar is just white sugar with molasses, and raw sugar is no longer available on the market. Blackstrap molasses is the only sugar with anything to offer of nutritional value. It does contain some minerals from the original sugar cane, plus calcium and iron from the processing.

People may become confused as they try to limit their sugar intake because manufacturers use various forms of sugar without listing the word "sugar" on the label. The following are all sugars:

- sucrose (table sugar, brown sugar, confectioner's sugar, raw sugar, turbinado)—contains equal parts of glucose and fructose
- glucose (dextrose, corn syrup, and glucose syrup)—a naturally occurring sugar
- fructose (fruits and honey)—a naturally occurring sugar

- honey—a natural syrup made of glucose, fructose, and water
- sorbitol—a naturally occurring sugar alcohol
- high-fructose corn syrup (liquid sweetener found in soft drinks)—some of the glucose in corn syrup is converted to fructose
- lactose—sugar found in milk

Most people would be wise to observe the following methods of decreasing sugar intake:
1. Drink fewer soft drinks (regular soft drinks average 8 teaspoons per 12 oz.)
2. Eat fewer baked goods and, when cooking your own, decrease the sugar content.
3. Read food labels and avoid foods containing added sugar.

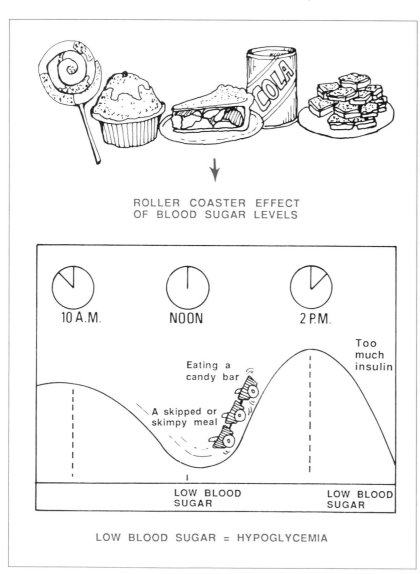

ROLLER COASTER EFFECT OF BLOOD SUGAR LEVELS

10 A.M.   NOON   2 P.M.

Too much insulin

Eating a candy bar

A skipped or skimpy meal

LOW BLOOD SUGAR   LOW BLOOD SUGAR

LOW BLOOD SUGAR = HYPOGLYCEMIA

Sugar Substitutes

How safe are artificial sweeteners?

Some manufacturers use non-nutritive sweeteners (sugar substitutes) that your body doesn't convert to energy or fat. Nutritive sweeteners contain about 20 calories in a teaspoon while sugar substitutes have few or no calories.

Currently there are three sugar substitutes approved by the U.S. Food and Drug Administration (FDA): aspartame, saccharin, and acesulfame K.

The chart on the next page describes each of these substitutes. The safety of artificial sweeteners being used as food additives is continuously being reviewed by the FDA because of the potential danger. In addition, they have limitations when used in cooking (see chart).

Selecting a sweetener

Here is a summary of different sweeteners. Each has advantages and disadvantages; no one is ideal. If you have diabetes, check with your doctor before using an alternative to table sugar.

Sweetener	What it is	Calories	Advantages	Disadvantages
Sucrose Other names: table sugar, brown sugar, confectioner's sugar, invert sugar, raw sugar, turbinado.	Produced from sugar cane or sugar beets; contains equal parts glucose and fructose.	Yes.	Excellent sweetening capability. Enhances baking process.	Adds "empty" calories. Causes fast and high rise in blood sugar. May aggravate high blood levels of triglycerides. Promotes tooth decay.
Glucose Used commercially as dextrose, corn syrup or glucose syrup.	Naturally occurring sugar. Carbohydrates break down into glucose during digestion.	Yes.	Good sweetening capability.	Causes fast and high rise in blood sugar. Builds up in the blood if diabetes is poorly controlled. Promotes tooth decay.
Fructose	Occurs naturally in fruit and honey; makes up 50 percent of table sugar.	Yes.	Doesn't require insulin initially to enter cells. May be used in well-controlled diabetes.	No help in weight control. May aggravate high blood levels of triglycerides. Promotes tooth decay.
High-fructose corn syrup	Liquid sweetener containing 42 to 90 percent fructose.	Yes.	None other than cost savings for manufacturers.	Not well-studied. Assumed to have similar effects as sucrose and fructose.
Honey	A natural syrup made up of glucose, fructose and water.	Yes.	Excellent taste.	Not appropriate if you have diabetes, because of high glucose content. Promotes tooth decay.
Sorbitol, mannitol and xylitol	Naturally occurring sugar alcohols.	Yes.	May be absorbed into blood more slowly than glucose or sucrose. May be used in well-controlled diabetes. Do not promote tooth decay.	Can cause diarrhea. Tolerance varies from as little as 10 grams of sorbitol (the amount in about five pieces of hard candy) to 30 grams.
Aspartame (NutraSweet and Equal.)	A combination of the amino acids aspartic acid and phenylalanine.	No.	No aftertaste. Doesn't promote tooth decay.	Loses sweetness in cooking or baking. Safety is controversial, but FDA and most doctors believe reasonable amounts are safe, except if you have phenylketonuria.
Acesulfame K (Sunette and Sweet One.)	White, odorless crystals derived from acetoacetic acid.	No.	No bitter aftertaste. Can use in cooking and baking. Doesn't promote tooth decay.	Doesn't give same texture to baked goods as sugar.
Saccharin (Sweet 'n Low, Sprinkle Sweet, Twin and Sweet 10.)	Chemical similar to acesulfame K.	No.	Fair sweetening capability. Doesn't promote tooth decay.	Bitter aftertaste. Doesn't bake well. Safety under review.

Reprinted from July 1990 *Mayo Clinic Health Letter* with permission of Mayo Foundation for Medical Education and Research, Rochester, Minnesota 55905.

Fiber

Fiber, or roughage or bulk, is that part of the foods we eat which is not digestible. Dietary fiber consists of all parts of the plant cell wall that are resistant to the normal digestive enzymes of the small intestine. Crude fiber is the term used for the fiber left in plant food after it has been subjected to acid and alkali breakdown in the laboratory for nutrient analysis. Crude fiber therefore includes only the most rugged cellulose and legume. Fiber absorbs water, swelling its size and creating the necessary bulk to stimulate proper functioning of the intestines. As fiber moves through the digestive system and the colon, it also performs a cleaning action to sweep with it the remains of undigested food and bile secretions. This action contributes to a more thorough elimination of digestive residue and is considered an important factor in the maintenance of good health. A low intake of dietary fiber has been associated with such problems as constipation, diverticulitis, appendicitis, and even cancer of the colon.

Fiber can be found only in plants—vegetables, fruits, seeds, and cereals—never in foods of animal origin. Good sources of fiber are vegetables such as tomatoes, celery, cucumber, green peppers, broccoli, and cabbage; and fruits such as plums, apples, peaches, oranges, raspberries, pears, and grapefruit. Other sources of fiber include dry beans, dry peas, nuts, whole grain breads, cereals, and bran. However, over processing and refining of foods lower the fiber content. For example,

THE TYPES, SOURCES, AND ROLE OF FIBER

Water Soluble	Gums	Pectins	Role
	oatmeal	squash	Binds with cholesterol-containing bile acids in gut preventing reabsorption, decreases blood cholesterol, also delays glucose absorption and gastric emptying
	oat products	apples	
	dried beans	citrus fruits	
	barley	cauliflower	
		green beans	
		cabbage	
		dried peas	Protective against heart disease and diabetes
		carrots	
		strawberries	
		potatoes	
Water Insoluble	Celluloses	Hemicelluloses	Role
	whole wheat products	bran	Absorbs water, increases stool volume and decreases stool transit time, dilutes concentration of bile acids
	bran	cereals	
	cabbage	whole grains	
	green beans	brussels sprouts	
	broccoli	mustard greens	
	brussels sprout		Protective against colon cancer, constipation, and diverticulosis
	peppers		
	apples		
	carrots		

Note: serving sizes 1/2 cup beans, legumes, barley, rice; 3/4 cup cereals, oatmeal, oat bran; 1 slice whole grain bread, 1 medium fruit.

a fresh apple contains 1.0 grams of fiber, apple sauce contains 0.6 grams and apple juice provides only 0.2 grams.

Actually, the types of fiber found in fruits and vegetables differ from those found in the cereal product. The fiber in whole wheat products, for example, is cellulose and lignin and is better at providing stool bulk than the small pectin substances in fruits and vegetables. However, the fiber in fruits and vegetables seems better at chemically reacting to cleanse the blood. Pectin discourages cholesterol absorption on a chemical level by rendering inactive the bile acids which are responsible for breaking cholesterol down into absorbable form. (See chart on page 84.)

The National Cancer Institute has released specific dietary guidelines for reducing cancer and cancer-related deaths. One specific guideline is to gradually increase fiber intake to 25-35 grams a day. It is recommended that the fiber be obtained from a variety of sources since fibers do vary. Some fibers are soluble and others are insoluble in our diet. Therefore a mix of whole grains, fruits and vegetables is the best approach.

Some of the advantages to increasing your fiber intake include:
- It is a natural laxative.
- It has been linked to a lower risk of colon cancer.
- By filling up with high fiber foods one eats more food with fewer calories, thus helping weight control and loss.
- It helps lower blood cholesterol, thus reducing risk of heart disease.

One should gradually increase the fiber intake by adding about 5 grams of dietary fiber per day. This can easily be done by adding the following sources of fiber:
- 2 slices of whole wheat bread
- 1 cup of whole grain cereal
- 1 large baked potato with skin

- 1/3 cup of cooked dried beans
- 1 large apple, banana, orange, or pear
- 1 cup of vegetables

A typical day's fiber intake to reach the goal of 35 grams per day might look like this:
- 2 large pieces of fruit (10 grams)
- 1/2 cup cooked beans or lentils or 5 prunes (7.5 grams)
- 1 baked potato with skin (5 grams)
- 1 cup cooked vegetables (5 grams)
- 2 slices whole wheat bread (5 grams)
- 1/2 cup whole grain cereal (2.5 grams)

The fiber source chart below provides values for other foods which one might consider including in the diet to increase fiber intake.

HIGH FIBER FOOD CHOICES

Vegetables	Grams
1/2 cup lima beans	8.3
3 oz. peanuts	8
1/2 cup peas	4.1
1/2 cup corn kernels	4
1 baked potato (medium)	3.9
1/2 cup zucchini	2.7
Legumes	
1/2 cup kidney beans	8-10
1/2 cup black beans	8
1/2 cup Great Northern beans	6
1/2 cup lentils	4
Fruits	
1 medium pear, orange, or apple	2-3
1 medium banana	3
2 prunes (dried)	2.4
1/2 medium grapefruit	1.7
1/2 cup strawberries	1.6
Grain Products	
1/2 cup All Bran cereal	12
1/2 cup Grape Nuts	7.5
2 large biscuits shredded wheat	5.6
1 bran muffin	4.2
1/3 cup oat bran	4
3 oz. spaghetti (uncooked)	3
3/4 cup oatmeal (cooked)	2.8
2/3 cup oat flakes	2.7
1/2 cup brown rice (cooked)	2.4

Proteins

Proteins are made up of amino acids needed to build, repair, and regulate the function of the body's cells. The body can manufacture some amino acids but not all. Those which must be supplied by the foods we eat each day are known as **essential amino acids.** Protein foods that contain all the essential amino acids are called **complete proteins.** Those protein foods lacking in certain essential amino acids are referred to as **incomplete proteins.** However, two or more incomplete proteins can be combined to form a complete protein.

These incomplete proteins are the plant protein sources rather than the animal sources of protein. Plant protein sources are less concentrated in protein and generally low in one or more essential amino acids. In order to meet the need for all the essential amino acids in the diet, a combination of plant sources should be used.

Three simple rules for selecting plant sources of proteins should be followed by those who do not eat animal sources of protein:

- Combine legumes (peas, lentils, dried beans, soybeans, garbanzos) with grains (rice, oats, rye, wheat, barley, millet).
- Combine legumes with nuts and seeds (sesame, sunflower, almonds, etc.).
- Combine dairy products with any vegetable protein source.

The key factor is providing the body with a variety of foods in a relatively balanced diet. If this occurs the body has the ability to accommodate wide variations in the type and amount of protein it receives and still meet its needs. As a rule, Americans actually consume too much protein.

If we do not get adequate amounts of protein in our

PROTEIN CONCENTRATION OF SOME COMMON FOODS

Food	gm. Protein/Serving
3 oz. serving of cooked, lean meat	20
1 cup cooked soy beans	
mature	20
immature	18
1 cup cooked navy beans	15
1 cup milk	9
1 cup noodles	7
1 oz. cheddar cheese	7
1/2 cup lima beans	7
1 egg	6
1/2 cup peas	5
1 tablespoon peanut butter	4
1 slice bread	2

Function	Sources	Calories per gram	Recommended % in diet
Important for growth, maintenance, and repair of tissue Also used to form hormones and enzymes; additional source of energy.	Complete proteins: cheese, eggs, milk, chicken, fish, meat Incomplete proteins: dried peas, beans, legumes, black-eyed peas, soybeans, black beans.	4	10-12%

diet, the body immediately begins to break down tissue, usually beginning with muscle tissue, in order to release the amino acids it needs. Protein needs vary with age and body size. The following formula can be used to determine specific requirements of the body: the recommended daily allowance for protein for both men and women is .8 grams per kg of body weight which translates to .36 grams per pound.

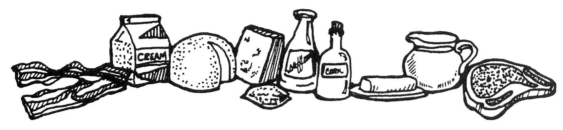

Fats

Some fats are needed by the body to fulfill several important functions. However, the typical American diet contains over 40% fat as compared to the 20-30% which is currently recommended. In addition, it is important to examine the types of fat included in your diet.

The basic building blocks of fats are fatty acids. The fatty acids combine with glycerol to form glycerides. When glycerol combines with three fatty acids it forms triglycerides. The classification of fats is also based on the number of hydrogen atoms combined with the carbon atoms. Saturated fats have the maximum number of hydrogen atoms, and they remain solid at room temperature. Hydrogenation is a process in which a fat or oil is made to react with hydrogen. This results in a more stable fat and is used to convert a liquid polyunsaturated oil to a more solid form.

Those fatty acids which the human body requires but cannot produce are called essential fatty acids. They are polyunsaturated fats and can be obtained primarily from vegetable oils. Linoleic acid is the most important essential fatty acid, and it should provide about 2% of the calories in the diet.

Actually, all fats are a mixture of satu-rated, polyunsaturated and monounsaturated fatty acids. But some foods are higher in one than the other and it is important to know these differences. Dietary rules recommend that only 10% of the calories in the diet come from saturated fats. So much "invisible" fat is in foods that many people are unaware of just how much they are getting. The amount of fats being consumed is now recognized as a major health problem; countries with a high rate of heart disease have diets rich in saturated fat and cholesterol. It has been found that saturated fat is the prime influence on blood cholesterol level—one gram raises it twice as much as an equal amount of polyunsaturated fat.

Another major health hazard is cancer. Studies now link six forms of cancer with dietary fat, including cancer of the breast and colon—two of the top cancer killers in the United States.

Fat has several important functions in the body. It serves as a secondary source of energy (after carbohydrates)—the fat deposits in body tissues serve as a reserve fuel supply. Fat provides the acids necessary for proper growth, healthy skin, and the metabolism of cholesterol. In addition, it aids in the transportation of the fat soluble vitamins (A, D, E, K) and insulates and cushions the body and its organs.

In determining which fats are best to use, a number of studies now indicate that monounsaturated fats are best for lowering your risk of heart disease. One recent study showed that those on a high monounsaturated fat diet had lower overall blood cholesterol and the HDL level increased. Two excellent choices of oils that are high in monounsaturated fats are olive oil and canola oil (sold as Puritan Oil).

Although polyunsaturated fats are better than saturated fats in lowering heart disease risk, there is some evidence linking them with increased risk of cancer. The American Heart Association therefore recommends that no more than 10% of the total calories in the diet be from polyunsaturated fats.

Not only are the saturated fats to be avoided (and limited to no more than 10% of the total calories in the diet), but also those fats that have been hydrogenated or par-

tially hydrogenated should be limited. Hydrogenation is a process used by manufacturers in which products with polyunsaturated fats have some of the fatty acids converted to saturated fatty acids. This makes them more solid, increases the stability of the fat, and extends the shelf-life of the product. The more solid the vegetable oil, the more hydrogenated it is, and the more it should be avoided. A good guideline is to use margarines that are labeled "diet" (contain more water and only half the fat of other margarines), tub or liquid "squeeze" margarines rather than stick margarines or butter.

One effective way of gaining control of the fat in your diet is to estimate your daily target fat rate. There are two ways to identify this rate. One is to use the formula and calculate your individual rate based on your daily calorie intake. A second way is to estimate your rate using a standard chart. See the following charts to utilize each method.

CALCULATING YOUR DAILY TARGET FAT RATE

Total Fat Intake

Total daily calories x 30% = $\dfrac{\text{daily calories from fat}}{9}$ = ____ g total fat

(Example: 2400 calories x .30 = 720/9 = 80 grams of total fat)

Saturated Fat Intake

Total daily calories x .10% = 240/9 = 26 grams of saturated fat)

Estimating Your Daily Target Fat Rate

Daily Calorie Level	Fat Calories Per Day	Total Fat (maximum grams allowed)	Saturated Fat (maximum grams allowed)
1,200	360	40	13
1,800	540	60	20
2,400	720	80	27
3,000	900	100	33

Source: Nutrition and Your Health: Dietary Guidelines for Americans. U.S. Department of Agriculture and U.S. Department of Health and Human Services, 1990.

EVALUATING OILS, BUTTERS, MARGARINES

Item	Mono-unsaturated Fat	Poly-unsaturated Fat	Saturated Fat	Cholesterol
Canola	62%	32%	6% 1.0 grams	0
Safflower	13%	77%	10% 1.0 grams	0
Sunflower	20%	69%	11% 1.5 grams	0
Corn oil	25%	62%	13% 1.5 grams	0
Peanut oil	49%	33%	18% 2.5 grams	0
Olive oil	77%	9%	14% 2.0 grams	0
Soybean oil	24%	61%	15% 2.0 grams	0
Butter	30%	4%	54% 7.5 grams	30 mg
Vegetable Shortening	43%	25%	25 5.0 grams	10 mg
Palm oil	37%	9%	49% 6.5 grams	0
Soft Diet Margarine	3%	2%	1% 1.0 grams	0
Soft Margarine (Tub)	19%	52%	29% 2.0 grams	0
Coconut oil	6%	2%	81% 12.0 grams	0
Margarine	48%	29%	18%	0

MAKING HEALTHY FAT CHOICES
Comparison of Percent of Calories Derived from Fat

Poor Choice (percent fat)
whole milk (48%)
cheddar cheese (72%)
deep fried chicken thigh (62%)
fish sticks, fried (65%)
french fries (47%)
tuna in oil (52%)
croissant (50%)
chocolate chip cookies (52%)
peanuts (74%)
vanilla ice cream (50%)
mayonnaise (99%)

Best Choice (percent fat)
skim milk (0%)
2% cottage cheese (20%)
chicken, broiled, no skin (24%)
fish, broiled (lemon & 1/2 tsp. oil) (25%)
baked potato with 1/2 tsp. margarine (16%)
tuna in water (11%)
bagel (11%)
ginger snaps (20%)
pretzels (10%)
sherbet (1%)
catsup (6%)

HIGH SATURATED FAT FOODS

1 oz. cream cheese	6	3 oz. lean sirloin steak	13
1 oz. whole milk cheese	5	4 oz. corned beef	16
8 oz. plain yogurt (whole milk)	5	1 cup soft ice cream	13
4 oz. creamed cottage cheese	3	1 ham and cheese omelette	13
1/2 cup shredded coconut	12	1 cup whole milk	5
1 tbsp. heavy cream	4	1 cup egg nog	11
1 tbsp. sour cream	1.5	1 frankfurter	5.5
1 oz. cheddar cheese	6	3 oz. peanut butter	7.2
1 oz. milk chocolate bar	8	3 oz. pork sausage	9.2

Fat Substitutes

A recent trend is the development of fat-free fat substitutes which are now being used in desserts, snacks, and condiments. These substitutes may help you reduce the fat calories in your diet, but there are some limitations as described below.

FAT SUBSTITUTES

Fat substitute	Source	Use	Limitations
Simplesse	Blend of egg white and milk protein	Frozen desserts (Simple Pleasures). In the future will be used in salad dressings, mayonnaise, margarine, etc.	Cannot be used in foods to be heated
Olestra	Chain of sugar and fatty acid links that cannot be digested	Replace up to 35% of fat calories in oils and shortening, and up to 75% of fat in commercially prepared foods	Not yet approved by FDA—may affect absorption of fat soluble vitamins
Cellulose gel	Gels, gelatins and plant gums	Nonfat ice cream (Sealtest Free) and frozen yogurt	
Oatrim	Oat bran	Being tested for use in non-heated foods	Not for foods to be heated

Function	Sources	Calories per gram	Recommended % in diet
Part of the structure of every cell Stored energy Supplies essential fatty acids Provides and carries fat soluble vitamins A, D, E, K	*Unsaturated:* Safflower oil, corn oil, sunflower oil, soybean oil margarines (made with vegetable oils) *Saturated:* Solid and hydrogenated shortening, coconut oil, cocoa butter, palm oil, butter, cheese, meat, milk *Monounsaturated:* Olive oil, peanut oil	9	20 10% poly-unsaturated

SOURCES OF FAT IN THE AMERICAN DIET

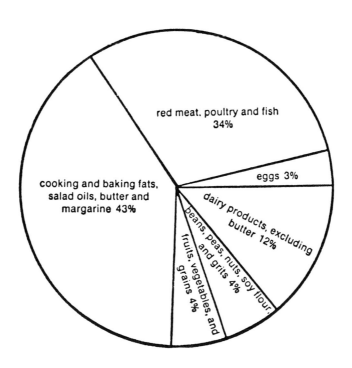

"Nutrient Content of the National Food Supply," R. Marston, L. Page. National Food Review, pp. 28-33, U.S. Department of Agriculture, December 1978.

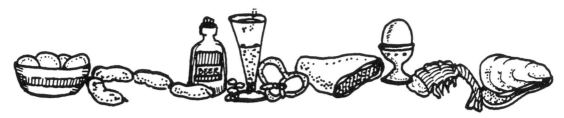

Cholesterol

Cholesterol is a waxy, fatty-like material utilized by the body in many chemical processes. Even though cholesterol has no calories as fat does, scientist often refer to it as a fat because it has similar effects on the body. Cholesterol has many important functions in the body: it is a key part of brain tissue, it helps protect nerve fibers, it is necessary for sex hormones as well as other hormones, it helps your body create and store Vitamin D, and it is necessary for the membranes of all body cells.

Cholesterol is carried through the blood by a series of molecules called lipoproteins. The **low density lipoproteins** (LDLs) pick up cholesterol that originates from our diet or is manufactured in the liver and deposits it in the cells for processing. If there is more cholesterol than is needed for daily metabolism, the LDLs may deposit this fatty cargo on the lining of the arteries. These deposits may narrow the arteries in the heart and cause a fatty plaque to build up along the artery. This not only causes the heart to strain in order to pump blood, but may cause a clot which dislodges from an artery and flows through the bloodstream. This clot may eventually lodge in a coronary artery causing reduction of blood flow to the heart muscle and perhaps death from a heart attack. However, **high density lipoproteins** (HDLs) float around in the bloodstream and pick up the excess cholesterol and carry it back to the liver for excretion from the body. Obviously, the goal is to try to increase the levels of HDL in the blood. Studies show this can be done by:

- vigorous aerobic exercise
- eating a low fat, low cholesterol diet
- not smoking
- avoiding obesity

The effects of consumption of dietary cholesterol vary from person to person. Some individuals may be lucky enough to maintain a low blood cholesterol level regardless of their diet, but these people are definitely the exception not the rule. Obviously many factors influence blood cholesterol level; we presently do not completely understand just how a change in this level can be brought about. It does not seem, for instance, that a high dietary intake will depress the body's synthesis of cholesterol to the point that it will cancel out the effect of diet. Some studies now reveal that stress causes an increase in cholesterol production and that a Vitamin C deficiency inhibits the removal of cholesterol from the body as it passes through the liver.

Regarding an optimal level for blood cholesterol, it seems that *below 180* (per 100 ml of blood) an individual's risk of heart disease is low. This risk starts to rise slowly with increasing blood cholesterol levels. Above a level of 250, the risk of heart attack jumps sharply. However, no blood cholesterol level can guarantee prevention of a heart attack. It is not possible to draw a line between safe and unsafe, though we can predict that the chances or odds of suffering a heart attack rise as the cholesterol level rises. (See Chapter 2 for additional information.)

Although we still have many unanswered questions, most research has shown that a low fat, low cholesterol diet may be the best way to prevent heart disease. The following agencies have determined that there is enough evidence to strongly advocate this diet for all Americans: U.S. Department of Agriculture, Department of Health, Education, and Welfare, Senate Select Committee on Nutrition and Human Needs, American Heart Association, American Health Association, National Heart, Lung and Blood Institute, and Center for Science in the Public Interest. The American Heart Association recommends that cholesterol intake not exceed 300 mg daily.

The only foods which contain cholesterol are those from animal sources. Therefore, a low cholesterol intake involves lowering our consumption of the following: eggs (no more than 3 per week), shrimp, caviar, red meat, all organ and gland meats. (See Chapter 7 for a more complete description of how you can lower your cholesterol.)

The chart which follows is a guide to the amount of cholesterol in common foods.

FOODS HIGH IN CHOLESTEROL

Item and quantity	Milligrams of cholesterol	Item and quantity	Milligrams of cholesterol
ham and cheese omelette - 1 serving	586	lemon meringue pie - 1 piece	137
lobster Newburg - 1 cup	456	ricotta cheese - 1 cup	112
calf's liver - 3.5 oz.	434	Boston cream pie - 1 piece	100
McDonald's scrambled eggs - 1 serv.	349	Arby's club sandwich - 1	100
custard - baked - 1 cup	278	spareribs - 4 oz.	96
egg salad sandwich - 1	262	lamb - roasted lean - 3 oz	89
egg - 1 medium	242	pork - 3 oz.	80
cream puff with custard filling	200	beef - 3 oz.	77
chicken a la king - 1 cup	170	chicken - no skin - 3 oz	76
tapioca cream pudding - 1 cup	157	turkey - 3 oz.	69

SOURCES OF CHOLESTEROL IN THE AMERICAN DIET

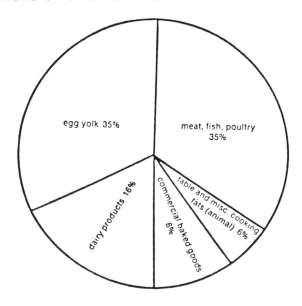

egg yolk 35%

meat, fish, poultry 35%

dairy products 16%

commercial baked goods 8%

table and misc. cooking fats (animal) 6%

CHOLESTEROL CONTENT IN SEAFOOD

Item and quantity	Milligrams of cholesterol
18 oz. Maine Lobster	310
3 1/2 oz. Squid	233
7 oz. shrimp	230
13 oz. Rock Lobster	200
3 1/2 oz. crayfish	139
16 oz. snow crab legs	130
13-19 oysters - raw	120
5 oz. mackerel	100
5 oz. swordfish	100
16 oz. Alaska King crab	100
5 oz. rainbow trout	90
5 oz. Haddock	85
5 oz. catfish	85
3 1/2 oz. blue crab	78
3 1/2 oz. Dungeness crab	59
3 1/2 oz. clams	34
3 1/2 oz. scallops	33

MAKING HEALTHY CHOLESTEROL CHOICES

Instead of.....	Substitute...
milk (whole) - 1 cup (34)	2% milk - 1 cup (22)
ricotta (whole) 1/4 cup (32)	ricotta (skim) (19)
ice cream - 1 cup (88)	yogurt (frozen) (10)
bologna - 1 slice (52)	ham - 1 slice (25)
shrimp - 11 large (96)	scallops - 3 oz. (45)
oysters - 16 (120)	clams - 5 large (50)
turkey (dark) - 3 oz. (87)	turkey (light) - 3 oz. (66)
butter - 1 teaspoon (12)	margarine (soft) 1 t (0)
cream cheese - 2 T (31)	cottage cheese - 2 T (8)
half 'n half - 1 T (6)	evaporated milk (skim) (.6)
mayonnaise - 1 T (9)	salad dressing - 1 T (0)
sour cream - 1 T (6)	yogurt (plain) (.9)
brownie - 1 (17)	fig bar - 1 (0)
coffee cake - 1 square (35)	angel food cake - 1 slice (0)
choc. raisins - 1/2 cup (9.5)	raisins - 1/2 cup (0)
Danish (plain) (17)	doughnut (plain) (7)
egg custard - 3/5 cup (165)	fruit salad (fresh) - 1 cup (0)

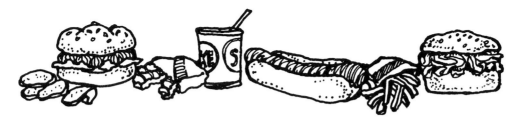

Fast Foods

Three primary problems are associated with eating too much fast food: salt, fat, and calories. Since salt is a leading cause of hypertension, which is a significant factor in heart disease, increased consumption should be avoided. Too much fat consumption elevates the cholesterol levels and also increases the risk of coronary artery disease. The typical fast food is not only high in calories but 50% of those calories come from fat, which is considerably more than recommended by nutritionist. For example, a "Whopper" with French fries and a milkshake total 1,215 calories—more than half of most people's daily need.

A junk food can be defined as anything edible that contains little or no essential nutrients except calories, and one that replaces nutritionally more important foods. Therefore, a "Big Mac" or a "Quarter Pounder" or a "Whopper" are not junk food. They are, however, a lot of calories and fat.

CALORIC AND NUTRITIONAL VALUES OF FAST FOODS

These statistics are compiled from the latest available information provided by the individual restaurants.

	Serving Size (g)	Calories	Protein (g)	Carbo-hydrates (g)	Fat (g)	Choles-terol (mg)	Sodium (mg)
BURGER KING							
Whopper Sandwich	270	614	27	45	36	90	865
Whopper w/cheese	294	706	32	47	44	115	1177
Double Whopper	351	844	46	45	53	169	933
Cheeseburger	121	318	17	28	15	50	661
Hamburger	108	272	15	28	11	37	505
Bacon Double Cheeseburger	160	515	32	26	31	105	748
BK Broiler Chicken Sandwich	168	379	24	31	18	53	764
Chicken Sandwich	229	685	26	56	40	82	1417
Chef Salad (no dressing)	273	178	17	7	9	103	568
French Fries (med. salted)	116	372	5	43	20	0	238
Croissan'wich with egg & cheese	110	315	13	19	20	222	607
with ham, egg & cheese	144	346	19	19	21	241	962
Bagel Sandwich (egg & cheese)	161	407	19	46	16	247	759
Biscuit with sausage	127	478	11	44	29	33	1007

(continued)

	Serving Size (g)	Calories	Protein (g)	Carbo-hydrates (g)	Fat (g)	Choles-terol (mg)	Sodium (mg)
DAIRY QUEEN							
Hamburger	148	360	21	33	16	45	630
Hot Dog	100	280	11	21	16	45	830
with chili	128	320	13	23	20	55	985
Fish Fillet	177	430	20	45	18	40	674
Chicken Breast Fillet	202	608	27	46	34	78	725
French Fries (large)	113	320	3	40	16	15	185
Cone, small	85	140	3	22	4	10	45
Cone, small dipped	92	190	3	25	9	10	55
Sundae, regular	177	310	5	56	8	20	120
Shake, regular	418	710	14	120	19	50	260
"Mr. Misty," regular	330	250	0	63	0	0	10
KENTUCKY FRIED CHICKEN							
Original Recipe							
Drumstick	57	146	13	4	9	67	275
Thigh	104	294	18	11	20	123	619
Side Breast	90	267	19	11	17	77	735
Center Breast	115	283	28	9	15	93	672
Extra Crispy							
Drumstick	69	204	14	6	14	71	324
Thigh	119	406	20	14	30	129	688
Side Breast	110	343	22	14	22	81	748
Center Breast	135	342	33	12	20	114	790
Lite 'n Crispy							
Drumstick	47	121	n/a	n/a	7	61	196
Thigh	79	246	n/a	n/a	17	80	386
Side Breast	76	204	n/a	n/a	12	63	417
Center Breast	86	220	n/a	n/a	12	67	416
Biscuit (1)	65	235	5	28	12	2	655
Mashed Potatoes & Gravy	98	71	2	12	2	0	339
MCDONALD'S							
Hamburger	102	260	12	31	10	37	500
Cheeseburger	116	310	15	31	14	53	750
Quarter Pounder	166	410	23	34	21	86	660
Big Mac	215	560	25	43	32	103	950
Filet-o-Fish	142	440	14	38	26	50	1030
McD.L.T.	234	580	26	36	37	109	990
McChicken	190	490	19	39	29	43	780
Chicken McNuggets, plain	112	270	20	17	15	56	580
Egg McMuffin	138	290	18	28	11	226	740

	Serving Size (g)	Calories	Protein (g)	Carbo-hydrates (g)	Fat (g)	Choles-terol (mg)	Sodium (mg)
(McDonald's, continued)							
Sausage McMuffin	117	370	17	27	22	64	830
with egg	167	440	23	28	27	263	980
Hot Cakes w/butter, syrup	176	410	8	74	9	21	640
Chef Salad	283	230	21	8	13	128	490
French Fries (med.)	97	320	4	36	17	12	150
TACO BELL							
Taco	78	183	10	11	11	32	276
Taco Bell Grande	163	335	18	18	23	56	472
Tostada w/Red Sauce	156	243	9	27	11	16	596
Chicken Tostada w/Red Sauce	164	264	12	20	15	37	454
Taco Supreme	92	230	11	12	15	32	276
Nachos Bell Grande	287	649	22	67	35	36	997
Nachos Supreme	145	367	12	41	27	18	471
Enchirito w/Red Sauce	213	382	20	31	20	54	1243
MexiMelt	106	266	13	19	15	38	689
Pintos 'n Cheese w/Red Sauce	128	190	9	19	9	16	642
Taco Salad	575	905	34	55	61	80	910
Bean Burrito w/Red Sauce	206	447	15	63	14	9	1148
Burrito Supreme w/Sauce	255	503	20	55	22	33	1181
Beef Burrito w/Sauce	206	493	25	48	21	57	1311
WENDY'S							
Hot, stuffed, baked potato							
plain	250	270	6	63	tr.	0	20
with cheese	318	420	8	66	15	10	310
with bacon & cheese	362	520	20	70	18	20	1460
Hamburger, plain, single	126	340	24	30	15	65	500
with everything	210	420	25	35	21	70	890
Wendy's Big Classic	260	570	27	47	33	80	1085
Grilled Chicken Sandwich	175	340	24	37	13	60	815
Fish Fillet Sandwich	170	460	18	42	25	50	780
Chef Salad	257	130	14	8	5	40	460
French Fries (small)	91	240	3	33	12	0	145
Chili (regular, 9 oz.)	255	220	21	23	7	45	750
BEVERAGES							
Coca-Cola Classic	12 oz.	140	0	38	0	0	15
Diet Coke	12 oz.	1	0	0	0	0	30
Sprite	12 oz.	140	0	36	0	0	15
Milk (2%)	8 oz.	120	8	12	5	18	130
Milk, whole	8 oz.	157	8	11	9	35	119
Orange juice	6 oz.	80	1	19	0	0	0

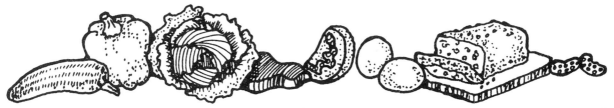

Vitamins

A vitamin is an organic substance essential for the body to perform its complex chemical reactions. Vitamins cannot be synthesized by the body and are not nutrients in the sense of supplying energy or building tissue, but they aid in the utilization and absorption of the nutrients. Each vitamin performs one or more specific functions in the body. The chart which follows describes each vitamin and gives specific information about its function, best sources, and daily requirements.

An important question many people ask is whether the use of a vitamin supplement is recommended. The following reasons have been given to support the need for a supplement:

1. The body's demand for vitamins may increase depending on the stresses and physical activities of the day.
2. One's intake of dietary vitamins may vary—particularly when eating away from home, smoking, and consuming alcoholic beverages.
3. The Recommended Dietary Allowance (RDA) cannot serve as an absolute indicator of the adequacy of a given intake for a given individual.

Vitamins can be divided into two groups on the basis of their solubility. The **fat-soluble** vitamins A, D, E, and K are those found in foods associated with fats (lipids). They are not destroyed by ordinary cooking and normally are not excreted in the urine but tend to remain stored in the body in moderate quantities. Due to such reserves, the body does not need a day-to-day supply.

The **water-soluble** vitamins, B and C, are transported in the fluids of the tissues and cells and are not stored in the body in appreciable quantities. These vitamins may be affected by cooking methods and can be lost in varying amounts by discarding the water in which the food was cooked or soaked. Some vitamins are lost in various types of food processing (milling flour, making "instant" potatoes, pasteurizing milk, etc.). However, all of the required vitamins can be found in a well-balanced diet.

The question of whether to take vitamin supplements must be determined by each individual. One theory supporting the use of a supplement is that, depending on the stresses and physical activities of the day, your body's demand for vitamins may increase. Even though all vitamins except C are stored in the liver and are available to meet an increase in requirements, it makes sense to keep these reserves well stocked. The intake of natural vitamins in your diet may vary, particularly when you eat away from home or if you consume alcoholic beverages.

Others disagree with this concept since any excessive ingestion of vitamins is usually excreted in the urine on a daily basis. Ingesting more vitamins than recommended will thus be of limited or no benefit and can actually be harmful. Those vitamins that are stored in the body can cause many problems and side effects if their level goes too high. Large doses of vitamins A and D can be particularly toxic. At the present time, there is no evidence to indicate a difference between vitamins derived from natural sources and those synthesized by a chemist.

VITAMIN INFORMATION

Vitamin	Food Sources	Deficiency Effect	Function	RDA (Adults)
A	Fish-liver oils, liver, butter, cream, whole milk, whole-milk cheeses, egg yolk, dark-green leafy vegetables, yellow fruits and vegetables.	Night blindness, eye inflammation, dry, rough skin, reduced resistance to infection.	Needed for normal vision. Protects against night blindness. Keeps skin and mucous membranes resistant to infection.	5000 IU
B Complex B₁ (Thiamine)	Pork, liver, organ meats, brewer's yeast, wheat germ, whole-grain cereals and breads, enriched cereals and breads, soybeans, peanuts and other legumes, milk.	Beriberi.	Promotes normal appetite and digestion. Necessary for a healthy nervous system.	1.5 mg.
B₂ (Riboflavin)	Milk, powdered whey, liver, organ meats, meats, eggs, leafy green vegetables, dried yeast, enriched foods.	Cracks at corners of mouth, inflamed, sore lips, inflamed, discolored tongue, dermatitis, anemia.	Helps cells use oxygen. Helps maintain good vision. Needed for good skin.	1.7 mg.
Niacin	Lean meat, fish, poultry, liver, kidney, whole-grain and enriched cereals and breads, green vegetables, peanuts, brewer's yeast.	Pellagra.	Aids metabolism of proteins, carbos, fats.	20 mg.
Pantothenic Acid	Present in most plant and animal tissue, liver, kidney, yeast, eggs, peanuts, whole-grain cereals, beef, tomatoes, broccoli, salmon.	(Rare) Gastrointestinal disturbance, depression, confusion.	Necessary for metabolism of proteins, carbos, fats.	10 mg.
B₆ (Pyridoxine)	Wheat germ, meat, liver, kidney, whole-grain cereals, soybeans, peanuts, corn.	(Rare) Inflamed mouth and tongue, depression, irritability, convulsions.	Maintains normal hemoglobin (carries oxygen to tissues).	2.0 mg.
Biotin	Liver, sweetbreads, yeast, eggs, legumes.	(Extremely rare) Inflamed skin, hair loss, lethargy, loss of appetite.	Coenzyme, functions in metabolism of major nutrients.	0.3 mg.

VITAMIN INFORMATION, continued

Vitamin	Food Sources	Deficiency Effect	Function	RDA (Adult)
Folic Acid	Widespread in liver, kidney, yeast, deep-green leafy vegetables.	Anemia, stunted growth, damage to lining of small intestine.	Maintains normal hemoglobin.	200 mcg (men) 180 mcg (women)
B$_{12}$ (Cyanocobalamin)	Animal protein.	Pernicious anemia, stunted growth.	Maintains normal hemoglobin.	6 mcg.
C (Ascorbic Acid)	Citrus fruits, tomatoes, strawberries, cantaloupe, cabbage, broccoli, kale, potatoes.	Scurvy.	Maintains cementing material that holds the body cells together. Needed for healthy gums. Helps body resist infection.	60 mg.
D	Fish-liver oils, fortified milk, activated sterols, exposure to sunlight.	Rickets, osteomalacia (loss of calcium from bones in adults).	Builds strong bones and teeth. Aids calcium absorption.	400 IU
E (Tocopherol)	Plant tissues, wheat germ oil, vegetable oils, nuts, legumes.	Unknown in persons eating normal, mixed diet.	Not fully understood. Works as anti-oxidant.	15 IU
K	Green leaves such as spinach, cabbage, cauliflower.	Excessive bleeding.	Aids blood-clotting.	80 mcg (men) 65 mcg (women)

Adapted from the following sources: 1980 Recommended Daily Dietary Allowances, Food and Nutrition Board, National Academy of Sciences — National Research Council; *Runner's World*, April 1981.

MDR and RDA

As a guide to an adequate intake of the various nutrients, the Minimum Daily Requirement (MDR) and Recommended Dietary Allowance (RDA) have been established. The MDRs were established by the Food and Drug Administration and are average levels, with a small safety margin, required to prevent symptoms of actual deficiency. The RDAs were developed by the Food and Nutrition Board of the National Academy of Sciences and are higher than MDRs. Actually, a reliable test for determining individual requirements has not yet been devised.

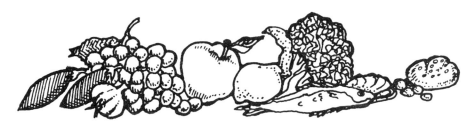

Minerals

Minerals are inorganic nutrients important in activating numerous reactions that release energy during the breakdown of carbohydrates, proteins and fats. Minerals needed in substantial amounts are called microminerals. Six microminerals are required in larger quantities than the others: sodium, potassium, chloride, calcium, phosphorus, and magnesium. These are needed in the diet in amounts of 100 mg. or more per day. There are 14 others, called trace minerals, which are required in amounts from 100 mg. per day to as little as a few micrograms.

Minerals are supplied by the foods we eat and the water we drink. Although the quantities needed are small, they are essential to human life and health.

The chart on page 102 describes each mineral and provides information about its function, sources, and RDA.

Salt

Salt is an essential mineral nutrient composed of sodium and chloride. We need the electrolyte, sodium, to help maintain a proper fluid balance in our blood and tissues and the acid base balance outside the body cells. However, an excessive intake forces the kidneys to work overtime and contributes to bloating, tissue swelling, and menstrual discomforts. In addition, the relationship of salt to the development of high blood pressure is now well documented. Studies show a worldwide correlation between the quantity of salt ingested and the incidence of hypertension in the population. In those countries where a low amount of salt is consumed, there is a corresponding low incidence of hypertension. While our actual physiological requirement for sodium is only 220 mg. (or about 1/10 of a teaspoon), the average American consumes 10-20 grams (the equivalent of 2-4 teaspoons) of salt per day.

A safe and adequate range of sodium intake per day is about 1100-3300 mg. for adults or the equivalent of 3/4-1 1/2 teaspoons of salt. (Note: 1 teaspoon of salt provides 2000 mg. of sodium.)

The problem is that we really can't tell how much salt is in the processed foods we eat. However, we do know that salt is needlessly added to many foods by the

MINERAL REQUIREMENTS

MINERALS	WHAT IT DOES	R.D.A.	GOOD SOURCES	
CALCIUM	Developing & maintaining strong bones & teeth — normal blood clotting, heartbeat, transmission of nerve impulses, & muscle contraction	800 mg.	milk & milk products green leafy vegetables, almonds	MACROMINERALS
PHOSPHORUS	Utilization of energy, muscle action, & nerve transmission. With calcium, essential for formation of bones, & teeth	800 mg.	meat, poultry, fish, eggs, & whole grain foods	
MAGNESIUM	Essential for energy conversions in the body. Helps control muscle contractions.	300 - 350 mg.	dark bread, nuts, green leafy vegetables, dairy products.	
POTASSIUM	With sodium it helps regulate the balance and volume of body fluids. Influences the contractibility of the muscles.	1875 - 5625 mg.	all fruits & vegetables, pecans & walnuts, wheat germ, soybeans, & molasses	
SODIUM	Found in blood plasma & other fluids outside cells — helps to maintain normal water balance	500- 2400 mcg.	meat, fish, poultry, eggs, and milk	
CHLORIDE (Mainly in compound form with sodium or potassium)	Regulates correct balance of acid & alkali in blood. Stimulates production of hydrochloric acid in stomach for disgestion	1700 - 5100 mg.	table salt, kelp, ripe olives & rye flour	
IRON	Red Blood Cell Formation	*15 mg-F 10 mg-M	eggs, liver, whole grains, dried fruits & legumes	TRACE
ZINC	Protein synthesis, growth, and development	15 mg.	fish, beef, chicken, whole grains, vegetables, & oysters	
IODINE	Functioning of thyroid gland (breathing rate of tissues)	150 mcg.	seafoods	
COPPER	Action of enzyme systems & normal functioning of central nervous system — Involved with storage & release of iron to form hemoglobin.	2.0 - 3.0 mg.	organ meats, shellfish nuts, & dried legumes	
SELENIUM	Functioning of kidneys, pancreas, and liver.	*55 mcg.-F 70 mcg.-M	organ meats, muscle and seafoods	
MANGANESE	Normal tendon & bone structure	2.5 - 5.0 mg.	peas, beans, nuts, fruits, & whole grains	

*F = female, M = male.

processors. This is why canned and ready-to-eat foods increase our sodium intake enormously. Therefore, follow these suggestions in order to reduce salt intake:

- Reduce use of salt in cooking and at the table.
- Choose foods that have not been processed (fresh fruits and vegetables).
- Reduce consumption of foods containing visible salt (potato chips, pretzels, salted nuts, corn chips, etc.).
- Reduce consumption of processed foods (canned vegetables, snack foods, frozen dinners).

Salt Substitutes

A salt substitute should be used only when recommended by a doctor. Many of these substitutes contain sodium; others are harmful to individuals with certain diseases. A better way to enhance the flavor of foods is to use spices and herbs.

Most salt substitutes contain potassium in place of the sodium, and its easy to overload your body with too much potassium if you make a one-to-one substitution for ordinary salt. Since potassium levels affect the body's chemical balance which regulates heartbeat, it can cause dangerous changes in heart rhythm when not balanced.

However, there are some salt substitutes which contain neither sodium nor potassium. These use a mixture of spices and herbs.

Water

Water is considered an essential nutrient even though it provides no energy. Even short-term loss of water may be hazardous to one's health and can prove to be fatal. It is the most important nutrient because most of the other essential nutrients can be used

by the body only because of their reaction to water—it provides the medium within which the other nutrients can function.

The amount of water needed depends on the body weight of the individual. The average adult needs about two liters (slightly more than two quarts) of water per day to maintain adequate water balance. This means normally drinking 6-8 glasses per day and even more during prolonged activity or when exercising in warm weather. Sources of water include beverages and foods. Most fruits and some vegetables (lettuce, celery) contain 90 percent water—others contain as much as 60 percent. Other solid foods such as lean beef (60% water), bread (33% water), and butter (15% water) contribute to our daily intake.

One's body weight is approximately 60 percent water. The water is stored in various body compartments and is mostly within the body cells. The amount found in body tissues varies with muscle tissue containing approximately 72 percent water and fat between 20-25 percent water. Since women generally have a higher fat composition, they have about 50 percent water. Other water is found outside the cells.

As an exerciser the proper balance of water and electrolytes is important. It also plays a key role in the regulation of body temperature. Water is the main component of sweat and when it evaporates from the skin's surface, it helps dissipate excess body heat.

While the feeling of thirst serves as a fairly accurate guide to the need for water most of the time, when exercising in hot, humid environments it may not be accurate. During this type of weather, the body can have enormous sweat loss amounting to a gallon or more during prolonged exercise.

The major electrolytes found in sweat are sodium, chloride, potassium, magnesium, and calcium. However, studies show that the concentration of electrolytes in the blood following an intense workout with heavy sweating is actually increased. This is due to a number of factors such as the comparative greater water loss. The studies indicate that even during marathons an electrolyte deficiency is not likely to occur. The body is stimulated to reabsorb more of these minerals and fewer are excreted in the urine. At times when it is needed, the body has an effective mechanism for conserving its mineral resources. The key factor is to replace the body water which is lost during exercise. Even over extended periods of intensive workouts, water alone is the recommended fluid replacement. By drinking water and eating a balanced diet, one can maintain proper electrolyte levels in the body. One might consider adding a little salt to meals, eating high potassium foods such as bananas and citrus fruits, and including foods high in iron content.

A question commonly asked is whether one should take one of the special commercial solutions referred to as glucose-electrolyte replacement solutions (or GES). Familiar brand names include Gatorade, ERG, QuickKick. Basically these products are mainly water with carbohydrates in the form of glucose and/or sucrose and some of the main electrolytes. Studies have shown that these fluids do not replenish body water during exercise more effectively than plain water and since electrolytes do not need to be replenished during the exercise, the need for such drinks is questionable. In fact, those with a higher concentration of glucose (sugar) may even slow the absorption of water by the body.

Caffeine

Caffeine is a stimulant that is commonly found in coffee, cocoa, tea, and chocolate.

In addition, caffeine is added to certain cola drinks, diet pills, aspirin, and cold remedies. As a stimulant we know caffeine stimulates the central nervous system which is why it tends to increase alertness.

While many claims have been made linking caffeine consumption with a variety of illnesses and health problems, to date very little actual proof of any link can be documented. For instance, the following claims are as yet unproven:

- Too much caffeine causes infertility.
- Coffee drinkers have a higher risk of cancer.
- Intake of caffeine during pregnancy causes babies with birth defects.
- Excessive caffeine causes high blood pressure.
- Avoiding caffeine helps relieve Premenstrual Syndrome (PMS).
- Increased coffee drinking increases the blood cholesterol.
- Caffeine can enhance athletic performance.
- Caffeine contributes to the formation of fibrocystic breast disease.

UNDERSTANDING NUTRITION LABELS

It is important for consumers to understand the information provided on food labels. The tremendous increase in processed foods makes it necessary for one to use the label in determining the nutritional quality of the food before purchasing it. In general, the consumer should look for foods that provide the greatest percentages of the USRDA for the major nutrients and for weight control those with the lowest calorie content. However, awareness of the fiber, fat, and cholesterol content is now of equal importance.

Unfortunately, the information provided on food labels in the past has been confusing and sometimes misleading. The greatest problem was the information that was not provided (about saturated fat, fiber, sodium, cholesterol). In addition, many foods did not even have labels with nutritional data or a list of ingredients. The consumer can expect to see some major changes in new food labels. The Food and Drug Administration (FDA) is implementing the following improvements:

- Nutrition labeling will be required on nearly all foods regulated by the FDA. Foods regulated by the USDA such as meat and poultry will not be covered. Nutritional information for fresh fruits and vegetables will be available in booklets or on the shelf.
- The information on serving size will be uniform and based on a commonly consumed portion determined by the FDA.
- The amount of saturated fat, fiber, and cholesterol plus calories from fat will be listed.
- A list of ingredients for nearly all FDA regulated products will be printed.
- Any health claims for a food must be supported by "significant agreement" about the scientific evidence. The U.S. Public Health Service will develop model messages that can be used by food groups.
- Specific definitions for terms such as "low fat" and "high fiber" will be required.

In evaluating the list of ingredients one should keep in mind that items are listed in descending order according to weight. It is also important to note the various names used to describe certain substances such as sugar (sucrose, fructose, maltose, corn syrup, honey) which can greatly increase the total quantity of that ingredient in the product. The total calories listed must be within 20% of the actual calorie count.

An informed consumer will take the time to read food labels and learn what the data means.

Label Terms You Should Know

Enriched—means that essential nutrients that were lost during processing have at least partially been replaced by the manufacturer.

Fortified—means that nutrients have been added that were not in the substance originally or were present in smaller amounts.

Sugar-free or Sugarless—The FDA refers

PROPOSED NEW FOOD LABEL INFORMATION

Nutrition Information

Serving Size	1/4 pizza
Servings per container	4
Calories	240
*Calories from Fat	63
Protein	9 grams
Carbohydrate	359 grams
*Dietary Fiber	2 grams
Fat	7 grams
*Saturated Fat	4 grams
*Cholesterol	15 milligrams
Sodium	640 milligrams

Percent of U.S. Recommended Daily Allowance

Vitamin A	15
Vitamin C	8
Calcium	10
Iron	6

Optional:
Thiamine
Riboflavin
Niacin

*Indicates this is a new item required on labels.

to sugar as sucrose (common table sugar). Therefore, companies can say their products are sugar-free even though they contain glucose, fructose, and sugar alcohols and as many calories as foods containing "sugars".

"90 Percent Fat Free"—merely a marketing gimmick since the consumer is mislead into believing it is low fat when it may not be. The important information is how much fat is in the product.

DID YOU KNOW????

(Check your nutritional IQ)

1. Both palm kernel and coconut oil are more than 80% saturated fat while beef fat is 50% saturated fat. Oils are found in a variety of snacks (crackers, chips, cookies, cake mixes, and granola bars) and in foods such as non-dairy substitutes.
2. A teaspoon of oil contains about 40 calories (9 calories per gram).
3. Margarine which lists water as the first ingredient on the label has half to one-third less fat than other margarines.
4. Premium ice creams contain considerably more fat than supermarket ice cream.
5. Stick margarine is higher in saturated fat than margarine in tubs.
6. Chicken is 64% protein and 31% fat but a T-bone steak is only 20% protein and 80% fat.
7. Honey is a blend of sugars—mainly fructose and glucose. It has few nutrients and is not significantly healthier than sugar.
8. Heinz Ketchup has more sugar than Sealtest Chocolate Ice Cream (29%—21%). Wishbone Russian Dressing has more sugar than Coca-Cola (30%—

8.8%). Coffeemate Non-Dairy Creamer has more sugar than Hershey's Milk Chocolate (65%—51%).
9. One quarter cup of sunflower seeds contains 140 calories and is 64% fat.
10. Fried chicken sandwiches at fast food restaurants have as much fat as a pint and a half of ice cream (42 grams).
11. One ounce of Kellogg's Corn Flakes has nearly twice the sodium as an ounce of Planter's Cocktail Peanuts (260 mg—132 mg). One-half cup of Jello Instant Chocolate Pudding and Pie Filling has more sodium than 3 slices of Oscar Mayer Sugar Cured Bacon (404 mg—302 mg). One-half cup of cottage cheese has more sodium than 10 potato chips (435 mg—200 mg).
12. Caffeine is found in many products:
    Brewed coffee — 110 mg per cup
    Instant coffee — 66 mg per cup
    Tea — 30 - 40 mg per cup
    Cocoa — 13 mg per cup
    Coca-Cola — 65 mg
    Dr. Pepper — 61 mg
    Tab — 49 mg
    Pepsi Cola — 43 mg
    Anacin — 32 mg
    Excedrin — 64 mg
    Empirin — 32 mg
13. A food labeled as "low calorie" must contain no more than 40 calories per serving. Reduced calories must be at least one-third lower in calories than the food for which it substitutes.
14. Many foods labeled as "natural" contain additives, preservatives, artificial coloring or other artificial ingredients. No federal standards regulate the use of the term "natural."
15. Packaged microwave popcorn contains as much fat as most cookies, high levels

of sodium and twice as many calories as regular popcorn. The message—pop your own using a hot-air popper.

16. You can save calories and fat in small ways that count at fast food restaurants.
Kentucky Fried Chicken:
Remove the breading and skin to cut the calories in half and the fat by two-thirds.
McDonald's:
Eliminate the mayonnaise and save 135 calories and 15 grams of fat.
Burger King:
Have a Burger King Broiler without the sauce and eliminate 90 calories and more than half the fat.
Wendy's:
At the salad bar, avoid the Cheddar Chips, pasta salad, potato salad, and cole slaw to save 110 calories and twice the fat.

17. Microwave cooking retains vitamins and minerals better than other methods of cooking if you don't overcook.

QUESTIONS AND ANSWERS

If I increase the calcium-rich foods in my diet, won't I take in added fat and calories?

While dairy products are higher in calories and fat content than some foods, there are many choices which provide the needed calcium without the high fat. Follow these tips:

- Select dairy products made from skim milk.
- Use ricotta cheese as a dip or spread.
- Use sesame seeds on vegetables, rice and salads.
- Use Parmesan cheese on vegetables and salads.
- Make salad dressings with yogurt, tofu, or skim milk cottage cheese.
- Include a dark, leafy vegetable in your daily menu.
- Eat sardines, salmon, and oysters.

And, of course, remember that exercise is important in preventing osteoporosis (see Chapter 11) and can help burn up those extra calories.

What about fish oil supplements?

Although much publicity has been given to the use of fish oil supplements that contain the omega-3 fatty acids to lower cholesterol and triglycerides, according to the American Heart Association, the American Medical Association, and many renowned scientists, these supplements do not work and are not recommended until their long-term effectiveness and safety have been established. Part of the problem is that the dosage of fish oil supplements that might work has not been determined, and some scientists are not convinced that the omega-3 fatty acid portion of fish is what serves as the heart's protector. Some physicians believe it may be a different component of the fish or a combination of components that work together. Others have stated that one would have to swallow about 50 capsules a day to receive the levels of omega-3 fatty acids which seem to be effective in reducing the risk of heart disease.

At this point, the best recommendation is to wait until further research has been conducted. Of course, substituting fish for meat in the diet is suggested to help lower the intake of saturated fats in the diet, and this does have an important influence on total blood cholesterol level.

Can too much protein be harmful?

Yes, it can. The danger is that excessive intake of protein puts a strain on the kidneys.

Surplus protein gets burned for energy or stored fat. Unfortunately, when the excess is burned for energy only about half is efficiently converted. The remainder becomes harmful toxins such as ammonia that the kidney must process and excrete. In addition, large amounts of water are needed to remove the waste products and thus there is a risk of dehydration. Another problem is that protein is usually accompanied by high fat content—beef and dairy products are sometimes 50% fat.

Since many women of reproductive age are deficient in iron, do you have any advice or tips to help?

Try the following:
— Consume turkey, chicken, lean red meat or shellfish three or four times weekly.
— Since coffee and tea can cut iron absorption by as much as 50%, eliminate them from your diet.
— Foods rich in Vitamin C will help your body absorb iron.
— Avoid hard physical workouts in high temperatures.

What is anemia, and how do I know if I am suffering from it?

Anemia is defined as a level below the normal amount of hemoglobin or red blood cells. The usual symptoms include paleness, weakness, fatigue, shortness of breath and palpitations of the heart. Iron-deficient women also have more trouble recovering from hard physical workouts because they accumulate more lactic acid and their bodies have more trouble eliminating it.

What is the relationship between diet and cancer?

According to the University of California Wellness Letter (Oct., 1987), about one-third of all cancers are in some way linked to what we eat. This link is related to the substances called free radicals which are suspected as cancer producing. Some methods of food preparation (e.g., foods that are grilled, barbecued, or fried at high temperatures) may release these highly reactive substances. On the other hand, substances such as beta carotene (which is transformed into Vitamin A by the body) and Vitamin C seem to gather these free radicals and neutralize their cancer-causing potential. The National Cancer Institute has identified certain foods which may serve as possible protectors against cancer. They include:

• Yellow, orange, and green leafy vegetables and fruit such as carrots, cantaloupes, broccoli, yams, spinach.
• Vitamin A food sources such as liver, butter, milk, cheese, fish oil.
• Vitamin C food sources such as citrus fruits, tomatoes, broccoli, strawberries, potatoes, peppers.
• Vitamin E food sources such as nuts, vegetable oils, whole grains, wheat germ, dried beans.
• Selenium food sources such as seafood, meats, grains, tomatoes.
• Fiber—plant foods such as fruit, vegetables, and whole grains.
• Cruciferous found in the cabbage family such as broccoli, kale, Brussels sprouts, cauliflower.

In addition, people are urged to avoid the possible cancer-causing foods: fats, alcohol nitrites (used to preserve bacon, hot dogs, sausages, etc.), and aflatoxins (poisons found in moldy peanuts, peanut butter, seeds, corn, etc.).

Are there any dangers in a vegetarian diet?

If you are a strict vegetarian and avoid all milk products as well as meat, there are potential problems. Unless care is taken, protein intake may be insufficient, a calcium deficiency may result, and Vitamin B_{12} intake may be inadequate. On the other side, vegetarians generally have a diet lower in calories, higher in fiber, and lower in fats.

Is bottled water safer from impurities and should I switch to it?

While lab tests now being required indicate that bottled water is safe and doesn't pose any health hazards, it is not necessarily any purer than regular tap water. Although most perceive bottled water to be healthier, studies show about 25% of bottled water comes the same municipal water sources as tap water but costs 300-1,200 times more per gallon. If you like the taste of bottled water better and don't mind the added cost that's fine, but don't be mislead into thinking It is necessarily better for your health.

What is tofu?

Tofu is soybean curds that are high in protein but also high in polyunsaturated fat. Four ounces of tofu has 5 grams of fat. And even though many consider tofu to be a health food, it is 53% fat.

How can I get nutritional advice that I trust?

The best way is to seek advice from a nutritionist who is a registered dietician. A professional nutritionist has the initials R.D. (registered dietician) and/or L.D. (licensed dietician) after his/her name. A quack may even have a Ph.D. in an unrelated field or try to impress you with a degree from a diploma mill, but he/she lacks the knowledge to be trusted. To locate a qualified nutritionist ask your physician, call the local or state American Dietetic Association, a hospital dietary department, or your local health department.

REFERENCES

Tufts University Diet & Nutrition Letter, Vol. 5, No. 7, September 1987.
Executive Fitness, Vol. 18, No. 10, October 1987.
University of California, *Berkeley Wellness Letter,* Vol. 3, Issue 9, June 1987.
Nutrition and Your Health: Dietary Guidelines for Americans. Consumer Information Center, Dept. 514-X, Pueblo, CO 81009

SUGGESTED LABS: 21, 22, 23, 24.

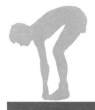

Controlling Your Weight

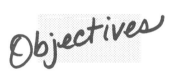

- Define the difference between obesity and overweight.
- Describe the health problems linked to obesity.
- Describe the causes of obesity
- Describe methods for calculating one's healthy weight
- Describe the importance of knowing one's BMR
- Describe qualities for weight control
- Describe a plan for eating healthy in order to lose weight without "dieting"
- Describe the dangers of a variety of popular diet plans
- Describe the risks of eating disorders.

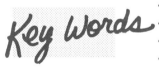

- Anorexia nervosa
- BMR
- Bulimia
- Calorie
- METS
- Obesity
- Set Point
- Spot Reduce

OBESITY VS OVERWEIGHT

One of the major health problems in the United States today is obesity. An obese person is one who has an excess accumulation of body fat. An optimal percent of body fat of the average person is estimated from 10-15% for men and from 15-20% for women. An individual who is overweight is generally defined as one who weighs more than 10% above the desired weight. Using these definitions, one could be obese without being overweight or could be overweight without being obese. It is not so much a question of how heavy a person is but how much excess body fat one possesses that is important in regard to health problems associated with obesity.

Why Worry About Your Weight?

Since every extra pound of fat forces the heart to pump blood through an extra two-thirds mile of blood vessels, if you are obese you are endangering your health. Unfortunately, a large segment of the American population is obese. The average American gains one pound of weight each year beyond the age of 25, and this gain is in the form of fat! Furthermore, there is a high relationship between obesity and increased risk of death from a variety of diseases. Studies show that obesity may not only increase the risk of developing some diseases but may aggravate diseases which are caused by other factors. Specifically, obesity has been linked to the following problems:
1. High blood pressure and heart disease.
2. Stroke and circulatory problems.
3. Increased level of cholesterol and triglycerides.
4. Many types of bone and joint disorders.
5. Diabetes.
6. Lower back difficulties.
7. Respiratory ailments.
8. Higher incidence of accidents, surgical and pregnancy complications.

Some life insurance figures have shown that the mortality rate of obese males is 150% higher than the normal mortality rate. Current estimates are that six out of ten of the leading causes of death in this country are diet related. There is little doubt that being overweight and obese is a threat to the quality and length of one's life.

The Causes of Obesity

An estimated 50% of adults in this country are considered overweight by the American Medical Association due to the following major reasons:
1. Lack of physical activity
2. Overeating
3. Emotional problems
4. Physiological disturbances

Other factors which may affect weight include heredity, environment and basal metabolic rate. Studies show that children of obese parents are likely to be overweight, and children whose parents are lean generally are the same. This relationship may also be caused by acquired family eating habits or culturally-developed attitudes toward weight.

The eating patterns that contribute to obesity are typically established early in life. Therefore, permanent changes in weight will require permanent changes in eating habits, such as food preparation, food selection, and manner of eating. In addition, the basal metabolism rate (BMR)—the rate at which the body uses energy to maintain itself while at complete rest without food—differs among people.

Human fat cells increase in number very rapidly early in life and, once formed, become fixed for life. Overeating by a young

111

child tends to rapidly multiply the number of fat cells. The child may even have difficulty controlling his or her weight throughout life. As individuals grow older, they become less active. This reduction of activity, along with a decline in the basal metabolism rate (BMR) means that eating habits must be adjusted. Otherwise, gains in weight or increases in body fat percentages will occur. After age 20, BMR decreases about 3 percent per decade.

Most nutritionists believe that inactivity is the most important reason for the high incidence of obesity in our modern Western societies. Our sedentary lifestyle—not overeating—has been the major cause of the problem. As a matter of fact, it appears that the majority of obese individuals do not eat any more than the non-obese. Clearly, sedentary lifestyles have contributed to the high incidence of obesity. We simply do not have a level of activity that will "burn up" the calories we take in each day. Therefore, the real key to controlling our weight and obesity is being active. We must include a planned exercise program as a part of our daily lives.

Keeping our weight at the optimal level is a lifetime activity and, for most of us, a lifetime of dieting cannot be successful. We must not think in terms of "going on a diet" but in terms of a change in our lifestyle to include increased exercise and improved eating habits.

How Much Should You Weigh?

In determining your correct average weight, the most common method is to refer to a published height-weight chart. A set of tables

which had previously served as a "standard" for many was the Metropolitan Life Insurance weight tables. However, in 1990 the U.S. Food and Drug Administration and the Health and Human Services Department issued new federal guidelines for body weight. One reason the Metropolitan scale was abandoned was the fact that it is based on a very select group of people (predominantly whites of higher socioeconomic status).

These new guidelines do not have separate charts for men and women but suggest a range by age and height with the higher weights in the range generally applicable to men and the lower weights to women. The chart also makes allowance for weight gain as one grows older. The current suggested healthy weight chart for adults appears below.

SUGGESTED WEIGHTS FOR ADULTS

Height	Weight in pounds 19 to 34 years	Weight in pounds 35 years and older
5-foot-0	97-128	108-138
5-foot-1	101-132	111-143
5-foot-2	104-137	115-148
5-foot-3	107-141	119-152
5-foot-4	111-146	122-157
5-foot-5	114-150	126-162
5-foot-6	118-155	130-167
5-foot-7	121-160	134-172
5-foot-8	125-164	138-178
5-foot-9	129-169	142-183
5-foot-10	132-174	146-188
5-foot-11	136-179	151-194
6-foot-0	140-184	155-199
6-foot-1	144-189	159-205
6-foot-2	148-195	164-210
6-foot-3	152-200	168-216
6-foot-4	156-205	173-222
6-foot-5	160-211	177-228
6-foot-6	164-216	182-234

Height is measured without shoes; weight, without clothes.
The higher weights in the ranges generally apply to men; the lower weights more often apply to women, who have less muscle and bone.
Source: Derived from National Research Council, 1989.

CALORIC VALUES

The calorie is the common unit of measurement used to express the potential energy of food and the amount of energy used by the body in performing various activities. The energy level required to keep the body functioning is influenced by body composition, body size, and age. Generally, men have a higher minimum caloric need than women due to a greater proportion of musculature and less fat and because they are larger. More energy is used to transform food to energy when more muscle tissue is present.

The approximate energy values of the basic energy-yielding food groups are carbohydrates, four calories per gram; proteins, four calories per gram; and fats, nine calories per gram. The body burns food calories to obtain energy for physical activities and to provide energy for all body processes from thinking to digestion. Caloric expenditure can be calculated by measuring the amount of oxygen used in performing the activity. It takes approximately one liter of oxygen to burn five calories of food. Therefore, a person who uses three liters of oxygen per minute in exercising, will burn up the equivalent of 900 calories for each hour of exercise at that rate. Energy expenditures for different activities vary according to body weight and skill level. Approximations have been prepared from actual measurements and are listed in Appendix D.

In determining the total number of calories needed, one must consider:
1. Those needed for basal metabolism.
2. Those needed for muscular activity.
3. Those needed to digest, absorb, and metabolize the food we eat.

As you increase your physical activity, the caloric need increases. There are various methods of measuring the caloric costs of activities. The following table indicates the approximate calories per kilogram of body weight and per pound per hour.

	CALORIES/KILOGRAM/HOUR	CALORIES/LB./HR
sedentary (sitting, studying)	0.23	.50
light activities (standing)	0.27	.59
moderate activities	0.50	1.10
active exercise (fast walking)	0.77	1.69
strenuous exercise (jogging, running)	1.09	2.39

METS is another measure of calorie intensity. A MET refers to the rate of energy needed at rest, or approximately 1.25 calories (about a quarter liter of oxygen.). The MET cost of an activity indicates the number of times above rest you have to increase your metabolism. If an activity is classified at 7 METS it simply means that it requires seven times more energy than at a state of rest. Seven METS are equivalent to 8.8 calories per minute or a little more than 1.75 liters of oxygen uptake—which would be at the high end of moderate exercise. Anything over 10 METS is considered very vigorous. Your maximum METS indicates the number of times you are capable of increasing your metabolism above rest. Obviously, the more you can increase your metabolism, the more exercise you can do. Therefore, the higher your maximum METS, the higher your level of physical fitness.

By calculating the number of calories consumed and the number expended through daily activities, you can determine if caloric balance is achieved. The diagram which follows reflects the importance of analyzing caloric intake and expenditure if you are to achieve and maintain the correct weight.

BMR

The Basal Metabolic Rate (BMR) is the rate at which one's body metabolizes (burns) food and nutrients to perform normal, minimal body functions at rest. The usual estimate is that the BMR requires one calorie per hour for each kilogram of body weight—for women this is approximately 1200 calories and for men about 1500 calories. However, because the rate can vary for different individuals, one can compute his/her particular rate using the following formula:

Women:	Men:
Weight (lbs)_____	Weight (lbs) _____
+ 0	+ 0
Subtotal_____	Subtotal_____
Weight (lbs)_____	2 x Wt. (lbs) _____
BMR _____	BMR _____
Example: (woman)	Example: (man)
Weight (lbs) 133	Weight (lbs) 168
+ 0	+ 0
Subtotal 1330	Subtotal 1680
Weight 133	2 x Wt 336
BMR 1463	BMR 2016

To adjust the BMR for age, reduce the number calculated by 2% for each 10 years of age over 20:

          30 years = 2% reduction   1200 BMR x .98 = 1176
          40 years = 4% reduction   1200 BMR x .96 = 1152

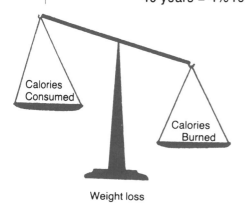

Weight loss

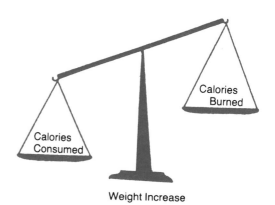

Weight Increase

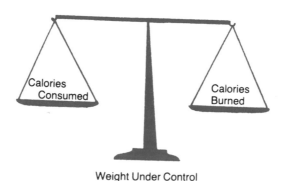

Weight Under Control

An important reason for knowing one's BMR is to use it in calculating the total caloric expenditure when determining the number of calories for a weight control program. The total calories expended in exercise plus the BMR equals the total number of calories one burns each day. Since the key to weight control is balancing calorie intake with the calories burned (through BMR and activity), knowing this value is important.

In addition, one should understand that the BMR drops when a person diets (therefore the body needs fewer calories to maintain its weight) and exercise raises the BMR (causing the body to burn more calories throughout the day).

GUIDELINES FOR WEIGHT CONTROL

The best strategy for a lifetime of successful weight control is a sound, nutritious diet combined with regular, vigorous exercise. The primary goal is not just to shed fat but to keep it off, or better yet, never to put it on. The key factor in weight control is that weight loss or weight gain depends on the ratio between calorie intake and calorie expenditure. Quick-reducing diets lack the balance of needed foods and may cause great harm. In addition, they seldom result in a permanent weight loss because they fail to bring about a change in basic eating habits and lifestyle. To be effective, diets must be considered from a long-range view and must result in the adoption of a lifetime style of eating that a person can live with every day.

In planning a diet, remember that *energy is the job of carbohydrates, and muscle repair is the job of proteins.* If you select a high-protein, low-carbohydrate diet, it can actually lead to a deterioration of muscle tissue as the protein exhausts itself trying to supply energy and maintain healthy tissue. In addition, low-carbohydrate diets can lead to such problems as kidney disorders, loss of muscle tissue, fatigue, and dizziness.

When designing a reducing program, the following factors should be considered:

1. The diet must produce a negative caloric balance. In order to "burn up" fatty tissue, more energy must be expended in calories than the energy consumed in food.

2. The diet must contain all the required nutrients from a variety of sources and provide a caloric intake not lower than 1200 calories per day.

3. The weight loss should be a gradual one which can be maintained. In a semistarvation diet, it is not fatty tissue that is lost, but lean muscle tissue and water.

4. Reducing plans should include an exercise program. Exercise will help develop muscle as it "burns" excess body fat. Combining diet with exercise will result in a weight loss of more fatty tissue. The exercise should burn a minimum of 300 calories per session.

5. Reducing plans must be adaptable to a lifetime of use, not just a short term. Therefore, foods should be those one finds acceptable in terms of taste, cost, and ease of acquisition.

6. The plan should include behavior modification techniques to identify and eliminate dieting habits that contribute to improper nutrition.

Since there are 3500 calories in a pound of stored body fat, one pound a week can be lost eliminating 500 calories a day from the diet, by "burning up" 500 more calories each day through exercise, or through a combination of eliminating calories from the diet and increased exercise.

Establishing Healthy Eating Habits

Your goal is to establish permanent healthful eating habits—those that you can and will maintain throughout your life. Through techniques of behavior modification you can bring about a change in your diet and eating habits.

Consider implementing the following habits:

1. Learn to control your eating behavior — be in control and establish new habits.
2. Eat slowly.
3. Space meals evenly throughout the day.
4. Plan snacks into your diet.
5. Don't skip meals.
6. Watch your progress.
7. Include exercise.
8. Make a food list when shopping and stick to it. Never shop when you are hungry.
9. Don't watch television or listen to the radio while eating.
10. Reduce recipes and fix only the amount needed for one meal.

No satisfactory fat reduction drug or quick weight-loss plan has been developed. There is no substitute for a long range diet and exercise plan. Set reasonable goals—don't expect to lose the weight overnight or even to change your "bad habits" quickly.

Losing Weight Without Eating Less

By simply substituting low fat foods for those that are high fat, one can lose weight and not eat less. Try this method of eating and see the difference in your weight.

- Switch to low fat and non-fat dairy products (i.e., milk, yogurt, cottage cheese, sour cream, etc.). This can cut back from 70-90 calories per serving.
- Choose lean cuts of meat or switch from meat to skinless poultry or fish.
- Eat lots of fresh fruits and vegetables and grains such as bread and pasta.
- Switch from a morning croissant to a bran muffin (every day)—reduce 10 pounds in one year.
- Replace your tablespoon of butter with a tablespoon of cream cheese and reduce 5 pounds in a year.

The chart below shows additional ways of saving calories.

SAVING CALORIES

Instead of...	(cal.)	Substitute these...	(cal.)	Save
milkshakes (chocolate or vanilla)	260	yogurt shake with fruit	140	120
brownie squares, with nuts—2 in.	300	Angel food cake, 1 slice	125	175
fruit pie, 1 slice	300	apple, baked	95	205
doughnut, glazed	235	muffin (corn, bran, berry)	135	100
fish, breaded and fried, 3 oz.	175	fish, broiled, 3 oz.	80	95
ice cream, 1/2 cup	175	ice milk, 1/2 cup	90	85

The "Apple" vs "Pear" Weight Loss Battle

While those whose fat is stored primarily above the waist and in the abdomen are at higher risk for heart disease, this type of fat is more easily reduced than the fat on the hips, thighs, and buttocks. Because the abdominal fat cells are so active, the turnover rate for abdominal fat is high, and when exercise is part of the weight reduction program, more fat is lost from the trunk than from the extremities.

Unfortunately, the fat cells in the lower extremities are more stubborn and exercise alone may not be effective in reducing the fat. It seems that one will need a more intensified approach that includes a low fat, reduced calorie diet, and considerable regular exercise. Even then studies show it is more difficult to reshape your figure if you are in the "pear" group.

A recent report in *The Physician and Sportsmedicine* magazine notes that obese men tend to be shaped more like "apples" while obese women tend to be shaped as "pears."

Diet Program Facts

- Regardless of how successful a particular weight-loss plan is, most people do gain back the weight. In addition, within five years people not only regain their original weight, they add three to four extra pounds.
- Research suggests that when weight is regained it tends to come back in the abdomen.
- For some people, the 1200 calories per day diet may be too restrictive (heavier people who are physically active).
- The importance of combining exercise with dieting is clear. If you diet without exercising your resting metabolic rate is lowered and you actually burn fewer calories during the normal day's activities. But more importantly, you may actually gain weight even faster when you stop dieting than if you had never dieted. By including exercise you maintain your metabolic rate and assure that the weight lost is mainly fat (not muscle). Exercise can even increase your total lean muscle mass which causes the body to burn more calories even at rest.
- The best exercise is that recommended for developing cardiovascular fitness: moderate aerobic exercise such as walking, jogging, swimming, bicycling, aerobic dancing, etc.

FAD DIETS

Fad diets are extremely popular because everyone is looking for a quick and easy way to achieve weight control. However, fad dieting ultimately leads to failure because it usually does not result in a permanent weight loss. The main shortcoming of fad diets is that they do not bring about a change in basic eating habits and lifestyle. Losing weight is not a temporary, short-term problem, so "going on" a diet (and, of course, eventually "going off") will not solve the problem. To be effective, a diet must help in establishing eating habits that will lead not only to weight control but to a healthy life. Therefore, the best strategy for a life time of successful weight control is a sound, nutritious diet combined with regular, vigorous exercise.

Actually, it is fortunate that so few people can stay on a fad diet. Most quick-reducing diets lack the necessary nutritional balance and may cause great harm if adhered to for long periods of time. In addition, fad diets tend to disturb the body's metabolic balance and returning to "normal" is difficult. The individual may deposit more fat than usual after going off the diet. Some diets even make the claim that they provide a special metabolic combination of foods which accelerates weight loss. There is no such magic combination, just as no one food can help break down fat. Also, remember there is no such thing as a "fattening food"—it is the total number of calories in all foods eaten that determines whether you gain weight. Fat deposits can result from excess calories from any source—carbohydrates, proteins, and alcohol, as well as fats.

Fasting

Some people mistakenly seek semi-starvation or fasting as a means of quick weight loss. The weight loss experienced with fasting and other drastic measures is mainly lean body mass or muscle. Fasting tends to confuse the body and it starts burning up the wrong tissues. Research clearly shows that when fasting only one-third of the weight loss is fatty tissue, while two-thirds is lean body tissue. The reason for this occurrence is that when energy intake is too low, the body maintains the blood glucose level by converting the available amino acids in muscle tissue to glucose.

Another problem arising from extreme caloric deprivation is that the body decreases its metabolic rate. Therefore, calories are burned more slowly and even an extremely small number of calories are sufficient to maintain one's weight. This also triggers the mechanism which causes the body to store fat more efficiently, thus a decrease in lean muscle tissue and an increase in fat storage, to say nothing of the potential health problems which an individual can suffer through a prolonged or consistent program of fasting. Fasting is certainly not recommended as an approach to effective and safe weight loss.

Diet Aids (Pills, Candy, Gum, etc.)

The basic problem with all diet aids is similar to that of fad diets—they do not meet the nutritional needs of the individual and they do not bring about a change in the basic eating habits of the individual.

The goals of such aids are to curb the appetite, numb the taste buds, or provide a feeling of fullness. Most pills contain a drug called phenylpropanolamine (PPA), which your body can build a tolerance to and which can lead to psychological dependence. Some pills have caffeine to relieve feeling of fatigue or diuretics which cause only water weight loss. The chewing gum or candy-type diet aids depend on benzocaine, a mild topical anesthetic, to numb your taste buds.

Just because a diet aid is sold over the counter doesn't mean it is completely safe. Certain individuals may be susceptible to a particular chemical, may unintentionally overdose on a drug which is found in other medications being taken, and some may develop other side effects. Obviously, however, the major drawback is that such an approach does not contribute to a permanent weight loss.

EVALUATING LEADING DIET PLANS

Description	Comments
Specialized programs: Weight Watchers, T.O.P.S.	
Nutritious food plans which emphasize lowering calories and increasing exercise. All basic nutrients are included. Some behavior modification techniques presented.	Group meetings are held to encourage maintenance of the program. A membership fee and fees for meetings are charged. Stresses a slow, permanent weight loss but requires following a fairly rigid meal plan.
Diet Pills (Dexatrim, Dietic, Dexedrine, diuretics)	
Pills used to suppress the appetite and/or increase fluid loss. May also increase the rate of metabolism.	Weight loss, if any, is due to water loss—not fat. Side effects such as nervousness, tremors, insomnia, hypertension, depression, and dependency are possible with heavy use. Not effective over long periods of time.
Meal Replacement Products or Liquid Formula Diets (Slim-fast, Dynatrim, Ultra-slim)	
Individuals drink a special formula of approximately 220 calories per day in combination with a snack and one nutritious meal. A total of 1200 calories per day is suggested.	Becomes boring and monotonous. Difficult to maintain over a long period and it does not teach healthy eating habits in order to maintain the weight loss. Dangerous if individual skips the recommended meal. Inappropriate use can lead to dehydration, electrolyte imbalance, and other problems.
Pritikin Diet Plan	
Extremely low-fat diet combined with exercise. Stresses intake of complex carbohydrates and high fiber foods.	Very strict in allowing no cholesterol, salt, or artificial sweeteners. Encourages the individual to adopt these new eating habits for the long term.
Fasting	
Only intake is liquids and vitamin and mineral supplements. Should only be used for grossly obese in a hospital setting.	Weight loss at first is very rapid, but it declines as the basal metabolic rate decreases. Most weight loss is lean muscle tissue rather than fat. Can be dangerous. Does not meet long term needs since the individual does not learn a new eating pattern.
Very Low Calorie Liquid Diet (Cambridge, etc.)	
Actually a modified fast with a person permitted a high protein liquid (350-660 calories per day) in a special preparation which may contain vitamins, minerals, carbohydrates, and proteins.	Weight loss at first is very rapid, but weight is likely to be regained quickly after the diet. Can be extremely dangerous due to lack of vitamins and minerals and roughage. Heart problems, diabetes, anemia, and even deaths from metabolic effects have been recorded. Does not lead to a change in eating habits.
Specialized Programs (pre-packaged foods—Jenny Craig, Nutri-System, etc.)	
Extremely low-fat pre-packaged foods, sold weekly to participants. Some behavior modification techniques presented, some counseling is involved. A maintenance program is available.	A membership fee is charged. Food is purchased each week and is fairly expensive.

EATING DISORDERS

Anorexia nervosa

Although we have stressed the importance of maintaining one's body weight at an optimal level and of the need for an acceptable body fat level, it is not healthy to become obsessed with weight loss to the point that extreme measures are employed. Some weight loss methods are extremely dangerous, can lead to serious health problems, and can even be life-threatening. The obsession to become thin and have a "perfect body" has led some to try a technique of starvation referred to as anorexia nervosa. This disease, which is particularly common among young women, is characterized by an intense fear of becoming obese—even when considerable weight has been lost.

The anorexic usually begins with a normal dieting program, begins to skip one or more meals a day, and then may not eat for several days. Some anorexics will eat a complete meal and then use self-induced vomiting. The individual may also try to speed up the weight loss by excessive exercising and overuse of laxatives or diuretics.

Characteristics of individuals who have anorexia nervosa are an usually stressful life, social rejection, loss of a boyfriend, poor self-esteem, depression, and obsessive/compulsive personality, a perfectionist attitude, and from a mother-dominated family.

Anorexia nervosa can cause the following health problems:
- menstruation ceases (as body fat loss becomes extreme)
- electrolyte imbalances which increase the risk of heart attack
- limited functioning of the immune system
- digestive disorders
- anemia
- mental confusion and inability to concentrate
- severe dryness of the skin

The anorexic will not accept the fact that his/her behavior is abnormal or harmful, and the problem goes unnoticed by family and friends until the condition is severe. Typically, the anorexic cannot overcome the disorder without treatment, and yet it is difficult to get the anorexic to accept help and seek treatment. Treatment should be by a trained counselor who can provide psychological and medical therapy to assist the individual in overcoming the disorder and hopefully begin to reverse the physical damage. Some individuals may require hospitalization and long-term treatment.

Bulimia

Another eating disorder which is particularly common among college women is bulimia. As with anorexics, bulimics are preoccupied with food and body image. However, it may be more difficult to identify an individual who is bulimic since the person typically maintains a body weight that is near normal.

The bulimic engages in binge eating in which the intake of calories may be between 1,000-20,000 in a one- or two-hour period, which is then followed by purging through vomiting, laxatives, or fasting.

Some of the typical health problems which can occur with a bulimic include:
- fluid and electrolyte imbalance
- erosion of the teeth from stomach acids
- irritation and tearing of the esophagus
- kidney and bladder problems
- ulcers and colitis
- irregular heart rhythm

As with the anorexic, early treatment by trained professionals is vital to overcome this dangerous eating disorder.

GAINING WEIGHT SAFELY

Some individuals have difficulty gaining weight and feel they are too thin or underweight. This may be an athlete who burns an excessive number of calories during workouts or just someone whose heredity or metabolism rate contribute to a lower weight. Although some individuals may be unhappy about being "underweight," if you are currently regularly eating a healthy selection of foods, it is important to be cautious in undertaking a program to gain weight. You may be unhappy about being thin now, but you naturally gain weight as you grow older and mature. Many overweight adults remember when they could eat anything and never gain an ounce, but now have great difficulty controlling their weight. In addition, you should avoid an increased intake of high-fat foods, which could lead to problems with your cholesterol level.

The following suggestions for gaining weight safely may assist you:

- Use muscle-building exercises to stimulate muscular development. Remember good muscular development contributes to a better looking physique and muscle is heavier than fat deposits.
- Substitute fruit juices and skim milk for beverages such as water, coffee, and tea that do not have calories. Fruit juices and frozen yogurt shakes can greatly increase your calorie intake.
- Drink a commercial nutritional supplement such as an instant breakfast (made with skim milk) or Ensure, Isocal, or Sustacal.
- Eat healthy snacks between meals—low fat fruit yogurt, hot or cold cereal, muffins, bananas, dried fruit, baked potatoes topped with cottage cheese, and vegetable pizza.

- Eat three meals per day consistently. Do not skip a meal—make meal time a priority.

BEHAVIOR MODIFICATION

Establishing a Healthy Eating Plan—Not a Diet Plan!

1. *Set reasonable, realistic goals.*

    Use your body fat measurement, body measurement index, height-weight tables, and the "mirror test" to determine whether or not you need to lose fat and as a guide to how much to lose.

    Remember slow, gradual weight loss is the only effective method. Take the number of pounds you want to lose and calculate how many weeks it will take if you lose one-half pound a week. Then do the same calculation for losing one pound per week. The date you reach your goal should be somewhere between these two projected dates. Don't rush and expect to reach your goal sooner.

2. *Evaluate your current eating habits and modify them to eliminate the bad habits.*

    Your goal is permanent weight loss so you need to look at your eating behavior and lifestyle and make changes that will ensure long-term success. Consider such things as why you eat what you eat, the amount you eat, and when you eat. A number of the diet analysis ideas in this chapter will help you make this evaluation. Once you know your problem areas you can begin to consider modifications. Use these ideas to make better food selections (lower fat and calories, increased complex carbohydrates, etc.). The key is to recognize your bad eating habits and do something to change them.

3. *Be certain you include exercise in your lifestyle.*

Studies confirm that those who exercise are more likely to lose fat and keep it off than those who try to "diet" only. Find an exercise you enjoy and can conveniently fit into your daily schedule (or at least three times weekly) for at least 20 minutes.

4. *Chart your progress.*

Using a tape measure (and body fat measures if possible) as well as the scale, keep track of your body changes. Remember increased muscle tissue may increase your total weight but lower your fat percentage. Don't be discouraged if you have your ups and downs. Stay with it through the setbacks.

Diet Analysis

One of the most revealing projects you can undertake is a thorough analysis of your current diet in terms of calories and grams of carbohydrates, fat and protein. Such an analysis, based on all food eaten for a given period, will enable you to determine your average daily intake of calories from each nutrient category and the percentage of each eaten.

The recommended daily intake percentages are as follows:

- Carbohydrates—68%
- Fat—20% (10% unsaturated, 10% saturated)
- Protein—12%

It is difficult to give precise figures on the percentage of protein, carbohydrate, and fat that should be included in a person's diet, but those stated are accepted as being preventative standards. Protein proportions should be in the higher range for pregnant women, young people still in the growing stages, and those in exercise programs aimed at increasing lean muscle mass, with a proportional decrease in fat.

See Labs 21-24 for a method of making a complete diet analysis.

QUESTIONS AND ANSWERS

How does exercise contribute to weight control?

Exercise can play an important role in your effort to regulate weight. Not only does the exercise burn calories but it also helps maintain muscle tone and shape. An added benefit can be improvement in the body's ability to burn fat. Vigorous exercise over a period of time enables the body to use its stores of fat more efficiently as muscle fuel. The body's ability to burn fat improves with exercise.

How can I tell if I am losing body fat?

Other than weighing yourself regularly, there is another simple way to determine if you are making progress in shedding body fat. The best way to do this is to keep a weekly record of the circumference of your upper arm or thigh.

Although most noncontractile fat is stored under the skin with the thicker layers around the waist, when you reduce your bodily percentage of fat it is reduced proportionately from all over the body and not from any one spot. Thus, you may have a one-inch layer of fat at your waist and one-fourth inch on the back of your arm. As you reduce your fat and the one-inch waist fat is reduced by 50 percent to one-half inch, the one-fourth inch of arm fat is reduced to one-eighth inch. The difference is that you had less there to begin with.

Authorities suggest the following rules for

recording weekly arm measurements:
- Take the measurements before a training session.
- Use the same cloth tape measure for every measurement. Relax the arm and take the measurement midway between the elbow and tip of the shoulder with the arm hanging away from the body. Record to the nearest sixteenth-inch.

What is set point?

Your set point is the weight you normally maintain, give or take a few pounds, when you are not consciously attempting to control it. It is the weight to which your body returns after dieting or overeating. Unless we change our set point, the battle against overweight is continuous and usually futile. Exercise is the most effective way to lower your set point. This is probably because we were all designed to be fairly active and fairly lean. However, inactivity and modern day sedentary lifestyle have raised the set point above what it would ordinarily be. Dieting will not decrease the set point.

Can I spot reduce?

It is now very clear that you cannot spot reduce. Exercising the muscles in a particular area will not cause the fat around the muscle to be broken down by energy. During vigorous exercise the muscles call upon fat storage deposits throughout the body for fuel. Heredity determines our particular distribution of fat deposits. This is the reason each of us gains weight in different areas. The best way to lose fat is to participate in vigorous activity that can be sustained for long periods of time.

How can I eliminate cellulite?

First of all, you must understand that there really is no such thing as cellulite. Over ten years ago the *Journal of the American Medical Association* clearly stated that "There is no medical condition known or described as cellulite in this country." The term is used frequently to describe fat that appears to cause ripples and bumps on the thighs and buttocks. However, fat is fat, and it is additional weight gain that causes the bulging look. Since women tend to store fat more in the thighs and buttocks ("pear shape"), they may be more likely to have this dimpled look. In addition, certain outer layers of skin are thinner in women than men and therefore are more likely to reveal the bulging fat cells under the skin. The many special cures which are advertised for cellulite (massages, scrubbing, creams, supplements, and injections) are not effective. The fat causing this dimpled look is lost just like all fat on the body—by burning more calories than you take in—by losing weight through diet and exercise.

REFERENCES
1. Bailey, Covert. *The Fit-Or-Fat Target Diet.* Boston: Houghton Mifflin Co. 1984.
2. Dusek, Dorothy. *Weight Management—The Fitness Way.* Boston: Jones & Bartlett Pub. 1989.
3. Cotterman, Sandra. *Y's Way to Weight Management.* Champaign, IL: Human Kinetics Pub. 1985.

SUGGESTED LAB: 25.

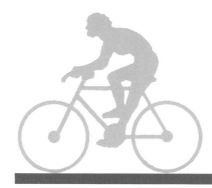

Exercise and Your Cardiovascular System

Objectives

- Identify the factors which tend to predispose people to heart disease.
- Identify ways to reduce blood cholesterol.
- Discuss the effects of physical training on the cardiovascular system.
- Trace the flow of blood through the cardiovascular system.

Key Words

- Angina
- Arteriosclerosis
- Artery
- Atherosclerosis
- Blood platelets
- Blood pressure
- Capillaries
- Cardiovascular disease
- Cholesterol
- Coronary arteries
- Diastolic
- High density lipoprotein (HDL)
- Low density lipoprotein (LDL)
- Pulse
- Red blood cells
- Systolic
- Varicose veins
- Veins
- White blood cells

Your cardiovascular system is comprised of the heart, blood vessels and blood. Essentially the heart is the pump which keeps the blood circulating to all parts of the body. This is accomplished by a vast network of blood vessels somewhat like a highway system that ultimately reaches even the smallest village. The blood carries the nutrients which keep tissues and all body parts supplied with oxygen, and on the reverse trip, removes accumulated waste materials. The reason the cardiovascular system is so important is because, in the long run, its efficiency can have a direct bearing on the quality and length of your life.

The Heart

Your heart is the most efficient machine known to man. This hollow, muscular organ, about the size of your fist, is so efficient that it is able to convert up to 50% of its fuel (food) into energy, while receiving only 10% of the body's oxygen and converting 80% of it. Imagine clenching your fist 72 times each minute 100,000 times a day without any rest. Or figured another way, imagine lifting a ten-pound weight three feet off the ground every 30 seconds for the rest of your life. This is about the equivalent work of a person's heart over a lifetime. What is amazing is that this beautiful machine does not complain more often!

The heart is composed of layers of muscles arranged in a circular fashion which, when contracted, cause the body's blood to be squeezed out of its chambers. This squeezing process is called **systole** and the relaxed phase is called **diastole.**

The efficiency of the heart (barring defects) is dependent upon how much it is used. Contrary to what you may have heard, there is no research which says that regular, progressive exercise is detrimental to the human heart. Increased demands on the heart serve only to cause an increase in size and power, thus allowing greater volume with fewer strokes. It is not uncommon for the heart of a highly-trained athlete to perform its function in 48 to 60 beats per minute, rather than the average 72 beats per minute.

Nourishment for the heart comes from a network of small arteries, called **coronary arteries**, which are located on the surface of the heart. These arteries carry the blood, oxygen, and food nutrients to the muscle fibers of the organ. Should blockage occur, as sometimes happens in later life, that portion of the heart muscle quickly dies.

Looking at Figure 7-1 on the next page, we see that the heart is divided into four separate chambers. The bottom two are called **ventricles** and the top two are called **atria**. The two top chambers are separated from the bottom chambers by valves, and the left and right chambers are divided by a wall of muscle called the **septum**.

The heart, then, is actually a double pump which moves blood from the right atrium and then into the lungs for oxygenation. The left ventricle pumps or squeezes the blood into arteries throughout all sections of the body.

Blood that has been "used" by the body comes to the heart via large veins called the **superior** and **inferior vena cava**. The superior vena cava drains blood from the head and arms, and the inferior vena cava services the blood from the lower sections of the body. The blood which nourishes the heart moves into the right atrium through the **coronary sinus**.

To prevent the "used" blood from surging back into the atrium when the ventricle contracts, the heart has a unique three flap valve called the **tricuspid valve**. When this valve is closed, the right ventricle pumps the blood into the **pulmonary artery**. This artery has branches extending into the lungs

125

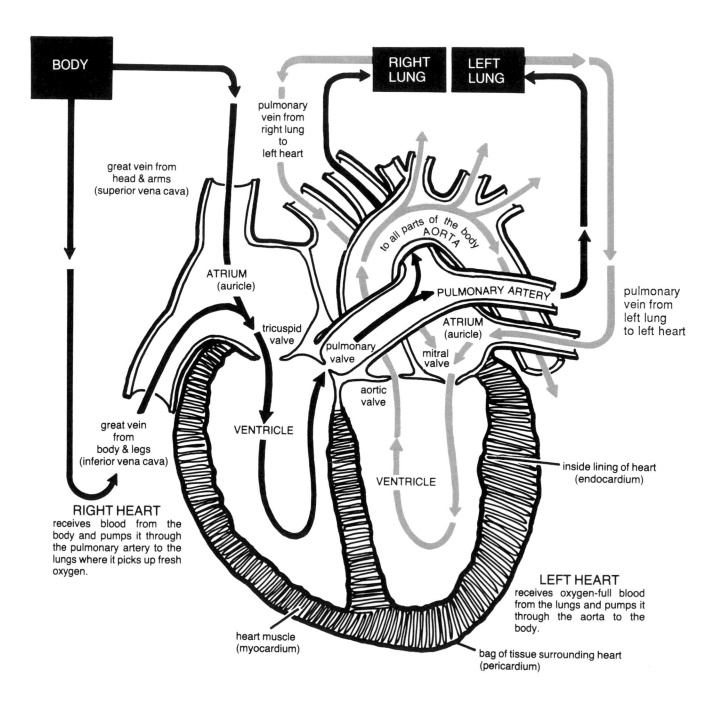

BODY

RIGHT LUNG

LEFT LUNG

pulmonary vein from right lung to left heart

great vein from head & arms (superior vena cava)

pulmonary vein from left lung to left heart

ATRIUM (auricle)

to all parts of the body AORTA

tricuspid valve

PULMONARY ARTERY

pulmonary valve

ATRIUM (auricle)

mitral valve

aortic valve

VENTRICLE

great vein from body & legs (inferior vena cava)

inside lining of heart (endocardium)

VENTRICLE

RIGHT HEART
receives blood from the body and pumps it through the pulmonary artery to the lungs where it picks up fresh oxygen.

LEFT HEART
receives oxygen-full blood from the lungs and pumps it through the aorta to the body.

bag of tissue surrounding heart (pericardium)

heart muscle (myocardium)

Figure 6-1. Your heart and how it works.
(Courtesy American Heart Association)

on both sides of the body, which moves the "deoxygenated" blood into the lungs where it picks up fresh oxygen and gives off carbon dioxide. This exchange involves millions of tiny air sacs called **alveoli** and the red cells of the blood.

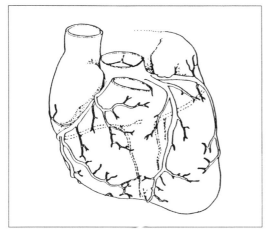

Figure 6-2. The heart receives its blood supply from the coronary arteries.

One of the characteristics of "oxygenation" is the change in color of the blood from dark red to a brighter color. The recharged blood then returns to the left atrium through the **pulmonary vein** and moves through another valve called the **bicuspid** and into the left ventricle chamber whose branches service all parts of the body.

Arteries and Veins

Vessels carrying blood away from the heart are called **arteries,** while those returning blood to the heart are called **veins.** See Figure 6-3 in which cross sections of an artery and vein are compared. Both arteries and veins have walls composed of three layers; however, the normal artery has a thick muscular wall which is elastic, thus enabling it to assist movement of blood throughout the body.

Capillaries

Arteries gradually reduce in size as they branch out in the body. The smallest of these branches are called capillaries. The function of the capillaries is to provide oxygen nutrients to the body cells and to pick up waste materials for the return flow to the heart. Thus, in effect, capillaries serve as bridges between arteries and veins (Figure 6-4).

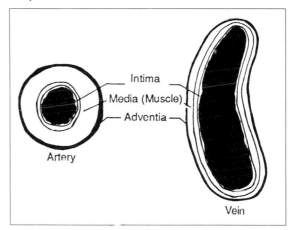

Figure 6-3. Cross section of an artery and vein. Notice the thickness of the arterial wall as contrasted with that of a vein.

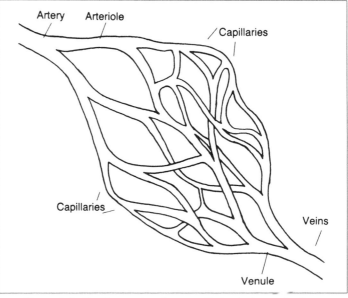

Figure 6-4. Capillary network connecting arteries and veins.

Since your body contains approximately 70,000 miles of blood vessels, they are small; so small, in fact, that the red blood cells must pass through in single file. The red cells are so tiny that if 3,000 of them were lined up the total length of the line would be less than an inch.

When the blood reaches these tiny capillaries it is traveling at a very slow rate of speed, thus allowing white cells, food and oxygen to leave the body by squeezing between the cells in the capillary walls. At the same time, carbon dioxide and other waste products enter the capillaries and are carried away.

There are two ways that the body's "used" blood is returned to the heart. One is a system of unique valves which allow the blood to flow in only one direction—toward the heart. The other method is the location of veins in relation to the muscles of the body. As the body muscles contract during movement, they squeeze the veins and thus push the blood along through the veins and toward the heart. When the muscle relaxes the blood is prevented from moving backwards by the venous valve system.

People whose jobs require that they sit or stand in one position for unduly long periods of time sometimes have difficulty with their circulation. Because of this, the veins may begin to lose their ability to function. This then causes a pooling or overaccumulation of blood in certain areas of the body, most notably in the lower extremities. This venous swelling, caused by too much blood, results in a condition called **varicose veins**. Heredity may also contribute to this condition.

Pulse

Your pulse is caused by the pressure of the blood in your body on the arterial walls. The best place to detect a pulse is in the neck at the carotid artery or at the radial artery in the wrist.

There are two "nodes" which control the rhythm of the heart. The **sinoatrial (SA) node** located in the atria provides the trigger which starts and regulates the approximately 72-80 heartbeats per minute. As this contraction spreads over the atria heart muscle, it stimulates an impulse in the **atrioventricular,** or **AV node,** which stimulates the papillary valve muscles and the two heart ventricles.

When something causes the heart rhythm to break down so that the muscle contractions become uncoordinated, the result is called **fibrillation**. Emergency care personnel almost always carry a machine called a defibrillator to restart or stimulate the heart.

YOUR BLOOD

The average person has approximately five to six quarts of blood. Essentially, blood can be separated into two main parts of which about 50 percent is a watery fluid called plasma. The remainder is made up of white blood cells, red blood cells, and platelets.

Red Cells

The average human body contains approximately 25 trillion red blood cells. And, since they last only about four months, the body is constantly reproducing them in its bone marrow. The red cells are unique in that they have the ability to change their shape to allow them to pass through an opening that is smaller than their own size. This is quite a feat when one considers that a hundred or so would fit nicely on the head of a pin.

The color of red blood cells is produced

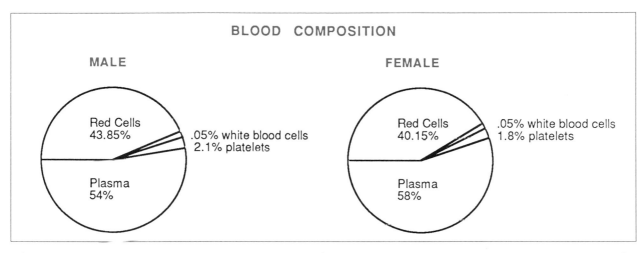

BLOOD COMPOSITION

MALE

Red Cells
43.85%

.05% white blood cells
2.1% platelets

Plasma
54%

FEMALE

Red Cells
40.15%

.05% white blood cells
1.8% platelets

Plasma
58%

by **hemoglobin**. It is hemoglobin that carries oxygen from the lungs to the capillaries for release to individual cells. This same hemoglobin attracts carbon dioxide, which it carries to the lungs to be exhaled.

Hemoglobin enables the blood to carry about sixty times as much oxygen as would be possible if the oxygen had to be dissolved in water or plasma. Hemoglobin is also found in the muscles of the body and provide a reserve of oxygen for sudden bursts of muscular energy. If our bodies did not contain hemoglobin, we would require over fifty times more blood just to survive.

Sometimes there are too few red blood cells or the red cells do not contain enough hemoglobin. When this condition occurs, there is a body deficiency in oxygen which keeps the muscles from burning all their fuel supplies. This results in a lack of body energy and is called anemia. Sometimes a hemoglobin deficiency can be improved by eating foods rich in iron, such as meat and eggs, and high in protein content.

White Cells

White cells, although fewer in number than red cells, still count in the billions. Proportionately they number about one white cell for every 650 red cells. White

cells are primarily responsible for defending the body against infection. They are able to move throughout the body and simply engulf and consume bacteria. The residue is a pus-like fluid which is composed of dead white cells, dead bacteria, and lymph.

Platelets

Blood platelets are another important part of our blood. Their primary role is to help the blood to clot whenever an injury occurs. This complicated process involves the creation of numerous tiny threads, called **fibrin**, which form a tangled mass which we then see as a blood clot.

Plasma

Blood plasma contains minerals (such as calcium, sodium, phosphorus, potassium), plus enzymes, plasma proteins, fats, sugars, and fibrinogen. The plasma also contains oxygen and carbon dioxide.

When whole blood is transfused into another person it must be carefully matched for compatibility. The main blood types are A, B, O, and AB. Lack of compatibility results in the formation of clumps within the blood, thus causing blockages in the smaller blood vessels.

129

Summary: Obviously, this elaborate distribution system, which we call the cardiovascular system, is a critical factor in the length and quality of human life. We must therefore develop and nurture it to the best of our ability.

THE FACTS ABOUT CARDIOVASCULAR DISEASE

Research concerning the values of exercise indicates that sedentary people are more prone to coronary heart disease (twice as frequent), low back pain (80% more frequent), diabetes, duodenal ulcer, and other internal conditions. Evidence also indicates that physically active people exhibit more resistance to mental stress, fatigue, aging, and neuromuscular tension; they also show less tendency toward obesity, are stronger and more flexible, have lower blood pressure, lower pulse rates and greater breathing capacity.

Despite available research, however, coronary heart disease continues to be America's number one killer, claiming approximately 550,000 yearly. Again, research indicates that, although the disease usually manifests itself in middle and later life, development occurs early in life.

In identifying factors which seemingly predispose persons to heart disease, the following are most frequently implicated:

1. **Heredity**—A family history of heart attacks before age fifty or sixty increases your risk of having heart problems.
2. **Inactivity**—Those who remain active have fewer heart problems than the sedentary.
3. **Obesity**—Excessive fat deposits put a direct strain on the heart and other systems of the body. There also is a direct relationship between diabetes and obesity.
4. **High Blood Pressure (Hypertension)**—This has been identified as a major cause of strokes and heart-related problems.
5. **Smoking**—There is a high correlation between smoking and cardiovascular problems.
6. **Stress**—Tension and stress place a strain on the heart and can lead to other types of diseases.
7. **High levels and type of cholesterol**—It has been proven that quantity and quality of cholesterol are directly related to cardiovascular problems.
8. **Diabetes**—There is definite correlation between diabetes and circulatory problems.
9. **Sex**—Males seem to have a higher incidence of heart disease; however, rapidly changing female lifestyles seem to be narrowing the differences between sexes.

THE PROBLEM

The heart, for all practical purposes, is essentially a large muscle about the size of a person's fist. The tissue, called the myocardium, requires a continuous blood supply, which is not supplied by the blood being pumped through the heart itself, but is delivered through the coronary arteries surrounding the myocardium.

It is not certain why the inner lining of the arteries, called the **intima**, thickens. However, it is widely believed that injury or trauma from smoking, high blood pressure, or even a viral infection may cause the initial harm. Naturally the smaller the vessel, the more potential for the problem, and since the coronary arteries are not large arteries, the rate and amount of blood nourishing the heart is diminished. In many cases the arterial passage narrows to the point that any clot (thrombosis) moving through the bloodstream is quite likely to lodge at this narrowed point. Of course, when this happens the heart muscle in that region quickly dies. Sometimes the blockage is not complete, but the heart muscle blood supply is decreased significantly, causing degrees of chest pain known as angina pectoris.

Extensive research conducted in the United States, Israel, England, Canada, Finland and elsewhere supports the concepts that greater morbidity and mortality occur among non-exercising groups as opposed to those who lead a more physically strenuous life.

THE EVIDENCE

The Early Studies

One of the earliest studies relating heart disease to inactivity was reported in 1954 by Morris (15) with other follow-ups reported in 1970. The initial study involved 31,000 drivers and conductors, age 35-64, who were employed by the London Transportation System. Most of the conductors were employed on double-decker buses, which required a considerable amount of walking and climbing. Results of the study showed a significantly higher annual incidence of heart attacks among those men having the least active jobs.

As a corresponding part of the study, sedentary postal clerks were compared to their more vigorous counterparts who delivered the mail. Among 100,000 subjects the same high incidence was found among the more sedentary. Also, the proportion of

men who survived a first attack was more than twice as great among heavy laborers as among those who engaged in only slight physical exertion.

In another study (14) Morris and Crawford analyzed autopsy reports involving approximately 4,000 non-coronary heart disease deaths. The evidence indicated approximately twice as many heart scars (indicating previous damage) among men who had jobs with little exercise as compared with those doing strenuous physical work.

In 1951 many San Francisco longshoremen, aged 35-64, underwent screening examinations for a long-range study. Sixteen years later, Paffenbarger (16) reported a follow-up on more than 3,000 of the original group. Of the total 888 deaths reported, 291, or 33 percent, were from coronary heart disease. Again, those men with more sedentary type jobs died from coronaries three times more frequently than those having more physically active positions. Other risk factors appearing were cigarette smoking and high systolic blood pressures.

Studies by Zukel and associates (20) comparing farmers to nonfarmers, indicated severe heart attacks occurring about half as much among farmers as in other occupational groups.

Taylor and others (18) looked at the relationship between heart attacks occurring in men aged 40-64 who were employed in the railroad industry. Jobs were classified as sedentary (clerks), moderately active (switchmen), and heavily active (section men). Adjusted death rates per 1,000 due to heart disease were as follows: clerks - 5.7, switchmen - 3.9, and section men - 2.8.

Frank (10) in 1968 found persons classified as "least active" physically had an initial myocardial infarction rate more than twice that of individuals classified "intermediate" and "most active." He also found being classified as "most active" did not seem to prevent initial infarctions, but did provide some additional benefits against early mortality.

The Framingham, Massachusetts study reported in 1971 by Kannel, Sorile, and McNamara (13), indicated that men classified most sedentary at all age levels had coronary problems approximately as frequently as those who were at least moderately active. The investigators implied that physical exercise may offer more protection against a heart attack causing death than against a less severe attack of angina pain or a nonlethal attack.

A nine year study conducted by Harvard's School of Public Health and Trinity College School of Medicine in Dublin, Ireland used 575 sets of Irish brothers, one of whom had emigrated to the Boston area while the other had remained in Ireland. The study found that the brothers who had remained in Ireland had lower blood pressure and lower levels of cholesterol. This was in spite of the fact that the Irish brothers ate 400-500 more calories per day and consumed a larger percentage of animal fat daily. Even though they consumed more calories than their American brothers, the Irishmen had less skinfold fat, weighed less and had lower levels of cholesterol. Smoking and drinking habits were much similar. There was only one possible reason why the Irish brothers had better health and hearts. The Irish brothers were generally active, while the American counterparts were generally sedentary.

Brunner and Manelis (4) classified Jewish men and women living in an Israel Kibbutzim into sedentary and nonsedentary workers. A sedentary worker was defined as one seated for at least 80 percent of working time. Included in this group were teachers, managers, clerks, treasurers, bus drivers, shoemakers, dressmakers, and workers in light industry. Non-sedentary workers were kitchen workers, gardeners, kindergarten teachers, industrial and farm workers.

The study was particularly significant since all participants engaged in a uniform way of life except for their occupation. Success or lack of it had no bearing on their income or standard of living.

The researchers found that sedentary workers had a rate of heart attacks from two to four times higher than did nonsedentary workers. In the words of the researchers: "The results of this study suggest that physical activity or work has a favorable influence on the prevention of ischemic heart disease in middle-age men and women or, perhaps it seems more fitting to indicate that the lack of physical activity has a promoting effect on the appearance of clinical heart disease."

Recent Research

In recent years the lack of high density lipoprotein (HDL) has been targeted as one of the greatest determinants of coronary heart disease. Numerous studies have shown that heart attack patients have significantly lower levels of HDL. There is now compelling evidence that physical activity can increase high density lipoprotein levels and thereby slow or retard the progression of coronary heart disease. It also has been documented that the greatest reduction of total cholesterol, and the greatest increases in HDL levels, occur when exercise is combined with a loss in body weight.

A few years ago the medical profession had proponents both for and against exercise as a value in prevention and control of coronary heart disease. Now the evidence is so voluminous in support of the value of exercise that arguments against have largely diminished. The arguments have now become how much exercise, how long, and what are the long-term effects?

Two recent seven-year longitudinal studies have helped to answer some of these questions. The first study was reported by the Washington University School of Medicine Staff, St. Louis. Appearing in the *Journal of the American College of Cardiology*, August, 1987, the study followed nine men with an average age of 57, all with coronary heart disease.

In the first year the men gradually built to an average jog of 18 miles per week and were working at 81% of predicted heart rate. Their average work capacity of the heart increased 44%. High density lipoprotein ratio changed significantly while total cholesterol showed no significant change.

In the following six years the men increased their oxygen use capacity slightly and increased their predicted heart rate to 85%. However, the most impressive part of the study was the continued increase in "good" HDL cholesterol: from an initial low of 38 at the beginning, to 45 at the end of the first year, to above 50. Through continued exercise, diet and body weight remained constant.

Of course, the problem is that many heart patients have neither the will and/or the physical ability to exercise at this level. The question then becomes, can the same benefits be gained with less effort and more enjoyment.

NORMAL
Lining (Endothelium)
Muscle
Lumen

EARLY INJURY
Platelets
Beginning Plaque

ATHEROSCLEROSIS
Plaque
Fat Deposits (Cholesterol)

VASCULAR PROBLEMS

Atherosclerosis

Atherosclerosis is a condition in which body arteries slowly narrow due to accumulations of fatty materials deposited in the inside arterial walls. As these deposits continue to enlarge, the arterial walls lose their elasticity and narrow. The condition usually begins as a lesion in the lining of the artery. As the fatty deposits gradually gather, the lesion expands in size and develops into plaque spreading across the artery. These deposits are cholesterol, fats, carbohydrates, fibrous tissue, and calcium residues. What is not fully understood is what causes the scar tissue to begin.

Blood clotting is a complicated series of events initiated by blood platelets passing against a rough surface. Therefore, as long as the inner arterial walls remain smooth there will be no clotting. However, if the plaque deposits continue to encroach upon the lumen of the artery, this roughness tends to cause clotting reactions to begin.

133

Once a clot has formed it will continue to move through the vascular system until it reaches an artery that is too small for passage. Consequently, tissues fed by this particular artery are deprived of oxygen and nutrients, causing loss of function to that tissue. When this occurs in an artery of the brain, the person is said to have suffered a stroke. The same occurrence happening to an artery of the heart causes a heart attack, or myocardial infarction.

Although it does not cause atherosclerosis directly, obesity does tend to increase the tendency to develop diabetes, abnormal blood lipids, and hypertension, all of which are associated with the development of atherosclerosis.

Hypertension increases the rate of cholesterol production in the liver and arteries. It also intensifies any atherosclerosis that may have stemmed from diet. It is interesting to note that hypertension can be the cause as well as the result of atherosclerosis.

A diet high in fat has been shown to increase the incidence of plaque formation (atherosclerosis). Refined sugars have also been implicated.

Arteriosclerosis, on the other hand, is the term used to characterize the many possibilities causing the artery wall to lose its elasticity and harden,

Heredity plays an important part. Some families show a high incidence of arteriosclerosis and/or atherosclerosis early in life. Other families seem to be almost immune.

Angina Pectoris

This term means "chest pain" and reflects a condition in which the heart muscle receives an insufficient supply of blood and oxygen. The pain, most often occurring in the chest, arms, jaw and neck, is frequently very heavy and will usually subside with cessation of all activity.

Congenital Heart Defect

This is any type of heart problem that a child has at birth. Problems range from a hole in the heart to defective valves or blood vessels. Most of these problems are now correctable by surgery.

Rheumatic Fever

Rheumatic fever can, and often does, damage the heart. Rheumatic fever is caused by a streptococcal infection, usually among children between the ages of 5-15. The disease may attack any part of the body, but when it scars the valves of the heart, it is called rheumatic fever.

Peripheral Vascular Disease

In general, this is a disease of the blood vessels affecting the legs, feet, arms, or hands. Problems range from varicose veins, to blood clots, or artherosclerotic deposits in the arteries of the extremities. In other cases, such as in Buerger's disease or Raynaud's disease, the tiny arteries of the fingers or toes close off for periods of time, because of vibration or cold.

Stroke

A stroke is what happens when the blood supply is cut off to a part of the brain. Strokes may occur because of atherosclerotic deposits in the arteries of the neck or brain, when a blood clot forms and closes off an artery (thrombus), or when a traveling blood clot (an embolus) lodges in an artery of the neck or brain (embolism). Another type of stroke occurs when a weak spot in a blood vessel of the brain ruptures

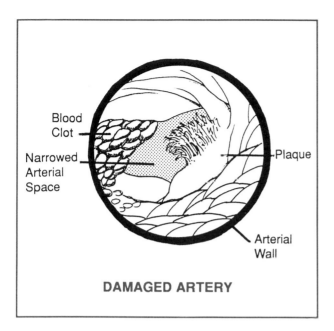

DAMAGED ARTERY

(Labels: Blood Clot, Narrowed Arterial Space, Plaque, Arterial Wall)

causing a cerebral hemorrhage. If the artery merely bulges but does not rupture, it is called a **cerebral aneurysm.**

Since the brain controls body movements, a stroke, depending on where it occurs in the brain, may affect any part of the body. Speech, memory, and any of the body muscles may be impaired. Recovery may range from little to none or it may be nearly total. Each case is different.

Sometimes there are warning signs. If the blood supply does not shut down all at once, but only partially, a person may experience what is called a little or minor stroke. Of course, persistent high blood pressure always facilitates cardiovascular problems, so this is one warning of impending problems. In addition, there are a few stroke signs which sometimes occur. They are:

- Dizziness or falling for no good reason
- Temporary loss of speech, comprehension, or memory
- Sudden numbness or weakness of the leg, arm, and face on one side of the body

- Temporary loss of vision or dimness of vision in one eye

Hypertension

Hypertension is simply another word for high blood pressure. What is alarming is that this problem is appearing much more often in younger people than in the past. Also, it is well documented that elevated systolic pressure of 160+ will increase the risk of heart attack four times, while diastolic pressures in excess of 95+ increase the heart attack risk factor six times.

Boyer and Kasch (3) report that high blood pressure is the most frequent disorder found in the practice of medicine. Stamler (17), in an extensive study of insurance company employees, found 20% of men in their forties and 25% of men in their sixties suffer from this condition.

Hypertension or high blood pressure is usually divided into three classifications as judged by the diastolic reading. They are:

Mild: 90-104
Moderate: 105-199
Severe: over 120

It must be emphasized that decisions for treatment are not made on the basis of a single reading. Physicians generally rely on three or four readings taken over a span of time before making a decision.

Fortunately, except for the most extreme cases, blood pressure can be controlled by reducing salt intake, exercising, and by controlling diet and weight. Extreme cases can and should be controlled with drug therapy. Although blood pressure tends to increase with age, most authorities agree that the standards discussed in Chapter 2 should be maintained for a healthy lifestyle.

Additional signs of high blood pressure. One of the reasons this disease is called the silent disease is that often there are no outward symptoms. In other cases, dizziness, headaches, and tiredness seem to be the most common signs. Of course, these are also symptoms of other diseases, so only a trained person can really diagnose.

Triglycerides

One screening test for cardiovascular disease is blood triglyceride level. Triglycerides constitute the storage package for fatty acids in the body. These fatty acids are packaged in threes with glycerol, thus the name triglycerides. Desirable levels of blood triglycerides will depend on a person's age and sex, but usually should be less than 100-120 mg. Elevated levels of triglycerides usually lead to other cardiovascular risk problems such as high blood cholesterol, hypertension, low levels of high density lipoprotein (HDL), diabetes and obesity.

Although heredity is important in determining a person's triglyceride level, there are a number of things that can be done to control the numbers. These include:

- Loss of body weight, particularly body fat.
- A reduction in dietary fat intake.
- Increase the complex carbohydrates and fiber in the diet, while reducing the amount of simple carbohydrates (sugars).
- Participate in an aerobic exercise program on a regular basis.

Cholesterol

Cholesterol is one of several lipids found in the blood. In order for the body to transport and use these lipids, they must first be combined with another molecule to make them soluble in the blood serum, the fluid portion of blood. This molecule is a protein, which combines with the fats to form lipoproteins, making possible the transportation and utilization of fats. Lipoprotein molecules appear in various sizes and weights, and the amounts of cholesterol and other lipids they contain vary according to the size and weight.

High Density Lipoprotein (HDL) — heaviest of these molecules; contains the highest proportion of protein.

Low Density Lipoprotein (LDL) — lighter than HDL; contains the largest proportion of cholesterol of any of the lipoproteins.

Very Low Density Lipoprotein (VLDL) — lighter still and is the fat-protein molecule in the blood stream which carries the largest amount of triglycerides.

Reducing Blood Cholesterol

Three proven methods of reducing blood cholesterol are:

1. **Dietary** — Decrease the daily caloric intake to no more than 24-27% fat, with approximately 10% allocated to saturated fats. Also increase the daily intake of fiber, pectin, and substitute vegetable protein for animal protein. The daily intake of cholesterol should be limited to 300 mg.
2. **Weight Control** — Reduce body fat.
3. **Regular Exercise Program** — Research indicates that even moderate aerobic exercise done regularly increases the body's HDL ratio.

Genetic factors are very important in determining an individual's amount and type of blood cholesterol.

Newborn children have high HDL cholesterol levels. The problem seems to be that as we grow older that ratio of good cholesterol tends to diminish. Authorities presently agree that the normal level for total cholesterol in the blood should be under

200 milligrams for 100 cubic centimeters and that roughly 60 percent of this total should be high density lipoprotein or "good" cholesterol (6).

Until recently, critics of exercise have contended that heart disease is a multifactorial disease and that there are many reasons for the significant decrease in deaths from heart disease since 1968. Yet nearly all now agree that a high percentage of HDL is probably the most important factor in determining whether coronary disease will occur.

Mounting evidence shows that exercise increases the amount of "good" or high density lipoprotein in the blood, regardless of diet. One of the more recent studies, conducted at Baylor Medical School, concludes that running more than eleven miles per week was associated with a significant increase in HDL blood cholesterol regardless of diet (12).

Another study found elevated high density lipoprotein levels among marathon runners. These researchers concluded that distance runners should have a lower risk of developing coronary heart disease than non-runners (1).

One of the most recent studies indicates that reducing total blood cholesterol through diet and medication substantially lowers the risk of heart attacks. The ten-year, $150 million study by the National Heart, Lung, and Blood Institute was conducted at twelve centers in the United States, and involved 3806 middle-aged men with no signs of heart disease. They were, however, considered high risk because cholesterol levels averaged 190 among them.

The study involved placing all the men on a moderate diet which reduced average cholesterol levels by 3.5%. Half of the men were given daily doses of cholestyramine, a cholesterol lowering drug. The other half were given a harmless, look-alike placebo.

Neither doctors nor patients knew who was getting the real medication.

The results were startling. Those who received the drug had an average drop in total cholesterol of 13.4% and also achieved a 20.3% reduction in low density lipoproteins (LDL) cholesterol. Finally, there were only 155 coronaries among those who took the drug compared with 185 among those men on the placebo. Additionally, men taking the drug developed fewer incipient heart disease symptoms. One conclusion of the study was that for each 1% drop in blood cholesterol level, a person might expect a 2% reduction in heart attack risk.

Both Dr. Michael Brown, Nobel Laureate, and Dr. Scott Grundy, Professor of Internal Medicine at the University of Texas, believe that as many as one-half to two-thirds of Americans have cholesterol levels that places them at risk for future cardiovascular problems.

What is known is that the liver produces receptor cells which act as a trap for low density lipoprotein or bad cholesterol. Once the LDL is trapped within the receptor cell it is broken down for use by the body.

Therefore a diet high in cholesterol overloads the liver with bad cholesterol thus limiting the amount of receptors or trap door cells it can produce. As the bad cholesterol increases in the blood stream it has to stay there longer, and the longer it stays, the more cholesterol it picks up, thus causing a vicious cycle leading to higher and higher levels of cholesterol.

Obesity causes an overproduction of very low-density lipoprotein, VLDL the worst kind. This then coupled with a diet loaded with high cholesterol leads to a very high level of LDL within a persons' blood—a problem not uncommon to many Americans.

The three most obvious means of control are diet control to reduce the quantity of cholesterol; exercise to control obesity; and

137

the use of certain drugs to increase the number of receptor cells produced by the liver.

Cholesterol and Aging

It has generally been accepted that total cholesterol increases with age. The question that has not been answered is why. A study of 2,000 men by Cooper at the Aerobic Center in Dallas, Texas has produced some startling information as reported in his publication Inside *Aerobics,* May, 1980.

"By studying this chart, you will notice that with increasing age, there is an increase in the total cholesterol comparable to what has been documented previously. Yet, the surprising finding is the fact that with age the HDL or good cholesterol remains nearly constant, whereas the LDL or bad cholesterol progressively increases. The total cholesterol-HDL ratio increased from 4.1 to 4.8. Is this simply a factor of aging or is there some other factor that correlated with this deteriorating lipid profile? We looked at several other risk factors and found that the best correlation was with percent body fat." (7)

Age (Years)	30	30-39	40-49	50-59	60+
Total Cholesterol	179	191	205	208	208
HDL Cholesterol	43	42	43	43	44
LDL Cholesterol	136	149	162	165	164
% Body Fat	18.1	22.0	23.5	23.8	23.0

Whereas younger men were relatively lean, that is, 18 percent body fat, men past forty had a high percent of body fat, and the correlation between percent body fat and the total and LDL cholesterol was much better than the correlation between cholesterol and age. In other words, as we grow older our percent body fat increases even though the body weight may remain the same. (Now you know why at age 40 your weight may be the same as it was at age 21, yet your waist measurement may be considerably larger.) But that doesn't have to occur. By maintaining a high level of physical fitness, you decrease the percent body fat and increase the muscle mass.

This increase in percentage of body fat appears to be another example of how we have accepted unequivocally the phenomenon of aging that in reality may not be physiological but simply adaptive; that is, as we grow older, our bodies start deteriorating rapidly, not so much because we are growing older but because we are less active as we grow older. Remember the statement of noted cardiologist Paul Dudley White, "It is fascinating to know that one can grow healthier as one grows older and not necessarily the reverse." Certainly, research is documenting this to be a true statement.

As you grow older, to keep the optimum total cholesterol, HDL, LDL, and total cholesterol-HDL ratio, watch your diet, your weight, and by all means keep exercising regularly! See Chapter 6 for a more complete discussion on weight control.

Awareness and Control of Elevated Blood Cholesterol

According to the December 1990 issue of the *Journal of the American Medical Association,* "great progress" has been made.

They cite these advances:

From 1983 to 1989, visits to doctors for high blood cholesterol treatment increased ninefold. This means that the general public is becoming knowledgeable and concerned.

At least six controlled studies have indicated that people who reduce their total blood cholesterol or the LDL (the bad type) by diet or drugs, can slow or possibly reverse the formation of deposits within their own arteries. This information has come about by improved techniques to take pictures of the arteries within the heart.

It is now known that LDL cholesterol sometimes combines with oxygen in the bloodstream, and may increase its ability to produce the arterial plaque which clogs arteries. This has raised the possibility that antioxidant nutrients as vitamins C and E, along with beta carotene, may assist in reducing the risk of heart disease. The ongoing Physicians' Health Study has produced some data, from a group of 333 men, which suggests that beta carotene found in orange, yellow, and green leafy fruits and vegetables (sweet potatoes, broccoli, carrots, and others) may influence the chance of heart attack and other coronary problems in men who already have heart disease.

Exercise and Prevention of Coronary Heart Disease

Although some researchers have claimed success in reversing the formation of fibrous plaque deposits, the issue still remains in doubt.

The medical profession believes that coronary heart disease can be arrested or prevented in most people by early identification of those most susceptible and by controlling the risk factors of obesity, high blood pressure, excessive anxiety, excessive salt intake, abnormal blood lipids and lack of exercise.

Smoking and the Heart

Research indicates distinct differences in the maximum exercise capacity of smokers and nonsmokers. Heart rate studies using both submaximal and maximal exercise tests have consistently shown that smokers develop faster heart rates at the same lower levels of exercise than nonsmokers. In other words, it costs more in terms of heart rate for a smoker to do the same amount of exertion as a nonsmoker.

QUESTIONS AND ANSWERS

How serious is coronary heart disease in the United States?

According to the National Center for Health Statistics, cardiovascular diseases yearly claim the lives of nearly one million Americans. (This is twice as many as die from cancer.) One in four Americans suffers from some form of cardiovascular disease. Heart attack is the leading cause of death, with nearly 550,000 deaths annually. Stroke is the second most serious cardiovascular disease, with about 500,000 Americans suffering strokes each year. And, finally, each year about 350,000 people die of heart attacks before reaching the hospital.

How early does heart disease begin?

Several studies have indicated plaque beginnings in the arteries of five-year-olds. Autopsies of children who have died in accidents have shown enough fatty deposits on coronary arteries of 15-year-olds to obstruct blood flow. Other studies have found as many as 40% of youngsters between the ages of 5-8 have at least one of the following risk factors for coronary heart disease: inactivity, elevated blood pressure, obesity, high cholesterol levels, and high blood pressure.

Can drinking four or more cups of coffee a day increase my chances for a heart attack?

The jury is still out on this one, with both yes and no research. Dr. Arthur Klatsky recently completed a study of over 100,000 patients undergoing general medical care at Kaiser Permanente hospitals in Northern California from 1978 through 1985. His findings indicated a greater chance for a heart attack. Several additional studies have denoted a difference between "boiled coffee" and the more common American filtered coffee made by dripping hot water on coffee and filtering through paper. The filtered type being the safest.

I have read that men who consume three or more drinks of alcohol per day are more likely to have high blood pressure. Does this also hold true for females?

Harvard researchers reported at the November 1987 meeting of the American Heart Association that middle-aged women who drink two cocktails or three glasses of beer or wine a day are 40% more likely to have high blood pressure than women who don't drink. This is the first large study (over 58,000 nurses) of the effects of alcohol on blood pressure in women. Interestingly, the study also indicated that two glasses of beer or wine a day, or less than one and one-half cocktails, had no effect on women's blood pressure.

I know that high blood pressure is a real problem with older people, but as a teen-

ager I don't have to worry, do I?

There are about 57.5 million Americans with high blood pressure and of this number more than 2 million young people between ages 6 and 17 also have the problem.

However, there are some things which anyone can do which often help. They are:
- Reduce salt intake—most of us consume 12-20 grams daily but we need only 2 grams per day.
- Lose weight—a 10 pound loss frequently helps.
- Eat more fiber.
- Increase calcium and decrease caffeine—two cups of coffee will decrease calcium absorption by 100 milligrams.
- Exercise regularly.

Are changes inevitable as a person ages?

They may not all be. The issue is still in doubt. One study used 62 healthy adults between the ages of 25 and 79, all of whom had no symptoms of heart disease, had normal blood pressure, and were maintaining moderate levels of exercise.

When the participants were studied by age, systolic blood pressure did rise, but there were no changes in cardiac output or heart rate at rest. While maximum heart rate did progressively decline with age, *cardiac output did not,* even in elderly subjects.

This study clearly suggests that, barring disease, age by itself does not reduce cardiac output either at rest or during exercise.

Does this mean that if I exercise I won't have coronary heart disease?

No. One highly-publicized case involved the death of a 54-year-old physician who had run two to four miles a day, three to six days a week for over twenty years. After he experienced chest pain, studies indicated a 90% obstruction of one of his coronary

140

arteries. His blood pressure was 130/78, his cholesterol count low, he was a non-smoker, and weighed 152 pounds at 5'8". He did have an extensive history of chest pain among family members in their forties and fifties.

Another recent case involved a world class runner and noted author on running. He too had an extensive family history and at least one prior attack before dying.

Even persistent exercise is no absolute guarantee; however, the majority of research indicates that sensible exercise programs do help protect against coronary heart disease.

Another piece of information substantiating the hypothesis that people who exercise regularly may develop extra collateral circulation in the heart muscle concerns the late astronaut Ed White, who died in a fire at Cape Canaveral in the late 1960s. Doctors performing the autopsy found that atherosclerosis had completely closed one of the major arteries leading to his heart. However, because of the intensive physical training that he had been subjected to he had apparently developed additional arterial circulation leading to the heart muscle and did not die when the main artery closed. They did know that he had been able to engage in high levels of fitness training without accompanying signs of heart trouble.

I have read that men in their fifties who exercise regularly have heart and lung functions about equal to that of sedentary men in their thirties. Would the same hold true for women?

Dr. Barbara Drinkwater of Seattle's Pacific Medical Center believes so. In a recent meeting of the American Medical Women's Association she stated: "While exercise won't cure disease, it does lower the risk for hypertension, diabetes, and obesity, all of which boost the odds of heart attack, the number one killer of U.S. women."

Her study involved 90 women ages 20-70 who exercised vigorously for at least 30 minutes three times weekly. Other findings included:

During the six-year study, the active women's percentage of body fat remained stable. The sedentary women, however, raised from an average of 28% to 35% body fat.

The "active women" showed no significant cardiovascular "effects of aging" until age fifty.

Someone told me that eating grapefruit could lower my blood cholesterol count. Is there anything to it?

Researchers at the University of Florida think so. Recent human tests at the University of Florida Health Science Center found that patients who ate about three tablespoons of pectin (the sticky substance found in the rind and fleshy part of the grapefruit) lowered cholesterol levels an average of 7.6 percent after eight weeks.

In addition to lowering overall cholesterol, James Carda, M.D. found that pectin also lowered the amount of low density lipoproteins (LDL), which is the major carrier of cholesterol in the blood.

Can regular exercise affect my cholesterol level?

There is no ironclad proof at this time which says that exercise increases the HDL or good cholesterol in our blood. However, present research has indicated that the ratio of total cholesterol to HDL cholesterol was consistently better in more fit men. One study found that running at least 11 miles per week was associated with a 35% increase in HDL. Another study found people who ran 50-60 miles per week to have higher levels of HDL than runners covering 12-15 miles per week. Active people having low levels of body fat tend to show the best total cholesterol/HDL ratio.

Since I do not wish to run marathons, what is the minimum amount of running necessary to effect a change in HDL vs LDL?

Hartung, of Baylor College of Medicine, published a study in the *New England Journal of Medicine* which concluded that if a person ran a minimum of 11 miles per week there would be an increase in the good or high density lipoprotein regardless of any dietary changes.

Another study, involved 32 sedentary middle-aged men with coronary heart disease. The subjects participated for thirteen weeks by exercising daily on an indoor track to elevate their pulse rate to 70-85% of maximal heart rate for 20-30 minutes. The men averaged 1-3/4 miles per session and their HDL levels increased an average of 10%.

Another program evaluated 83 men who had suffered heart attacks. Their HDL cholesterol levels increased 11.7% during a 27 week period. (9)

A Finnish study arrived at approximately the same results by evaluating 100 asymptomatic middle-aged men. The group experienced an 11% increase in HDL by participating in 3-4 weekly sessions for 16 weeks.

While most people believe that aerobic conditioning is essential to the acquisition of the protective benefits of physical exercise, Goldberg et al. (11) found that weight training over a 16-week period also reduced the total cholesterol/HDL ratio.

Can the total cholesterol be too low?

Cooper (7) and others believe it can. Research has indicated that some bodily functions may be impaired since the production of some hormones and vitamins such as D are dependent upon certain amounts of cholesterol.

What is a good "moderate" level of cholesterol?

Obviously no two people are identical. However, Cooper believes that total cholesterol should be between 160 and 200 mg./dl., and the cholesterol/HDL ratio less than 4.5 with an even smaller amount for women. (6)

If the cardiovascular system is so important, how can I improve mine?

Oxygen is a body fuel most people take for granted. As we now know, the more oxygen the muscles receive, the more energy produced. The oxygen is carried to individual cells by hemoglobin in the blood. Thus, the amount of blood pumped throughout the body correlates with your capacity to do work.

One way to increase your oxygen supply is to exercise the muscle that serves as the pump. Since the heart is a muscle it responds to training as do all other muscles of the body. To develop the heart muscle, you must push it beyond its normal range and make it pump more blood with each beat (stroke volume).

As you begin to exercise, the heart beats faster and with greater force causing blood output to be greater with each beat. This increased heart rate is caused by an increased oxygen demand by the muscle cells. The heart rate reaches a plateau within a few minutes. It will continue at this level until you increase the pace. To maintain a balance between oxygen demand and oxygen supply is therefore the ultimate goal of the cardiovascular system. Fortunately, it is not necessary to exercise at your maximum level to overload the heart. This means that exercise or work performed at a comfortable pace is a sufficient workload.

REFERENCES

1. Adner et al., *Journal of American Medical Association,* Feb. 8, 1980.
2. Benditt, E., "The Origin of Atherosclerosis," *Scientific American* 236 (2) 74-85, 1977.
3. Boyer, J. L., and Kasch, F. W., "Exercise Therapy in Hypertensive Men," *Journal of American Medical Association* 211, No. 10 (March 9, 1970) p. 1668.
4. Bruner, D. and Manelis, G. "Physical Activity at Work and Ischemic Heart Disease." *Coronary Heart Disease and Physical Fitness,* edited by O. A. Larsen and R. O. Malmborg. Baltimore: University Park Press, 1971.
5. Cantwell, J. D., Quinton Exercise Stress Testing Seminar, Atlanta, GA, 1978.
6. Cooper, Kenneth, *Inside Aerobics,* Vol. 1, No. 1, April 1980.
7. Cooper, Kenneth, *Inside Aerobics,* Vol. 1, No. 2, May 1980.
8. Enger, S. C., Hjermann, I., Foss, O. P. et al. "High-density lipoprotein cholesterol and myocardial infarction or sudden coronary death: a prospective case-control study in middle-aged men of the Oslo Study." *Artery* 1979: 5 (February):170-181
9. Erkelens, D. W., Albers, J. J., Hazzard, W. R. et al.: High-density lipoprotein-cholesterol in survivors of myocardial infarction, *Journal of American Medical Association,* 1979: 242(Nov. 16):2185-2189.
10. Frank, C. W. "The Course of Coronary Heart Disease: Factors Relating to Prognosis." *Bulletin of the New York Academy of Medicine* 44:900, 1968.
11. Goldberg L., Elliott D. L., Schultz, R. W. et al.: "Changes in lipid and lipoprotein levels after weight training." *Journal of American Medical Association* 1984:252 (July 27), 504-506.
12. Hartung, G. H., *The New England Journal of Medicine* (302) (7), Feb. 14, 1980.
13. Kannel, W. B., Sorlie, P., and McNamara, P. *The Relation of Physical Activity to Risk of Coronary Heart Disease: The Framingham Study on Coronary Heart Disease and Physical Fitness.* O. A. Larsen and R. O. Malmborg, Baltimore, MD.: University Park Press, 1971, p. 256.
14. Morris, J. N. and Crawford, M. D. "Coronary Heart Disease and Physical Activity of Work," *British Medical Journal* 12:1485, 1958.
15. Morris, J. N. and Crawford, M. D. "Coronary Heart Disease in Transport Workers." *British Journal of Industrial Medicine* 11:260, 1954.
16. Paffenbarger, R. S. et al. "Work Activity of Longshoremen as Related to Death from Coronary Heart Disease and Stroke." *New England Journal of Medicine* 20:1109, 1970.
17. Stamler, J., "Epidemiologic Studies on Cardiovascular Renal Disease," *Journal of Chronic Diseases* 12 (1960), p. 480.
18. Taylor, H. L. "Coronary Heart Disease in Physically Active and Sedentary Populations," *Journal of Sports Medicine and Physical Fitness,* 1962.
19. Williams, P. T., Wood, P. D., Haskell, W. L. et al.: "The effects of running mileage and duration on plasma lipoprotein levels," *Journal of American Medical Association* 1982; 247 (May 21); 2674-2679.
20. Zukel, W. J. and Associates. "A Short-term Community Study of the Epidemiology of Coronary Heart Disease: A Preliminary Report of the North Dakota Study," *American Journal of Public Health* 49:1630, 1959.

SUGGESTED LABS: 3, 4, 20, 26.

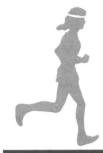

Your Respiratory System

Objectives
- Describe the process of respiration
- Discuss how exercise can improve respiration
- List the effects of smoking on the breathing process

Key Words
- Aerobic metabolism
- Alveoli
- Anaerobic metabolism
- Cilia
- Diaphragm
- Lung capacity
- Maximum oxygen uptake
- Oxygen debt
- Passive smoke
- Residual volume
- Steady state
- Trachea
- Vital capacity

Even when our bodies are at rest, the tissues need a constant supply of oxygen. Physical activity increases our oxygen needs, and the more strenuous the activity, the greater the demand. Since the body cells are not in direct contact with the external environment, the respiratory and cardiovascular systems play vital roles in the functioning of the body and especially in its ability to produce a high energy output.

DESCRIPTION OF THE SYSTEM

The respiratory process involves three separate but interrelated functions:
1. **External respiration**—the exchange of gases between the environment and the lungs.
2. **Cardiovascular transport**—the transport of gases between the lungs and various tissues.
3. **Internal respiration**—the actual exchange of gases between the blood and tissue fluids.

The effective functioning of all three processes is an important limiting factor to the nature and amount of activity that the body can perform.

Breathing is, of course, the process of external respiration by which oxygen in the air is brought into the lungs and into close contact with the blood which absorbs it and carries it to all parts of the body. The oxygen intake is dependent upon the maintenance of a free airway and the proper diffusion of gas to the cells throughout the body. This phase is critical because pulmonary obstruction or any other abnormality which impairs the proper passage of air to the lungs will disturb the gas diffusion, and consequently can leave arterial blood with insufficient quantities of oxygen and at the same time fail to rid the circulation of carbon dioxide.

The breathing action itself is not produced by the lungs. The lungs are entirely passive and dependent upon the contraction and relaxation of the muscles which surround them. The **diaphragm** is the strong wall of muscle that separates the chest cavity from the abdominal cavity. When the diaphragm muscle contracts (moves downward), it creates suction in the chest to draw in air and expand the lungs. When the muscle relaxes, the chest cavity decreases and the air is pushed out.

Air enters the lungs by traveling down the **trachea** (windpipe), which branches into two tubes called **bronchi**, one leading to each lung. The bronchi then branch into smaller and smaller **bronchioles**. The smallest bronchioles eventually terminate in a cluster of tiny air sacs which are called **alveoli**. The capillaries are the blood vessels that are imbedded in the walls of the alveoli where the gas and waste exchange takes place. The blood contains a chemical, called hemoglobin, which attracts oxygen when the blood flows through regions where oxygen is plentiful and attracts carbon dioxide, which is produced when the body cells burn their fuel and it is plentiful. In normal situations, the blood is about 98% saturated with oxygen when it leaves the lungs. When at rest, about 30% of this oxygen is removed at the cellular level, but during heavy exercise, this value can be increased almost three times. Oxygen uptake is the amount of oxygen extracted from the circulating blood in one minute and, when measured during maximal exercise, it is termed maximum oxygen uptake. Because maximal oxygen uptake represents the ability of the body to mobilize all its systems during physical stress, it is considered the best single indication of one's level of physical fitness.

145

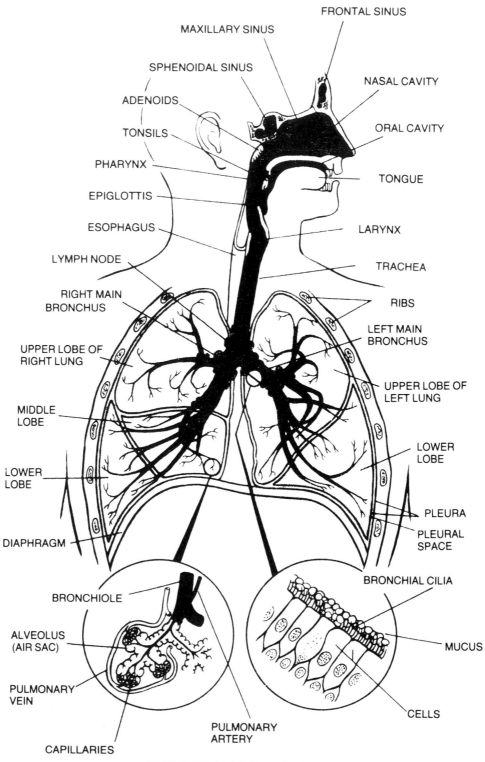

THE RESPIRATORY SYSTEM
(Courtesy American Lung Association)

The lungs are soft, spongy, and highly elastic. The right lung is divided into three lobes or sections and the left lung is divided into two lobes. The bronchial tubes leading to the lungs are lined with very small hairs, called **cilia**, that have a wave-like motion. By this motion the cilia carry mucus upward and out into the throat, where it is either coughed up and spat out or swallowed harmlessly. The mucus catches and holds much of the dust, germs, and other unwanted matter that has invaded the lungs and thus aids in eliminating it.

The respiratory system is exceptionally responsive to the oxygen needs of the body. The lungs have the ability to respond and are capable of providing more than enough oxygen. Therefore, the failure to meet increasing demands during physical activity is usually related to a problem existing elsewhere in the oxygen transport system. Improvement in the level of cardiorespiratory fitness usually depends on increasing the strength and efficiency of the heart and the oxygen-dispersing circulatory system.

Oxygen Consumption

The following terms relating to the respiratory system will enable you to gain a more complete understanding of its functioning.

Lung Capacity. Total lung capacity is the entire volume of air that can be contained in all the air passages. A normal adult lung holds approximately 6,200 to 7,400 milliliters of air.

Vital Capacity. The largest volume of air that can be exhaled after the deepest possible inhalation is vital capacity and is about 4,500 to 6,000 ml for men and between 3,000 and 4,500 ml for women.

Residual Volume. The air remaining in the lungs after a complete exhalation is residual volume. Generally, about 1,200 ml of air cannot be exhaled.

Tidal Volume. The amount of air breathed in and out in ventilation is termed tidal volume. During normal breathing while a subject is at rest, this amounts to approximately 500 ml. This amount will increase considerably during exercise.

Maximum Oxygen Uptake. The maximum oxygen consumption that one can attain and the amount of oxygen utilized during exercise.

Oxygen Uptake. The amount of oxygen extracted from circulating blood in one minute.

Oxygen Debt. The volume of oxygen consumed during the recovery period following exercise that is in excess of the volume that is normally consumed while at rest. Oxygen debt can be associated with even low levels of exercise. This occurs because oxygen consumption requires several minutes to reach the required or steady-state level even though the requirement to perform the exercise is constant from the very start of the exercise.

Oxygen Deficit. The initial period of exercise when the oxygen consumption is below the steady-state or required level is called oxygen deficit. The deficit is calculated as the difference between the amount of oxygen required and that which is actually consumed.

Aerobic Metabolism. When adequate oxygen is supplied to the cells during an activity.

Anaerobic Metabolism. The process called into effect when one engages in work that demands more than 50% of the aerobic capacity. This allows continued performance but only for a short time due to the rapid buildup of lactic acid.

Steady State. When a balance between supply and demand of oxygen is reached.

147

The oxygen transport system is able to supply adequate amounts of oxygen to the working tissue and heart rate, ventilation, and oxygen consumption can be maintained at a constant level for indefinite periods of time.

EFFECTS OF EXERCISE

Exercise and training programs can improve the efficiency of breathing. The well-trained individual can lower the rate of breathing and increase the depth. In addition, at a given level of submaximal exercise, a trained individual is able to achieve an oxygen uptake with less overall respiration. Thus, the trained person is able to extract a greater proportion of oxygen from the air breathed than the untrained person. In short, training enables the air to reach a wider alveolar area at rest and during exercise.

An immediate effect of exercise on the respiratory system is an increase in the rate and depth of breathing in response to the body's need for more oxygen and the removal of increased levels of carbon dioxide. In addition, there is an increased flow of blood to the tissues of the respiratory muscles and throughout the lungs themselves. As the depth of breathing increases, the number of alveoli utilized also increases.

Improved pulmonary ventilation can be accomplished by an increase in both the tidal volume and in the respiratory frequency. The tidal volume can increase from a resting average of 0.5 liters per minute to 2.5-3.0 liters per minute during maximal exercise. One can increase the respiratory frequency from 12-16 breaths per minute at rest to 40-50 breaths per minute during maximal exercise.

An individual at rest has an oxygen consumption of approximately 0.25 liters per minute or about 3.5 ml/kg/min. The VO_2 value (oxygen consumption) is influenced greatly by size, age, and level of fitness. It is frequently expressed relative to body weight to account for individual difference in size: ml. of oxygen per kg. of body weight multiplied by minutes.

Average individuals who are untrained generally have a maximal oxygen consumption ranging from 20-38 milliliters of oxygen per kilogram of body weight per minute. It is possible to train individuals to reach optimal levels of fitness of 38 to 85 ml/kg/min.

One's scores for maximum oxygen consumption can be placed on a continuum from the lowest known value of about 15 ML/KG/MIN to the highest known value of 94 ML/KG/MIN. Table 1 is an illustration of the continuum for maximum oxygen consumption.

Unfortunately, changes do occur as we age. One change is a reduction in our

TABLE 1
OXYGEN CAPACITY CONTINUUM

Low	Average	High
15 ML/KG/min	40-50 ML/KG/min Young adult males	94 ML/KG/min
Resulting from: lung disease sedentary habits old age circulatory disease poor nutrition	35-40 ML/KG/min Young adult females	Resulting from: good genetic stock participation in endurance activities excellent nutrition

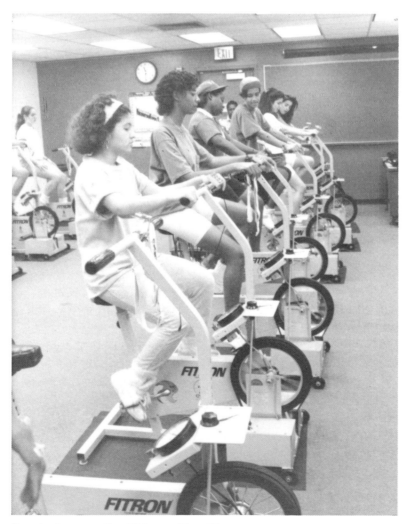

Exercise improves the efficiency of breathing.

maximum attainable heart rate, with a progressive reduction in the target zone (See Chapter 3 for suggested maximal heart rates and target zone for ages 25-70).

Studies have shown that individuals can improve their performances after reaching their VO$_2$ maximum ceiling by developing the ability to work at a higher percentage of capacity for prolonged periods of time. This is termed the **anaerobic threshold**—the point in an exercise of increasing intensity at which the body starts increasing anaerobic metabolism above resting levels. For instance, anaerobic threshold is expressed in terms of the percentage of VO$_2$ maximum which would indicate a greater performance potential for the same VO$_2$ maximum than one of 45% of VO$_2$ maximum. A higher anaerobic threshold percentage indicates that the individual can work at relatively higher levels of metabolism before having to rely on the inefficient, limiting process of anaerobic metabolism.

Adult women generally have a maximum aerobic capacity approximately 75% of that of men. The main difference in VO$_2$ maximum of men and women is related to hemoglobin and number of red blood cells. Men have approximately 15% more hemoglobin and 6% more red blood cells, indicating a greater oxygen carrying capacity. Men also have a larger number of capillaries which facilitate supplying oxygen to the cells and a larger heart and lung surface.

Research indicates that males and females respond to aerobic training with similar increases in VO$_2$ maximum, so sex is not an important factor in predicting improvements as long as other factors, especially the type of training, are equal. However, in most cases regular training can only increase the VO$_2$ maximum 10-20%. Some training adaptations may occur in approximately 4-6 weeks, but other changes may take considerably longer.

To achieve a high level of fitness, you must have healthy lungs and an efficient respiratory system. Without an adequate supply of oxygen, you will not be able to do extremely active exercises for long periods of time. As a matter of fact, the efficient functioning of the heart and lungs is required for optimal enjoyment of practically all activities.

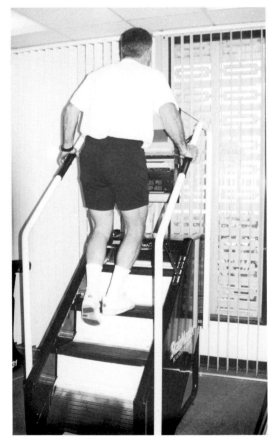

Stair climbing machines are a popular, efficient way to exercise aerobically.

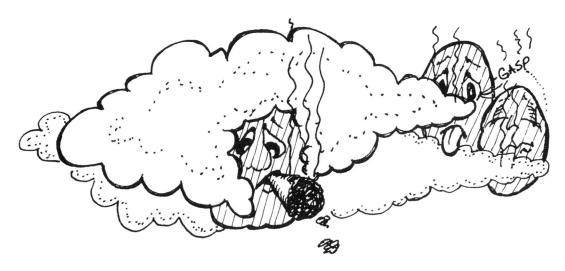

EFFECTS OF SMOKING

Overwhelming evidence indicates that smoking is one of the most dangerous habits engaged in by humans. For instance, smoking just one pack a day causes a much higher incidence of heart disease. The risk is slightly more than three times that for a nonsmoker.

Cigarette smoking has a profound effect upon the respiratory system. People who smoke commonly experience shortness of breath, nagging smoker's cough, and an elevated heart rate. Smokers also have higher risk of health problems such as chronic bronchitis, emphysema, obstructive pulmonary disease, heart disease, and cancer of the lung, oral cavity, larynx, and pharynx.

The most immediate effect that smoking has on the respiratory system is a reduction of the capacity for diffusing oxygen due to the tars deposited in the lungs. In addition, carbon monoxide in smoke reduces the oxygen capacity of the blood by displacing some of the oxygen that ordinarily would be combined with hemoglobin in red blood cells. The nicotine in tobacco causes the adrenal glands to release epinephrine which causes constriction of blood vessels that elevates the heart rate.

When the need for oxygen increases during exertion or exercise, the smoker is faced with greater breathing resistance and an obstruction of the air passageways when the glands in the bronchial tubes increase secretions. A lung disease which is caused by the destruction of the alveoli sacs is emphysema. This irreversible and incurable disease limits an individual's ability to acquire oxygen. Many pathologists state that small emphysematous changes occur in the lungs with even light smoking and progresses as long as the individual smokes. Smoking also contributes directly to more than 80% of all deaths from lung cancer.

Mention should also be made of the effects of smoking marijuana. Since marijuana contains greater amounts of tar and possibly other harmful substances than tobacco, and since marijuana smokers tend to inhale deeper and hold the smoke in the lungs longer, the risk associated with its use is even greater than that of tobacco smoking. Another significant problem is that it takes as long as thirty days for the major ingredient of marijuana to be eliminated completely from the body. Thus a frequent user may never be completely free of the toxic substances in the marijuana. According to the American Medical Association, marijuana can harm the user, has the potential for serious physical damage, and directly impairs the brain's functioning.

In the final analysis, if you are serious about improving your health and fitness, you must realize that smoking of any kind makes it impossible to reach your optimal fitness level. To undertake a vigorous exercise program while continuing to smoke is counterproductive to your efforts. The evidence is clear that young people who begin smoking will suffer more illness and earlier deaths than those who do not smoke. Cigarette smoking is clearly the most significant preventable cause of premature death and disability in the United States today.

Smoking Cessation

When people first begin to smoke, they usually believe they can quit anytime they choose. However, deciding to stop smoking becomes more difficult as the habit becomes more ingrained. The dependence on smoking becomes very similar to addiction to alcohol and drugs, with both psychological and physiological factors involved. Most smokers attempt to quit several times before succeeding; after quitting, relapses are not uncommon. Studies indicate that older adults are more psychologically dependent on cigarettes than younger smokers. Thus, the younger you are when you undertake a cessation program, the more likely you are to succeed in breaking the habit.

The smoker who decides to quit may either go "cold turkey"—i.e., stop all at once—or taper off gradually. The cold turkey method has proved to be the most successful. In addition, most ex-smokers managed to quit on their own without special products or special treatment programs. However, for those who need help in quitting, numerous resources are now available. Such agencies as the American Cancer Society, the American Heart Association, and the American Lung Association offer cessation kits and smoking cessation programs at little or no cost. Most such programs are designed to help the smoker understand why he or she smokes, how smoking affects the body, and provide motivation and support for quitting.

Many smokers believe that quitting will result in weight gain; however, this can be avoided by stocking up on low-calorie, healthy snacks (see Chapter 6) to satisfy what psychologists call an "oral need." In addition, exercise should be a vital part of any cessation program.

When you quit smoking, your body begins immediately to repair damage to your lungs and to restore the normal healthy condition of lung tissue. In addition to the physical benefits, you will gain self-confidence from your ability to exercise self-control and will join the growing majority of people who have chosen not to smoke.

QUESTIONS AND ANSWERS

Would raising the cost of cigarettes and banning all tobacco advertising lower the rate of consumption in the U.S.?

An interesting question. We may be different than our Northern friends, the Canadians; however, Canada banned all tobacco advertising in January 1989, and since then tobacco sales have significantly decreased. In 1989 sales dropped about 7%, and then dropped another 10% in the first four months of 1990. Of course, a pack of cigarettes in Canada is much more costly than in the United States.

Are we making any progress in reducing the number of people who smoke in the United States?

According to the Surgeon General's 1989 Report on Smoking we are making great progress. For instance: In 1965 approximately 40% of American adults smoked while in 1987 the number had decreased to about 29%. It is estimated that if the trend continues, about 22% will be smokers by the year 2000. Male smokers have shown the greatest decline, down from 50% to approximately 32%. The decline in smokers has been much slower among minorities, young women, blue collar workers, and the uneducated.

What about smoking and exercise?

As noted earlier, smoking only one pack a day increases the risk of a heart attack three times over that of a nonsmoker.

Smoking also seriously diminishes your maximum exercise capacity. McHenry at the Indiana University School of Medicine reports that when a group of state policemen were divided into three groups and exercised to maximum capacity, the non-smokers were able to exercise the longest. In this experiment, subjects were classified into three groups: smokers, former smokers who had quit at least one year, and nonsmokers. Other findings were as follows:

1. Nonsmokers had lower systolic blood pressure levels than smokers.
2. Smokers developed faster heart rates at the same level of exercise than do nonsmokers.
3. Former smokers had approximately the same blood pressure levels as non-

smokers, although those with previous history of very heavy smoking were not able to exercise as long as the non-smokers.

Is it true that premature facial wrinkling is linked to smoking?

It is if you believe researchers at the University of Utah. They reported their study in *Annals of Internal Medicine* and they contend that smoking more than triples the average person's likelihood of premature facial wrinkling. Dr. David Kadunce, author of the study, contends that skin tissue is similar to lung tissue, and is subject to the same kinds of stress as placed on smoker's lungs. The study included 109 white smokers and 23 white non-smokers between the ages of 35 and 59. The smokers had smoked between three to fifty pack-years, a pack year being equal to smoking one pack a day per year. Subjects also were asked to estimate the number of hours spent in the sun. The experts found that the degree of wrinkling increased with the number of pack-years. For non-smokers, sun exposure of 50,000 hours or more (about what the average outdoor worker or outdoor exerciser experiences) increased the risk of wrinkling eight times. However, when the smoking factor of as little as one pack-year was combined with the sun factor, the risk jumped to 12 times.

The researchers believe that direct exposure of the skin to tobacco smoke and known changes in the blood vessels supplying facial skin were the factors which increased wrinkling. So if you are concerned about looking old before your time, and are a smoker, you may wish to consider these findings.

I know that expectant mothers should not smoke because of possible harm to

the baby, but how dangerous is it?

According to researchers with the March of Dimes, women who smoke have twice the chance of miscarriage or stillbirth compared to women who do not smoke. In addition, there is a greater chance that the baby will be smaller at birth and more often premature.

Is it true that "residual or passive smoke" is nearly as bad for you as active smoking?

A number of studies have associated the involuntary inhalation of cigarette smoke to all kinds of respiratory problems in children. A new study, reported in *Pediatrics,* the journal of the American Academy of Pediatrics, indicates that non-smoking teenage athletes who were exposed to at least two hours of cigarette smoke per week developed increased coughing and decreased lung function. The group was composed of 193 healthy males and females from five New York high schools. The results indicated that while boys were exposed to passive smoke more often than girls, the effects were more pronounced on girls.

Can women reach maximum physiological levels commonly reached by male athletes?

One of the best indicators of cardiovascular efficiency and athletic success is maximal oxygen intake. Generally, maximum VO_2 of males exceeds females by 20-25%. This difference is probably attributed to the larger maximum cardiac output common to males and the quantity of O_2 extracted from a measured volume of blood as it circulates through the body tissues.

I have heard that some runners have "exercise induced asthma" (EIA). How

can I tell if this is my problem?

Actually about 33 million people have either confirmed or potential exercise induced asthma problems. The warning signs usually occur three to fifteen minutes after beginning exercise and include:
- Tightness in chest, difficulty in breathing, or coughing.
- Inability to keep up with other runners of equal age and ability.
- Exhaustion after exercise, requiring twenty to thirty minutes or more for recovery.
- Stomach ache.
- Decrease in quality performance in bad weather.

Most of the medical profession feel that most asthmatics should do regular aerobic exercise thirty to forty minutes three to four times a week. For those types of asthma induced by exercise, cold air, and atmospheric smog, swimming in a warm indoor pool will often help to alleviate these problems. Most long-term asthmatics have some lung damage resulting in a diminished aerobic capacity. This makes it all the more important to increase and efficiently utilize lung capacity.

What effect does exercise have on my respiratory system?
- Greater chest expansion.
- The depth of the chest is increased.
- Breathing rate is slower at rest.
- There is an increase in alveolar air space.
- Blood is exposed to oxygen over a greater area.
- The muscles of respiration are strengthened and consequently there is a reduction in resistance to air flow which ultimately facilitates the rapid flow of air in and out of the lungs.

- In performing similar work, an individual who exercises takes in smaller amounts of air and absorbs oxygen from the air in greater amounts than the individual who does not exercise. It is believed that the increased number of capillaries in the lungs and an increase in alveolar air space resulting in more blood being exposed to more air at any given time are responsible for this economy in respiration. This increase in efficiency results in an increase in maximum oxygen uptake. This is believed by exercise physiologists to be the best single indication of physical fitness.

SUGGESTED LAB: 17.

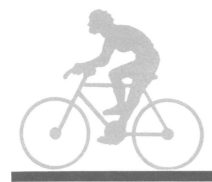

Your Muscular System

Objectives
- Identify the different classifications of muscles
- Identify and describe types of muscle contractions
- Discuss the effects of training on the muscles
- Discuss the effects of exercise on the muscular system

Key Words
- All or none principle
- Cartilage
- Fast-twitch muscle fibers
- Ligaments
- Mitochondria
- Myofibrils
- Myoglobin
- Sarcolemma
- Sarcoplasm
- Slow-twitch muscle fibers
- Tendons

An understanding of your muscular system is important in gaining the knowledge necessary to achieve your optimal health and fitness potential. All movements of the body depend on the functioning—contraction and relaxation—of muscle tissue. Although your cardiovascular system may be able to deliver large quantities of oxygen to the muscles, this will not ensure that the oxygen will be utilized. In addition to the functioning of the delivery system, the ability of the muscles to absorb oxygen from the blood in sufficient quantity to meet the energy demands of the activity is important.

When performing work, especially that of a continuous nature such as jogging or cycling, the muscles demand a steady supply of oxygen to continue production of energy. The amount of work which can be performed and how long it can be continued are dependent on the amount of oxygen which can actually be consumed and, therefore, the amount of energy which can be created.

By learning how and why a muscle functions as it does, you will be able to plan more effectively a program for greater muscular strength and endurance. Chapter 4 gives more specific information on developing a training program.

THE MUSCLE STRUCTURE

Very simply, a muscle can be described as a band of contractile fibers held together by a sheath of connective tissues. Muscles attach to bones by means of tendons or fibrous sheets which stem from the connective tissue sheath. Muscle tissue is composed of a number of muscle fibers or cells. Each fiber is composed of **myofibrils** which are the contractile units responsible for muscle shortening or lengthening. Two major categories of muscle fibers are the fast-twitch (or white) fibers and the slow-twitch (or red) fibers. Recent studies also reveal that there are two subtypes of fast-twitch fibers and that they respond differently to training.

Cartilage is a tough, elastic tissue that acts as a shock absorber or buffer between bones. **Ligaments** are connective tissue that bind bones together. They are extensible but not elastic. Healing of sprains does occur, but the stretched ligaments never completely return to their former length.

The **sarcolemma** is the cell membrane of the muscle cell, and **sarcoplasm** is the more fluid part of the cell. Running longitudinally within the sarcoplasm are slender column-like structures called myofibrils.

The absorption of oxygen from the blood into the muscle cells is made possible by the presence of a substance within the muscle cells called **myoglobin**. Myoglobin is an iron-containing protein similar to hemoglobin. The myoglobin is also responsible for the storage of oxygen within the muscle cells. Once absorbed into the myoglobin, the oxygen then combines with the nutrients (fats and carbohydrates) and enters the mitochondria of the muscle fibers. The **mitochondria** are tiny structures within the muscle fibers where oxygen and chemical substances are brought together to produce a series of chemical reactions which provide most of the energy required for muscular endurance activities.

Each individual varies in the number of **fast-twitch** and **slow-twitch** muscle fibers in their muscle tissue. The particular ratio you have is determined at birth and cannot be altered. Therefore, it is clear that those who inherit a predominance of slow-twitch fibers have an advantage in the performance of endurance-type activities and a greater

157

potential for the development of superior cardiorespiratory fitness. They will, of course, have a disadvantage in activities requiring speed and power. The individual with more fast-twitch fibers will tend to excel in speed or power sports but will not perform as well at long-term efforts which require superior aerobic capacity. The potential for a high level of cardiorespiratory fitness is also reduced. Recent studies do indicate that training can bring about improvement in aerobic capacity and glycogen content of the muscle. Therefore, even though genetics play an important role, training and conditioning must be considered in achieving sport success.

Diagram of a Joint

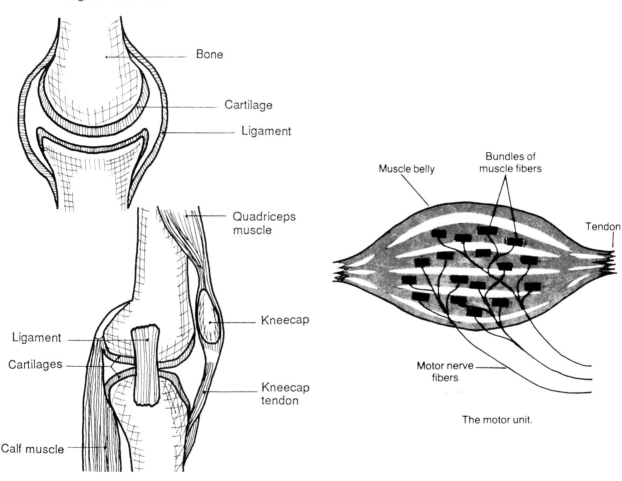

Bone

Cartilage

Ligament

Quadriceps muscle

Ligament

Cartilages

Kneecap

Kneecap tendon

Calf muscle

Muscle belly

Bundles of muscle fibers

Tendon

Motor nerve fibers

The motor unit.

The Motor Unit

A motor unit is a group of muscle fibers. Each motor unit may consist of as few as three muscle fibers (such as the muscles of the eyes) or as many has a hundred or more (such as the thigh muscles), depending on the degree of precision required for the task.

Each motor unit contracts as an entire unit. The reason for this is that all the muscle fibers in the unit are activated simultaneously by one motor nerve. If a delicate, precise movement is needed (such as in the fingers, eyes, or lungs), there may be only a few muscle fibers. When large movements are called for (such as in the thigh, back, or abdomen), each motor unit will consist of many muscle fibers. The nerve fiber with its branches and the muscle fibers stimulated by them form a complete motor unit.

The minimal threshold of excitability is specific to each motor unit. The muscle fibers in some motor units contract with only a small stimulus and some will not contract unless a very strong stimulus is given. A greater number of total motor units become activated as the nervous stimulus increases in intensity.

Whenever a muscle fiber contracts, it contracts maximally. This is referred to as the all-or-none principle of muscular contraction. Variations in the strength are therefore determined by the number of motor units stimulated. A muscle might contain numerous motor units, but the units may not all contract simultaneously. One factor is that the work load to be performed is evaluated in the brain, which stimulates the appropriate number of motor units.

Another factor determining the strength of the muscular response is the frequency of stimulation—the number of times per second that each motor unit is stimulated.

One reason a warmup is recommended as preparation for strenuous activity is that when a muscle contracts repeatedly, the first few contractions are each progressively greater until the maximal response is reached. A weak muscular contraction can result not only if the muscle is cold but also if it is fatigued or the needed nutrients are not present.

The number of muscle fibers and motor units does not change throughout life. An increase in strength is due to the individual muscle fiber becoming stronger.

The Muscle Fiber

The basic unit of the muscular system is the muscle fiber, and basically there are two types of muscle fibers.

Fast-twitch fibers are thick, strong, and able to produce a full contraction in one tenth the time it takes a slow-twitch fiber to respond. With aerobic training the "intermediate" fast-twitch fibers become more like slow-twitch fibers without actually changing their appearance. Unfortunately, the reverse is not true—you cannot make a sprinter out of a marathoner!

Slow-twitch fibers have a high "oxidative capacity" or ability to make ATP (adenosine triphosphate) in the presence of oxygen, while fast-twitch fibers have low oxidative capacity and produce ATP primarily anaerobically.

The *slow-twitch* fiber is slow to contract but has the ability to continue contracting for long periods of time. The slow-twitch fibers have a rich blood supply and high level of myoglobin and are important for endurance and activities such as marathon running and long distance swimming. Because they have a high mitochondrial content, they are able to make good use of oxygen for the production of energy.

The second major type of muscle fiber is the *fast-twitch* fiber which is best suited for fast, short-term contractions. However, there are two different categories of fast-twitch fibers: fast-white fibers and fast-red fibers. The fast-white fibers are not as well supplied by blood vessels, have a lower content of myoglobin and mitochondria and therefore a reduced capacity for processing oxygen. These fibers are utilized in fast, short burst activities like sprinting and shot putting. The fast-red fibers have a better blood supply and a higher content of myoglobin and mitochondria which enables them to process oxygen a little better. They are used in activities of high intensity but moderate duration such as middle distance running. The fast-red are still not the equal of the slow-twitch fibers in usefulness during a long term physical effort.

Energy Production

Contraction of muscle fibers is initiated when the muscle fiber is stimulated by impulses arriving via nerve cells.

Energy is required to initiate and continue the work of the muscles. The immediate source of energy is a chemical substance known as ATP (adenosine triphosphate) which releases energy when split into ADP (Adenosine diphosphate) and phosphate. There is only enough ATP available to sustain an individual for a few seconds—it must be continually reproduced.

The body must replace its local store of muscle ATP for as long as muscle contractions occur. The source of energy for the reconversion of ADP to ATP comes from the food we eat. But this method requires a constant supply of oxygen and is therefore called aerobic.

A second method of producing ATP can occur without oxygen through the breakdown of carbohydrates stored in muscle and liver. With this method less ATP is synthesized and a toxic substance known as lactic acid is produced. When lactic acid accumulates in the muscles and the bloodstream, it produces the sensation of fatigue and muscle soreness. High levels of lactic acid actually block the formation of more ATP and eventually may lead to the halting of muscle contractions altogether. This second type of energy production is referred to as anaerobic.

The **anaerobic threshold** is that level of work which leads to the accumulation of lactic acid in the muscles and body fluids. Very sedentary individuals exceed their anaerobic threshold at intensities representing a very low percentage of their maximal oxygen consumption. Highly trained marathoners have been able to work near 90% of their maximal oxygen consumption before exceeding their anaerobic threshold.

For the trained athlete the threshold for lactic acid buildup, the anaerobic threshold, occurs at a higher percentage of the athlete's aerobic capacity.

The source of energy varies according to the type of work. In bursts of all-out work, carbohydrates are used exclusively as fuel. Submaximal work which extends for an hour relies on an approximately 60-40 ratio of fat and carbohydrates. Longer work calls for an increasing importance of fat as fuel.

TYPES OF MUSCLES

Muscular tissue is much like an elastic band—it can be stretched and return again to its normal resting length. Muscular tissue has extensibility and elasticity. The contractibility of the muscle is its ability to become shorter and greater in circumference.

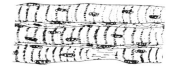

Striated muscle

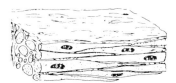

Cardiac muscle

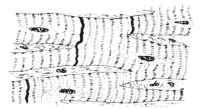

Smooth muscle

There are three major types of muscles in the body:

1. **Striated Muscle.** These muscles are the body's skeletal muscles, which provide force for moving the bones and stabilizing body parts. The striated muscles are composed of long, cylindrical fibers.
2. **Cardiac Muscle.** This muscle is found only in the heart, and it consists of a criss-crossing network of striated fibers.
3. **Smooth Muscle.** These muscles are found in the blood vessels and the hollow walls of the internal organs are smooth muscles.

The involuntary nervous system controls the smooth muscles, and the skeletal and certain other smaller striated muscles are called voluntary muscles. The cardiac muscle contracts rhythmically and automatically, without outside stimulation.

Types of Muscle Contraction

There are three basic types of muscular contraction: shortening, lengthening, or maintaining a static position. Each of these is described below.

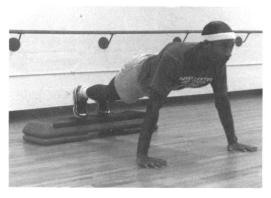

1. **Shortening or Concentric Contraction.** While one end of the muscle remains stationary, the other end pulls the bone and turns it about the joint. This is the usual type of contractor required for physical activities such as push-ups, sit-ups, and work with weights.
2. **Lengthening or Eccentric Contraction.** This is a gradual releasing of the contraction, as when one lowers a weight slowly. The muscle utilizes an eccentric contraction when lowering the body during a push-up or chin-up. The term "lengthening" is misleading since the muscle does not actually lengthen. It merely returns to its resting or original length.

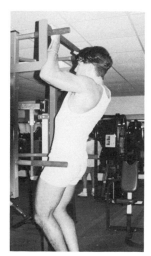

161

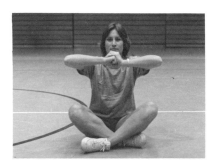

3. **Static Contraction.** During a static contraction, the muscle remains in a partial or complete contraction without changing its length. This type of contraction is performed when muscles which are antagonistic to each other contract with equal strength, thus balancing each other or when the muscle is held in partial or complete contraction against another immovable force.

Not all muscular action is for the purpose of causing motion. In nearly every movement of the body, some muscles have other functions. These functions include steadying and supporting a part, stabilizing a bone to which another muscle is attached, or neutralizing the unwanted action of a muscle which normally causes several movements. Therefore, we can classify muscles according to the types of contributions to a movement which they make: movers, stabilizers, and neutralizers.

The muscle converts glycogen and fat into the energy needed for work. In order to burn these fuels efficiently, oxygen is needed. Oxygen is delivered to the muscles by the red blood cells within the bloodstream. However, it is not possible for a muscle to take in enough energy producing food products during exercise to replace what is being used up. Therefore, your endurance will increase if you begin an activity with a greater amount of glycogen stored in your muscles.

EFFECTS OF EXERCISE ON THE MUSCULAR SYSTEM

As a muscle functions, the blood flow to it is increased through the capillaries into the muscle tissue. Therefore, depending on the type and extensiveness of the activity, there will be a temporary increase in the size of the muscle. Another effect is that additional motor units which may normally not be activated are called into action. A rise in body temperature is brought about due to the increased metabolic activity in the muscle tissue which increases the production of heat. The increased temperatures of the muscle causes the muscle to become more pliable, to be able to contract and relax more easily, and to contract at a faster rate.

Endurance exercises will also increase the production of red blood cells and stimulate the development of additional capillaries providing a richer blood supply to the muscle fibers. Studies also show that endurance training can increase the amount of myoglobin in the muscles and double the amount of oxygen that can be absorbed and stored. These and other changes can greatly improve the muscle tissue's ability to utilize oxygen and increase its capacity for long term physical activity.

EFFECTS OF TRAINING ON THE MUSCLES

When strenuous exercise is pursued over a prolonged period of time and is engaged in regularly, the blood vessels within the muscular tissue increase in number. This increase is due partly to the number of old capillaries which, when combined with new capillaries, may increase the circulation as much as 400%. This increased circulation gives a much greater supply of nutrients and oxygen to the muscle, thus increasing its endurance. Generally it takes about 8 to 12 weeks for this increase to take place. As we become older, a longer period is required to produce the changes.

Training provides some adaptations which enable the muscles to conserve glycogen and substitute fat for energy during competition. Specifically, the muscle capacity to burn fat is enhanced and the mechanism for breakdown and release of fat from fat cells is reinforced.

Muscle cells continually need energy, even in the resting state, because energy is expended in merely keeping cells alive.

Occasionally, extensive overuse or incorrect use of a muscle may lead to minor ailments. One such problem is bursitis—when the bursa becomes irritated and inflamed. The bursa is a protective sheath around the tendon, shaped like a sac, which has a slippery fluid on its inner walls.

Another ailment which can occur is a muscle cramp. A cramp occurs when a muscle contracts and will not relax again. This can happen during vigorous exercise, when the muscle is fatigued, or when it is subjected to cold. A muscle strain is the result of continuous use of certain muscles for an activity. This causes the muscles and tendons to ache but they recover after a period of rest.

However, a well-planned training program not only improves circulation, but it can develop the capacity of the muscle to function more effectively. Each individual needs to seek a training pattern that will lead to the greatest possible improvement of this important system.

QUESTIONS AND ANSWERS

Do people of the same sex have the same potential for muscle size?

No, your potential for muscular size is primarily influenced by the length of your muscles, and you didn't have much control over what you were given. Individuals who are blessed with longer muscle bellies have a greater potential for muscular size.

What is so called high-intensity exercise?

Most people consider high-intensity exercise to be the repeated performance of a movement against resistance which is done to a point of muscular failure. This means that you should do one set of each exercise at least eight but no more than twelve times. If you can do more than twelve, the resistance is not heavy enough, and if you cannot do at least eight repetitions, then the resistance is too heavy.

I frequently have sore muscles, but why is it sometimes delayed following a very strenuous workout?

One of the causes of muscle soreness is an inadequate blood flow which in turn deprives the muscle of oxygen and causes an accumulation of metabolic waste products within the muscle. Delayed muscle soreness sometimes occurs after exercise stressing eccentric contractions or muscle-lengthening exercises—for example, slowly lowering yourself after a chin on the high bar.

What are the effects of training on the muscular system?

1. Increase in muscle size (greater cross-section area). It is believed that muscle fibers increase in size but do not

increase in number. This is directly related to strength.

2. Proliferation of capillaries. The result is a better circulation of blood to the muscles and an increase in muscular endurance.

3. The sarcolemma of the muscle fibers becomes thicker and stronger.

4. The amount of connective tissue within the muscle thickens.

5. Nerve impulses travel more readily across the motor end plate.

In summary, the muscle becomes stronger, increases in endurance, reacts more quickly and efficiently, and is less prone to injury.

SKELETAL MUSCLE: STRUCTURE AND FUNCTION

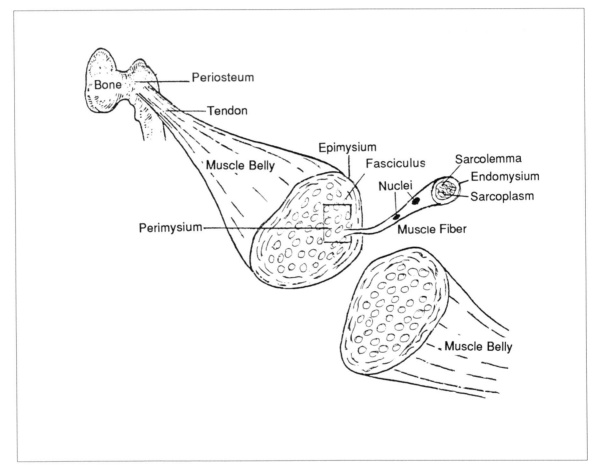

Diagram of a cross section of skeletal muscle, cut through the muscle belly, showing the arrangement of connective tissue wrappings. Individual muscle fibers are covered by the endomysium. Groups of fibers (fasciculi) are surrounded by the perimysium; the entire muscle is wrapped in the epimysium, a fibrous sheath of connective tissue. The surface of each muscle fiber is covered by the sarcolemma, a thin, elastic membrane, and the cytoplasm inside the sarcolemma is called the sarcoplasm.

SUGGESTED LABS: 9, 17.

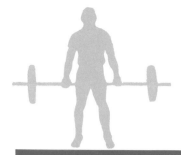

Handling Stress

Objectives

- Define stress, stressor, eustress, distress.
- Describe the stages of the general adaptation syndrome.
- Describe the short-term and long-term effects of stress on the body.
- Identify the role of exercise in managing stress.
- Describe how various relaxation techniques may be used to cope with stress.

Key Words

- Distress
- Eustress
- General Adaptation Syndrome
- Homeostasis
- Stress
- Stressor

According to Dr. Hans Selye (1), noted stress researcher, **stress** is a non-specific response of the body to any demand made upon it. This means that the body reacts in a similar manner regardless of the nature of the **stressor** or stimulus. These stressors can be physiological, social, or psychological in nature and affect the **homeostasis** (the body's attempt to maintain physiological balance) of the body, resulting in stress.

When we react to positive stressors it is called **eustress** and we experience improved performance and health. **Distress** is our response to negative stressors and is accompanied by deterioration in performance and health.

GENERAL ADAPTATION SYNDROME

Selye described the three phases with which the body responds to a stressor as alarm, resistance, and exhaustion. This three-phase pattern is known as the general adaptation syndrome.

During the **alarm phase,** the homeostasis of the body is disturbed as the brain perceives the stressor and the body prepares for action, known as the "fight or flight" syndrome. As our emotions take over, the stimulation of the autonomic nervous system and the endocrine glands result in the following physiological changes:

- Blood vessels in the skin and internal organs constrict, thus decreasing blood flow to these areas. At the same time, blood vessels in the skeletal muscles dilate to accommodate the increased blood flow.
- Cardiac output is increased due to increased heart rate and stroke volume.
- Systolic blood pressure is increased.
- Rate of respiratory ventilation is increased.
- The changing of glycogen to glucose is increased to facilitate muscular activity.
- Digestive functions are decreased as blood is diverted to the skeletal muscles.
- Muscular tension is increased.
- There is an increase in the breakdown of adipose tissue triglycerides.
- Perspiration increases.
- All senses become sharpened.

Hypothalamus sends signals through endocrine and autonomic nervous systems. Brain activity increases.

Pituitary gland dumps ACTH into bloodstream, stimulating adrenal glands.

Stress chemicals speed up heart rate; cardiac output increases, blood pressure increases.

The changing of glycogen to glucose is increased to facilitate muscular activity. Under extreme or prolonged stress, fats and proteins break down to provide energy.

All senses become sharpened; eyes dilate.

Rate of respiratory ventilation increases.

Muscular tension is increased.

Perspiration increases.

Digestive functions decrease as blood is diverted to skeletal muscles.

In the **resistance phase** the body attempts to adjust to the stressor and appears to return to homeostasis, as the heart rate and respiration return to normal and perspiration decreases. Hormones are secreted which give the body energy to cope with the stressor. This phase may be of very short duration and may only use a small amount of energy which is easily replaced. However, if intense or long-term stress exhausts the amount of stored energy available and adaptation does not occur, the **exhaustion phase** is entered. The endocrine system cannot produce a sufficient amount of hormones to counter the chronic stressor. Long-term stress, occurring over weeks or even years, may affect the heart, blood pressure, stomach, muscles, joints, and cause headaches and fatigue. Proper use of stress management techniques can alleviate these problems before serious physical and/or psychological disorders occur.

WARNING SIGNS OF STRESS

Your awareness of stress signals is the first step in learning how to cope with stress. Short-term effects of stress on the body are usually easy to observe and may include:
- elevated heart rate
- rapid breathing
- diarrhea
- constipation
- dry mouth
- lower back pain
- shortness of breath
- fatigue
- headaches
- dizziness
- sleep disturbances

Stress can also affect your memory and ability to concentrate, as well as cause you to be moody and irritable. It can also lead to excessive eating, drinking, and drug use.

Long term effects of stress may occur when a person has not effectively dealt with the stressor over a period of a few weeks to years. Hypertension, heart disease, stomach ulcers and severe headaches are among the physical conditions which can result from long-term distress. In addition, other indicators may be depression, weight control problems, ineffective use of time, excessive smoking, and drug and alcohol abuse. Chronic stress can cause the body to be less resistant to disease as it affects the immune system. Interferon, which is one of the body's defenses against virus infections and possibly cancer, is suppressed under some conditions of emotional stress. (2) Excess adrenaline not used up by physical exertion can play a part in the accumulation of cholesterol in the blood vessels that leads to heart disease.

Findings from a recent study, reported in the New England Journal of Medicine (3), suggest that those people under high levels of stress are more likely to catch the common cold when exposed to the cold virus. Three different measures were used to determine the stress level of the subjects: the number of stressful life events during the previous year, ranging from a spouse's death to celebrating Christmas; the subject's perception of stress; and the subject's level of negative emotions.

Dr. Kenneth Cooper suggests that if you feel stressed that you should check your resting heart rate early in the morning and then re-check it later in the day while at rest. A normal increase would be about 10 beats per minute; however, if your heart rate is increasing 20-30 beats per minute, this suggests a manifestation of stress.

To help you determine your own level of stress, the authors have developed a simple game called Stresso (Lab 28).

167

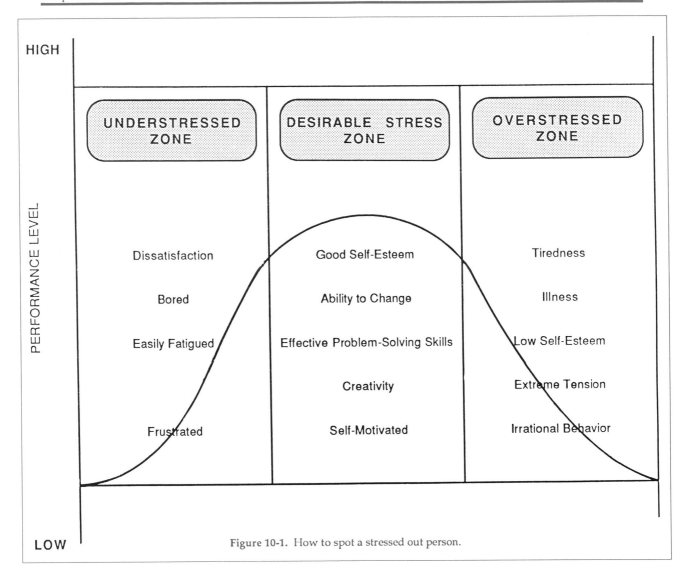

Figure 10-1. How to spot a stressed out person.

RECOGNIZING SOURCES OF STRESS

The first step in dealing with stress is recognizing that stress is a problem in your life; then you need to try to identify the stressors.

Minor hassles are experienced frequently by everyone, such as losing your keys, having to wait in lines, and being stuck in traffic. Instead of worrying about these annoyances which are beyond your control, realize that you have to put up with them and relax. Look around and see how tense other people are getting, and be proud of the fact that you can control your emotions.

Major events or changes in your life can be positive stressors such as graduation, marriage, birth of a child, or a job promotion which cause eustress. Negative stressors, such as the death of a loved one, suspension from school, or loss of your job can result in distress.

Results of a study by Bolger et al. (4)

showed that interpersonal conflicts are the most upsetting of daily stressors and that conflicts with other persons are more distressing than those with family members. Most conflicts with others were with friends, neighbors, or people at work.

Modern computer technology places new demands on people and thus is a new source of stress in many people's lives. Brod (5) describes this modern disease of adaptation as "technostress," which is caused by an inability to cope with the new computer technologies in a healthy manner.

MANAGING YOUR STRESS

It is sometimes possible to eliminate or reduce certain stressors in our lives, but often there are many variables in life that are impossible or difficult to control. The management of stress comes down to making choices in learning to cope or adapt to our problems. People with a strong sense of commitment and the belief that they have a lot of control over events in their lives tend to be able to withstand much stress without becoming ill (6).

- Establish challenging and attainable goals. Be realistic when setting your goals; you don't want to add to your frustration by not accomplishing them as quickly as you would like.
- Time management techniques can be very helpful. Keep an appointment book or calendar to organize your time and remind yourself of important dates and events. Learn to say "No" and set priorities. Allow yourself time in each day to relax.
- Make time for fun. Play is just as important to your well-being as rewarding work is. Everyone needs a break from their daily routine to just "have fun" and relax. "Having fun" means different things to different people. The key is finding what is fun for you.
- Crying is not all bad. A good cry provides emotional release, and when not taken to excess, can help to provide a safe and satisfying release of emotions.
- Laugh! Eustress may play a part in helping the body heal itself. Laughter causes endorphins to be released, which may play a part in reversing some of the distress damage.
- Sharing stress. Just talking to someone about your concerns and worries often helps. A family member, counselor, teacher, or friend will often help you to view your problem in a different light.

Sometimes we might perceive a situation as threatening when in reality it is not. We might feel that we are being pulled in many directions and become overwhelmed or depressed. In these instances, it might be wise to seek professional help. Some possible sources are your physician, school counselor or psychologist, and local or state health agencies.

SLEEP AND STRESS

Although most people spend approximately one-third of their lives in sleep, we still know very little about this complicated process. However, scientific observations have been recorded and we know that the following does occur:

- Physiological functions decrease during sleep—decreased blood pressure, pulse rate, body temperature, rate of breathing, and a decrease in muscle tone are examples of this phenomenon.

169

- The regeneration of body cells, while a continuous process, occurs more rapidly during sleep. A person's rate of growth, therefore, influences his or her need for sleep. Young people who are growing rapidly, and older people (whose recuperative powers are less efficient) often require more sleep.

Insomnia is a common complaint of stressed and tense people. Repeated and frequent experiences probably indicate a need for a medical checkup; however, there may be factors other than those previously mentioned which could help or contribute to the problem.

Factors such as room temperature, darkness, retiring at approximately the same hour each night, quietness, and the comfort of one's regular bed, all contribute to acquiring one's necessary rest. Of course, having a good day free of abnormal problems also contributes to having a good night's sleep.

Interestingly enough, scientists have found that the most important factor in falling asleep at night is whether or not your temperature is dropping. Your body temperature is at its lowest level in early morning, and usually is highest in early evening, and as it starts to fall you become sleepy. Many people who have difficulty in falling asleep at night have temperature cycles that aren't dropping when they go to bed.

Insomniacs who like desserts will love this suggestion. Some researchers have suggested that you should eat your desserts one hour before bedtime. The reasoning being that foods rich in carbohydrates cause an elevated blood sugar which moves the amino acid tryptophan to the brain. Tryptophan converts to a brain messenger which says you are sleepy. Warm milk, which also contains tryptophan, will also do the job.

Other Factors Contributing to Inability to Sleep

- Eating habits, being hungry, eating too much, taking stimulants such as coffee or certain beverages late in the day, all of these affect some people. The test is your own personal experience.
- Exercise. Mild, light exercise induces sleep somewhat; however, excessive exercise and accompanying fatigue can cause insomnia for others.
- Psychological tensions, brought about by social or economic problems.
- Excitement, such as an impending trip or abrupt change in living habits.

Loss of sleep is not always harmful. Out of necessity, men and women have often gone 48-72 hours without sleep and have recovered with no apparent ill effects after only twelve hours sleep. The longest that a person has been known to go without sleep and survive is nine days.

Since no two humans are alike, the best that can be said about sleep is that it is a highly individual matter. Most adults sleep 6-8 hours a day, but some require more. The test of whether you are acquiring enough sleep is whether you awaken each morning with a feeling of being ready for what the day has in store for you. Of course, the first half hour or so doesn't count since some people are "slow starters."

EXERCISE AND STRESS

Much evidence exists that physical exercise has significant value in reducing stress. According to Selye (1), people who are regular exercisers are able to resist stressors better, and stressful situations do not represent as much harm to the trained person as to the sedentary person.

Devries (7), working with mentally ill patients, verified that moderate physical activity had value in reducing tension. Patients involved in a rhythmic-type exercise such as jogging, cycling, walking, and bench stepping, using 20-60% of maximum heart rate levels of five to thirty minute duration, achieved significant levels of relaxation.

In addition, Michael (8), in a study titled "Stress Adaptation Through Exercise," found that moderate exercise seemed to cause a mild type of stress on the adrenal glands. This conditioning process seemed to strengthen the adrenals so that more severe stress was handled more effectively. It was concluded that repeated exercise caused an increase in adrenal activity resulting in the formation of an increased reserve of steroids, which are effective in counteracting stress.

Cooper believes that aerobic exercise can provide a powerful factor in dissipating the stress one has accumulated during the course of a hectic day. He believes that as adrenal secretion builds during a pressure-filled day, the body becomes chemically unbalanced; therefore, relaxation is impossible until the situation is corrected. Unfortunately, alcohol sometimes seems to help by depressing the body senses; thus, many people turn to this form of artificial assistance. A much better method is to exercise, allowing nature's natural waste removal process to operate by burning off the overaccumulation of excess secretions. In other words, exercise uses up the fight or flight response.

Pollock suggests that our attitudes while exercising may make a difference between alleviating stress or adding to stress. If you view exercise as yet another difficult thing to get through, or if you're angry or upset while exercising, exercise probably will seem like hard work and won't necessarily relax you. If you approach exercise with positive expectations, then it will potentially have a more positive effect on how you feel afterward.

It is also important that you choose a type of exercise that is enjoyable for you and doesn't add to your stress. According to Paul J. Rosch, M.D., President of the American Institute of Stress in New York, "the feeling of being out of control is uniformly distressing; what may be even more important is not the technique that you choose to lessen the effects of stress, but developing a sense of control to prevent stressful responses."

Another level of stress reduction is the ability of the body to deal with stress situations as they arise. We know, for instance, that the average unconditioned male and female have resting heart rates of 70-72 and 75-80 beats per minute, respectively. We also know that a conditioning program can drop this rate some 20-30 beats per minute. The important thing, however, is that in addition to a lower resting heart rate, the rate tends to remain lower, elevate more slowly, and recover more quickly in a conditioned person when unexpected anxiety arises or when the person increases the level of physical exercise.

This is partially due to the increased stroke volume of the trained person's heart, but it is also due to the fact that the trained cardiovascular system tends to provide a "governor" effect on the influence that adrenal secretions have on the heart. There have been numerous instances where a rapid acceleration in heart rate caused by intense physical or emotional stress has triggered a lethal heart attack, and the record books are full of reports of 35-45 year old people succumbing to such situations.

Research has shown that alpha wave activity in the brain is stimulated by aerobic activity. The same alpha waves are also seen during periods of relaxation and meditation. In addition, vigorous exercise causes the pituitary gland to release endorphins, morphine-like substances which act as painkillers and are associated with the feeling of euphoria that frequently occurs during and after exercise. Endorphins may be the reason why athletes sustain injuries during a contest yet continue to compete, not realizing they have sustained a major injury until later. Cooper identifies one such instance as follows:

In the 1982 Boston Marathon, Guy Gertsch, a runner from Salt Lake City, apparently sustained a stress fracture to his thigh bone at the seventh mile. Even though the bone was completely fractured, he completed the 26.2 mile race before collapsing. Then, several hours of surgery were required to stabilize the bone with a steel rod running from his hip to his knee. The surgeons theorized that the thigh muscles in this 38 year-old man were so powerful that they acted as splints for the bone during the run; and obviously the endorphins were a factor in enabling him to tolerate the pain and continue running at a 6:30 pace.

It is also known that endorphin levels of pregnant women tend to be much higher and this perhaps explains how women are able to withstand the pain associated with childbirth. The fact does suggest the possibility that the conditioned female quite likely would have a higher endorphin threshold than her unconditioned counterpart, and thus should have a less painful experience.

Cooper also believes that reasonably high endorphin levels are also present in the body even after relatively mild exercise sessions, such as running approximately three miles at a 7:30 to 9:00 minute pace, and says that these runners have at least a partial feeling of euphoria. It has also been speculated that the "second wind" phenomenon may occur as a result of the endorphin factor.

Relaxation Techniques

Progressive Muscle Relaxation is a very effective technique developed by Dr. Edmund Jacobsen which involves tensing and relaxing all the muscle groups in the body. It makes us aware of what high levels of muscular tension feel like and teaches you how to relax your body at will and release tension from the muscles. It can be used by athletes and other performers to control pre-competition anxiety and can also help us sleep better.

At least twenty minutes should be devoted to the relaxation exercises and it is preferable if they are conducted in a warm, dark room. The exercise sequence can be memorized, read to the person, or played on a tape recorder. The progressive relaxation technique is most effective if the person is lying down on his or her back, with a pillow or blanket under the head and/or knees. It may also be done sitting in a chair, but it is necessary for the chair to be high enough to support the head. The arms and legs should be uncrossed. Each contraction should be held for five seconds and then the muscle should totally relax, with special attention paid to these sensations. Perform each contraction twice.

Meditation is an easy relaxation technique to learn; it requires no special equipment and once learned, can be practiced almost anywhere. The relaxation

The following is an example of a progressive muscle relaxation sequence:

1. Point your right toe downward, then left toe, then both toes.
2. Pull your right toe up, then left toe, then both toes.
3. Contract your right thigh, then left, then both.
4. Push your right heel into the floor, then left, then both.
5. Contract your buttocks as you raise your hips slightly.
6. Contract your abdominal muscles.
7. Contract your stomach and lower back muscles and try to press your lower back into the floor.
8. Make a fist with your right hand, then left hand, then both hands at once. Feel the tension in your forearms.
9. Flex the right elbow by bringing the hand to the shoulder, then left elbow, then both elbows.
10. With your palms up, push on your right forearm until you feel your triceps tense, repeat with left, then both.
11. Shrug both shoulders as high as possible.
12. Push your head back gently, tensing the muscles in the back of the neck.
13. Bring the head forward towards the chest.
14. Tighten the muscles around the mouth, then eyes, then forehead. Stick your tongue out.
15. Take a deep breath, hold, and exhale slowly.

response brought about by meditation is believed to cause a decrease in heart and respiratory rates, blood pressure, and muscle tension and helps the body counteract the biochemical changes that cause stress.

Sit in an upright position in a chair with your hands resting on the arms of the chair or in your lap. Close your eyes and repeat the word *one* to yourself each time you inhale and word *two* as you exhale. Try to practice meditation for 15-20 minutes, twice a day if possible. Don't be concerned with the exact time or you will defeat the purpose of meditation.

Imagery can help you deal with stressful situations. Relax, close your eyes, and concentrate on a beautiful, peaceful scene such as a forest, lake, or mountain. Look with your mind at the details of the scene; pay attention to the smells, sounds, and colors. This process can be continued as long as you wish and can help you achieve relaxation of your mind and body.

Deep Breathing Exercises can be used to relieve stress by concentrating on breathing and increasing oxygen to the body. They may be performed in any position, but an effective position is sitting with the eyes closed, inhaling slowly and deeply through the nose and slowly exhaling through the mouth. Repeat about ten times.

There are many other relaxation

techniques that you may wish to explore, such as biofeedback, yoga, autogenic training, and massage. Everyone reacts to stress differently and you may want to try various techniques to see which one or combination of two or more works best for you. Remember, it is not the stressor that makes people ill, it is the way in which they react to the stressor. Take the time to learn some of these techniques; when you learn to control the stress in your life, you will enjoy a healthier and happier life.

QUESTIONS AND ANSWERS

How about sleeping pills?

Don't! In rare cases, and on the advice of a physician, they might be necessary. However, pills are a crutch which inevitably will be abused. What you might try, however, is a preliminary relaxation of mind and body. There are various techniques which, when practiced, contribute to relaxation. Such things as a warm bath, reading, listening to relaxing music, breathing deeply, and attempting to consciously relax the muscles, assist many people in the sleep process.

Does taking tranquilizers reduce stress?

No. Tranquilizers are addictive and their side effects can be worse than the stress they are supposed to treat.

I have heard that the so-called Type A personality, the aggressive, tense, competitive person, is more prone to heart attacks. True or not?

What was once taken for dogma is no longer taken so seriously. Doctors Richard Brand and David Ragland of the University of California at Berkeley recently completed a 22-year follow-up study on some middle-aged men. They have concluded that Type A behavior is not related to heart attack deaths. High blood pressure and smoking were much greater risks than behavior or personality. There are several studies, however, which suggest chronically angry and suspicious people are two times more likely to have coronary blockages. It is the frequent hostility, frustration and depression that these Type A people possess that may cause them problems, not the challenge-seeking aspects of Type A behavior. Workaholism need not be hazardous to your health, as long as you are good at the work and enjoy it.

REFERENCES
1. Selye, H. *The Stress of Life*. 2nd Edition. New York: McGraw-Hill Book Co., 1978.
2. Seliger, S. "Stress Can Be Good for You." *New York,* August 2, 1982.
3. Swartz, M. N. "Stress and the Common Cold." *The New England Journal of Medicine,* 325:654-656, 1991
4. Bolger, N., DeLongis, A., Kessler, R. C. and Schilling, D. "Effects of Daily Stress on Negative Mood." *Journal of Personality and Social Psychology,* 57:808-818, 1989.
5. Brod, C. *Technostress: The Human Cost of the Computer Revolution.* Reading, MA: Addison, Wesley, 1984.
6. McCutcheon, L. E., Lummis, G., and Ellis, E. L. "A Re-examination of the Line Between Stress and Performance." *Perceptual Motor Skills* 69:323-330, 1989.
7. DeVries, H. R. "Physical Education, Adult Fitness Programs: Does Physical Activity Promote Relaxation?" *Journal of Physical Education and Recreation* 46:53-54, 1975.
8. Michael, E. D. "Stress Adaptation Through Exercise." *Research Quarterly* 28:50-54.
9. Kaufman, E. "How to Thrive Under Pressure." *Self,* 1989, 165-168.
10. Miller, L. "To Beat Stress, Don't Relax: Get Tough." *Psychology Today,* 23:62-63, 1989.
11. "How to Stop a Cold: Lighten Up and Avoid Stress, Study Says." *The Miami Herald,* August 29, 1991.

SUGGESTED LABS: 27, 28, 29, 30.

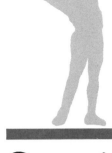

Special Concerns about Exercise and Fitness

Objectives

- Identify ways to prevent exercise injuries
- Recognize the symptoms and treatment of extreme heat and cold problems associated with exercise.
- Recognize and know how to treat minor exercise injuries

Key Words

- AIDS
- Anabolic steroids
- Heat exhaustion
- Heat stroke
- HIV
- Osteoporosis
- RICE
- Shin splints

It should be clear that achieving a high level of fitness or wellness involves more than following a good exercise program or eating healthy foods. There are many habits and lifestyle choices that affect one's level of total fitness. This chapter will address many of these special issues and the common injuries that sometimes occur during exercise.

PREVENTION OF INJURIES

At this point, you should be convinced of the necessity and pleasures that can occur from a vigorous activity or exercise program. Unfortunately, some people feel that injuries must accompany the pleasure and benefits of exercise. What most "weekend warriors" do not understand is that 80% of all exercise injuries can be prevented through knowledge, common sense, and a good five- to ten-minute stretching warmup prior to working out. What is certain is that the estimated number of 17 million people who yearly limp in to see their favorite doctor could be reduced. Knowing what the most common injuries are in your sport, and knowing how to handle them should they occur, will make your exercise program more enjoyable and safer.

1. Exercise should be avoided in the following situations: when it can aggravate an existing injury or illness, when one is not feeling well, and after eating a heavy meal.

2. Strenuous exercise can be hazardous in certain weather conditions—extreme heat and humidity or extreme cold.

3. One should use caution in the use of hot showers, sauna baths and steam rooms following an exercise session. Anything that inhibits the removal of heat which has built up during exercise can be dangerous.

4. It is important to become acclimatized to the weather in which you will be exercising. Acclimatizing is a process of gradually preparing the body for the environment by slowly exposing it to the unusual stresses whether it be hot, humid temperature or extreme cold. Gradually increase the time and pace of your workouts and realize it may take up to two weeks for the bodily functions to adapt. During hot weather it is best to exercise during early morning or evening hours.

5. Replacement of fluids lost through evaporation when exercising during hot weather is extremely important. The best method is to drink large quantities of water before, during, and after exercise.

6. Wearing the proper clothing for the specific weather conditions is a key factor. For instance, in hot weather you should wear light-colored clothing made of cotton or mesh material. As much area of the skin should be exposed as possible to speed the evaporation process. In cold weather, wear layers of thin clothing that can be removed one layer at a time as you exercise. Wearing a hat, gloves and covering for the ears and nose will help prevent rapid heat loss.

7. Be certain you identify your weak areas—the muscles, tendons, and ligaments which are vulnerable to injury—and do exercises to strengthen them.

8. An important key is to observe the body's warning signals—the muscles, joints, and bones.

9. Maintain a regular training program. Remember that long periods of inactivity lead to reconditioning, and you must

resume activity slowly and cautiously.

10. If you are using some sort of protective exercise equipment, make certain it is the proper type; i.e., helmets, guards, gloves, pads.

11. When working out at high altitudes (above 10,000 feet) the intensity of the workout should be reduced to maintain approximately the same cardiovascular training effect that one experiences at sea level. This is necessary because the lower atmospheric pressure makes it more difficult to deliver oxygen to the working muscles of the body.

12. Be aware of those symptoms that result from exercise which can be corrected through changes in your training program:

    a. Rapid heart rate during the 5-10 minutes of recovery—reduce the intensity of your workout.

    b. Nausea or vomiting after exercise—avoid eating for two hours or more before the workout and reduce the intensity of the program.

    c. Prolonged fatigue up to 24 hours after exercise—reduce the duration and intensity of the workout.

If you are injured, it is important to determine the cause of injury and try to correct its occurrence. Look for the following:

1. Overtraining—pushing yourself beyond your limits—overdoing it.

2. Poor training methods—increasing the intensity or duration too rapidly.

3. Some sort of structural problem which is putting added stress on muscles, tendons, bones, joints, etc., such as unequal leg length, bow legs, knock knees, exaggerated back curve.

4. Lack of flexibility may cause injury to certain muscles.

5. Muscle imbalance—one muscle which is stronger overpowers a weaker one.

If Injuries Occur

In the past 20 years sport medicine has gradually evolved away from the concept of using cold only during the acute phase of injuries such as sprains, and then replacing the cold with heat. Cold is now used during both first aid and rehabilitation of serious injury.

As a painkiller, cold provides relief by blocking or slowing the passage of pain messages along the small, slow conducting nerve fibers. This analgesic effect relieves pain in the same manner as acupuncture—by preventing pain messages from reaching the brain and by stimulating the production of endorphins. Cold also decreases muscle spasms which often accompany serious injury.

Cold affects the blood vessels, thereby limiting swelling and tissue damage. What many people do not know is that these benefits continue for approximately 10-16 minutes after injury. However, if cold is continued longer than 16 minutes, the small arteries in deeper tissues may rapidly dilate. This effect is similar to that of heat; i.e., a distinct increase in local blood flow and a temperature promotes healing and increases the carrying away of damaged tissue materials.

There are some potential dangers in using cold, however. Ice applied over a superficial nerve, such as the peroneal in the outer knee, can cause partial paralysis. Also, some people seem to have undue sensitivity to the cold, so caution is advised.

Water frozen in a Styrofoam cup provides an excellent means of application. Rub the cup for seven to ten minutes or until you feel a burning sensation and eventually an aching numbness. At this point, treatment should cease. As an added thought, if you choose to immerse a foot in ice water, try leaving the toes out. It feels better.

One easy way to remember the above information pertaining to the treatment of most new injuries is to remember the word RICE.

R — Rest the injured part.

I — Ice the injured part by using cold packs or ice cold water. Apply immediately, and continue for 10-16 minutes. Thereafter, reapply every two waking hours for the next 24-48 hours.

C — Compression. Pressure reduces blood flow and swelling to the injured part. An Ace bandage is excellent, but care must be used to insure that circulation is not completely cut off.

E — Elevation will always decrease blood flow. This is particularly true if the injured part can be elevated higher than the heart.

Muscle Problems

Muscle soreness is unfortunately one of the universal outcomes of vigorous exercise. This is particularly true when the exercise occurs after a prolonged period of inactivity. Although the causes of muscle soreness are not yet fully understood, some researchers believe that an over-accumulation of lactic acid in the tissues, brought about by fatigue, somehow triggers the pain symptom. Another factor is the accumulation of lactic acid in the affected muscle which causes pressure on nerve endings. Another hypothesis by DeVries is that muscle soreness may be caused by "tonic spasms"; i.e., small, continuous muscle contractions.

Limited activity in the form of gentle stretching and usage is probably the best means of dispelling the symptom. However, gentle massage and warm baths seem to give some relief, although the effects may be more psychological than physiological.

Muscle spasm, or **cramps,** are sudden, violent, involuntary muscle contractions that can be excruciatingly painful. Cramps may occur while engaging in activity or may occur during rest or sleep. There are two distinct types of cramping. The **clonic** type is characterized by repeated contractions and relaxation of the muscle, while the **tonic** type is continuous and steady contraction.

The cause of cramps is sometimes difficult to determine. However, the onset of fatigue, depletion of body fluids and minerals, and loss of reciprocal muscle coordination are all contributing factors.

When a cramp occurs in the body, the best thing to do is to stop immediately and alleviate the spasm by the application of constant pressure. Should it occur in the leg or foot, sometimes just putting body weight on the limb will help. When the cramp has dissipated, an easy gradual stretch of the part of the body affected will usually help. Moist, warm heat will also assist in relaxing muscles.

Muscle pulls or tears frequently occur to the unconditioned or "weekend athlete." While evidence concerning the warmup period is controversial, most coaches and athletes feel that a warmup is necessary to their well-being. It is certain that an adequate conditioning program decreases the number of such injuries.

Most authorities feel the best treatment is the immediate application of cold packs for several hours with repeated applications for up to 24 hours. After 24-28 hours most trainers prefer whirlpool baths, ultrasonic, and deep heat treatments. These injuries are very slow to heal and require much reconditioning.

Leg and Foot Problems

It is usually best to run on soft surfaces, such as grass, as this reduces the stress on joints and connective tissue. Proper footwear will greatly aid in absorbing the shock of running. Beach running is quite popular with many people because of its cooling and refreshing effect on the body.

Prolonged running on hard surfaces sometimes causes an inflammation and tearing of the muscles and tendons of the lower leg. This condition, commonly called **"shin splints,"** usually responds best to complete rest of the legs for a period of time.

Distance runners, soldiers, and others who put prolonged stress on the feet sometimes acquire a fracture of the long bones (metatarsals) of the foot. The injury causes swelling and pain, and can only be diagnosed by x-ray. Stress type fractures can be prevented by the use of a broad-soled running shoe with sufficient cushioning.

The most common pain complaint among runners is **knee pain.** Since most chronic knee pain is due to biomechanical problems in a runner's stride, the knee does not respond well to rest and the pain usually returns whenever a runner reaches a previous level of distance and intensity.

Podiatrists long ago determined that knee and hip problems are usually related to either foot problems, leg length, and/or weak quadriceps, and since the knee must absorb forces three to four times greater than body weight, it is not surprising that problems arise in this anatomical part of our body.

Since some problems may be caused by badly worn shoes, check these first. Some knee problems are caused by minor differences in leg length, and a felt pad or sponge wedge placed under the heel of the shorter leg might solve your problem. Of course, if you have a severe problem you may have to visit a podiatrist to be fitted with an orthotic (an insert fitted to your foot and shoe which will place your foot in a neutral plane).

In any event, once you have determined your problem, you can help prevent reoccurrences by strengthening the quadriceps, which in turn helps to stabilize the knee.

Heel pain, sometimes called a "stone bruise," usually occurs in the center or outer edge of the fat pad of the heel. The injury occurs because of repeated pounding of the heel on a hard surface, causing a swelling of the bursa lying between the fat pad and the bone of the heel. The best way to prevent this problem is to avoid running on hard surfaces and to wear shoes that are adequately cushioned. Also, ice applied immediately after running will reduce swelling, and a special heel cup will reduce shock to the heel area. This injury does not heal quickly.

Another painful foot problem is **plantar fascitis.** It is most noticeable when you arise in the morning and begin to take those first few steps of the day. The pain radiates from the heel area into the midsection of the foot. The pain gradually eases in walking and running as the plantar fascia muscles begins to loosen and stretch.

The major cause is an inward pronation of the foot which places an undue stretch on the plantar fascia muscle. Poorly fitting shoes, soft heel counters, misshapen shoes, or shoes with excessive wear under the heel usually contribute to this condition. Ice massage after running and customized orthotics usually alleviate this problem.

Sprains are injuries to ligaments surrounding a joint or to the capsule-like sac that surrounds a joint. While severe sprains may not be distinguishable from a more serious fracture except by x-ray, certain steps, if followed, will reduce pain and speed

recovery. They are as follows:
1. Stop activity—remove weight.
2. Elevate limb and apply an elastic (ace) bandage, taking care it is not applied too tightly.
3. Apply ice water or cold packs intermittently for 24 hours.
4. Apply prudent use of gentle exercise and warm soaks after damage has healed.

Friction blisters may be caused by poorly-fitting shoes, a wrinkle in a wet sock, or excessive use of feet that are not calloused. If pressure can be relieved until fluid is absorbed, this is probably the best course of action. However, this often cannot be done. In such cases, thoroughly scrub the part with soap and water, then sterilize a needle by holding it over a match flame, and make a small opening at the base of the blister. Drain the fluid and apply a sterile dressing. The area sometimes can be protected from further irritation by applying a small felt or rubber pad with a hole (doughnut) cut in the center to protect the blister. This will take the pressure off that particular spot.

Achilles tendonitis, a relatively common occurrence, usually begins with tenderness and soreness around the Achilles tendon, located at the back of the heel. This inflammation of the tendon within its sheath sometimes causes swelling and crepitus (a grating sound produced through use.) It is usually caused by strong pushing off movements associated with speed work and hard hill training.

Remedies include a heel pad to prevent the heel from dropping down and over-stretching, and preventive stretching exercises once healing has occurred.

A more serious injury caused by a violent contraction of the calf muscles sometimes results in a tearing away of the Achilles tendon at the back of the heel. If the tear is only partial, rest and support with an elastic bandage may alleviate the problem. However, if the tendon is severely damaged, medical help is a necessity.

Heat and Cold-Related Problems

Your body temperature is very important because about 80% of the energy metabolized during exercise in a hot environment is cast off as heat in active muscles. If this heat is not removed from the inner body, a possible dangerous rise in body temperature can occur. The body removes excessive heat by evaporation, convection, or radiation. Radiation and convection are caused when warm blood moves to and through the skin. Evaporation occurs when the body sweats and the fluid evaporates from the skin.

As you become dehydrated your blood volume decreases, causing less blood to be pumped to the skin. This decreases heat loss by radiation and convection and is of particular significance in hot, dry climates, since evaporation accounts for 80-90% of heat loss during upright exercise.

The body needs time to adapt to hot weather conditions. Even though you might be physically fit, you can only increase your tolerance to heat by exercising regularly in hot weather. Therefore, the following steps are recommended:
1. Plan your workouts for the coolest part of the day, such as early morning or early evening after the sun has gone down.
2. Cut back on your workouts—duration and intensity—until you become adapted to the heat.
3. Drink plenty of fluids—especially water.

4. Dress in lightweight, loose-fitting clothing.
5. Never wear rubberized clothing, plastic suits, sweatshirts or sweatpants.

Heat stroke is a body response to heat characterized by extremely high body temperature and disturbance of the body's sweating mechanism. Heat stroke symptoms are (1) hot, dry skin; (2) high body temperature; and (3) frequent unconsciousness. First aid measures include cooling the victim with cool water and prompt removal to a hospital. This is an extremely dangerous condition once symptoms develop.

Heat exhaustion is a response to heat characterized by fatigue, weakness, and collapse due to inadequate intake of fluids to compensate the loss of body salts and fluids through sweating. Heat exhaustion symptoms are pale skin, profuse perspiration, nausea, and frequent urination with body temperature normal. First aid measures include moving the victim to a cool area and protection from chilling.

Since a person can lose as much as three or four quarts of water in an hour of hard exercise, it is important to drink fluids before, during, and after intensive exercise. Research indicates that cool drinks (40-50 degrees) are absorbed faster than lukewarm drinks. If exercising in very hot weather, you should drink at least 16-20 ounces of fluids about two hours before exercising, and another 8 ounces just before engaging. And while exercising, drink 3 to 8 ounces every 10-20 minutes. After exercising, be sure to drink enough fluids to replace the fluids lost through sweating. About one pint for each pound should do the job.

Cold Weather. It is important to dress appropriately when exercising outside on cold days. Generally the following rules

should be observed:
1. Wear one layer less of clothing than you would if you were outside but not exercising.
2. Wear several layers of light clothing rather than one heavy layer.
3. Protect your hands by wearing mittens, gloves, or cotton socks.
4. Wear a head covering. Up to 40% of your body's heat is lost through the neck and head.

A brief warmup before going outside is also beneficial.

The Sun and Cancer

The sun is a very serious problem for those of us who either work outdoors or who engage extensively in outdoor sports. The American Cancer Society states.

- One serious sunburn early in life doubles the chance of developing skin cancer later in life.
- One in every seven Americans will develop skin cancer in their lifetime.
- Three-fourths of all deaths from skin cancer are caused by malignant melanoma.

The records indicate that the incidence of melanoma cancer has doubled in the last ten years. And, if current rates continue, one out of every 100 Americans will be diagnosed with this potent form of cancer.

The American Cancer Society has a simple diagnostic tool for early detection— they call it the ABCD way.

- A stands for Asymmetry—one half of a mole does not match the other half.
- B stands for bleeding or border irregularity. The edges of the skin mole are not definitive.
- C stands for color. The color of the mole is not a uniform black or brown, but may be shades of red, white, tan, brown,

181

blue or black.

- D stands for diameter or size. Any sudden increase in mole size indicates a problem.

Those with a higher risk of skin cancer include:

- People who sunburn easily.
- Those with fair skin and red or blonde hair.
- Those who spend a great deal of time in the sun.
- Those with a family member who has been diagnosed with melanoma cancer.

The depletion of the earth's protective atmosphere—the ozone layer—is increasing the rates of skin cancer. Since fewer dangerous rays are being filtered out, the sun is getting stronger and poses a greater risk to the average person. Therefore, it is recommended that you wear a sunscreen whenever you will be outdoors. A sunscreen with a SPF (sun protection factor) of 15 is adequate to allow exposure to the sun for up to seven hours. The sunscreen should be applied at least an hour before going into the sun and again after swimming or perspiring. It is important to wear a sunscreen even when it is a cloudy day and to realize that the rays can penetrate into three feet of water. Avoid the direct sun at midday because the sun's rays are strongest between 11:00 a.m. and 2:00 p.m.

ALCOHOL ABUSE

The abuse of alcohol is a significant problem in the United States. Reports indicate that as many as 3 million teenagers may have a drinking problem, that nearly 18 million adults are problem drinkers, and over 10 million drinkers suffer from alcoholism.

Even those who do not abuse the use of alcohol should be aware of its negative effects on fitness and athletic performance. According to a report by the U.S. Department of Health and Human Services, alcohol consumption either directly or indirectly affects every system of the body. Specific effects of alcohol on the body include:

- Liver: About one in three heavy drinkers develops scars on the liver associated with cirrhosis (a disease in which liver cells are destroyed and liver function is impaired). Even moderate drinkers have an increased risk of developing cirrhosis.
- Brain: Heavy use of alcohol causes a loss of cells in the brain and disrupts connection between nerve cells.
- Stomach: Alcohol stimulates the stomach to secrete gastric acids which inflame the lining of the stomach leading to peptic ulcers.
- Heart: Chronic abuse of alcohol frequently causes hypertension increasing the risk of heart attacks and strokes.
- Reproductive system: Alcohol is a major cause of male impotence. Drinking by women during pregnancy poses serious problems for the fetus.
- Digestive tract: There is increased risk of cancer of the digestive tract with long-term alcohol abuse. Cancers of the liver, stomach, and colon are also more common in alcoholics than the general population.

There are a number of factors which affect the blood alcohol level in your body:

- Speed of drinking. Faster drinking increases the blood alcohol level from a given amount of alcohol.
- Food in the stomach. Food will slow the absorption of alcohol.
- Body weight. A heavier person will have a lower blood alcohol level from a given amount of alcohol.

- History of drinking. Experienced drinkers have higher tolerance (more alcohol is required for the same effect).
- Body chemistry. Individual differences cause the rate of absorption to vary with certain people

If you choose to drink in moderation, you must take charge of your drinking habits to insure that you are drinking in a responsible manner. Some guidelines for responsible use of alcohol are:

- Drink slowly and space your drinks (no more than one per hour).
- Dilute your drinks with water, juices, or soda.
- Eat before or while you are drinking.
- Know your limits and learn to say no.
- Don't drive after drinking.
- Don't drink alone.
- Realize that one drink is equivalent to:
    5 oz. wine
    12 oz. beer
    1 1/2 oz. whiskey
    1 highball or cocktail
All have the same alcohol content.

ANABOLIC STEROID USE

A serious problem among athletes and non-athletes is the use of anabolic steroids to increase muscle mass and strength. Once you know the facts about the dangers of steroids, it should be clear that there is no substitute for implementing a well-designed strength problem.

One of the reasons we hear so much about steroids is because the *Journal of the American Medical Association* (December 1988) published the results of a study revealing that 6.6% of male high school seniors have used steroids to improve appearance and performance.

Those who take steroids are risking a variety of side effects that cannot make it worth the potential gain in muscle size and strength. In addition, athletes can now be barred from athletic competition if the use of steroids is detected. Several studies have reported the link between the early deaths of many athletes and the use of steroids:

- 25 Soviet athletes have died since the 1980 Olympics.
- The last 85 professional football players have died at an average age of 37.
- The average age of death of professional football players has decreased from 72.4 in the 1920s to 54.3 in the 1950s.

Anabolic steroids are synthetic versions of the male hormone testosterone (the primary male sex hormone). Although these hormones can promote muscle development and tissue growth, they have dangerous, undesirable side effects.

Male Side Effects:
- Increase in facial hair and body hair.
- Continued use can lead to impotence.
- Prolonged use can lead to shrinking of the testicles thus causing sterility.
- Development of feminine characteristics—enlarged nipples and increased breast size.

Female Side Effects:
- Development of irreversible masculine characteristics.
- Decreased breast size, increased facial and body hair.
- Menstrual irregularities.
- Deeper voices, darker facial and body hair.

Side Effects for Both Sexes:
- In childhood and adolescence, bone growth is retarded.
- The risk of liver disorders is greatly

increased.

- Increased cardiovascular risks include high blood pressure and artery blockage.
- Many experience dizziness, headaches, sleep disorders, fatigue, irritability, and depression.
- Severe mood swings and aggressive behavior are common.

OSTEOPOROSIS

Osteoporosis is a condition in which the bones have lost so much calcium content that they become weakened and may break easily. With osteoporosis the bones are "thinned out" from the loss of calcium and protein. The bones are the same size but the walls of the bone become thinner and the holes in the spongy bone become larger.

Osteoporosis is a major problem in the United States which primarily affects women over the age of fifty. A report by the *Physician and Sportsmedicine* magazine estimates that approximately 1.2 million fractures occur each year as a result of osteoporosis.

Early symptoms of osteoporosis are a loss of height, back pain or soreness, and a slight curvature of the upper back. The major factors believed to cause the development of osteoporosis are:

- small bones
- not enough calcium
- lack of exercise
- smoking
- not enough estrogen after menopause
- white or Oriental race

Osteoporosis is a special concern for women. A woman's bones are smaller and lighter than a man's, so a greater part of a woman's total bone is lost than a man's. A woman also loses bone faster than a man does, especially after menopause. The reason for this is that at menopause the ovaries

stop making estrogen and the levels of estrogen in the body decrease.

Preventing Osteoporosis

The most successful prevention methods should be started before a woman reaches menopause or, if the ovaries are removed, at that time. The following methods are suggested:

Diet

Calcium intake—If the calcium in the blood falls below a certain level, calcium will be removed from the bones to supply the rest of the body. Calcium also protects the bones by slowing the rate of bone loss. Women need 1000 mg of calcium per day before menopause and 1500 mg after menopause. Vitamin D can aid the absorption of calcium from the stomach.

Vegetable intake—A vegetarian diet is very healthy for the bones.

Meat intake—Eating too much protein found in meat can also lead to excessive bone loss.

Exercise

The bones need to be used to keep them healthy and strengthened. Weight-bearing activities such as walking, aerobic exercise to music, and jogging help slow the rate of bone loss and may also be able to start the growth of new bone.

Avoid Risks

Since cigarettes, alcohol, and caffeine increase bone loss, use of these substances should be limited or stopped. Some prescription drugs can also increase the rate of bone loss. If you are taking drugs such as thyroid medications, diuretics, corticosteroids for arthritis, or anticonvulsants, check with your doctor on how to reduce your risk of bone loss.

UNDERSTANDING AIDS

One's health, wellness and fitness is a personal responsibility that requires the making of choices about a number of issues (i.e., nutrition, exercise, smoking, etc.). One must also take responsibility for avoiding risks that can contribute to a loss of fitness as well as a loss of life.

For instance, there is a great deal you can do to avoid the risk of acquiring AIDS. AIDS stands for Acquired Immune Deficiency Syndrome. This complex illness interferes with the body's ability to fight off disease or infection. Basically, the disease attacks the body's immune system and leaves a person vulnerable to cancers and life-threatening infections.

It is caused by a virus which attacks certain types of white blood cells which play an important role in defending the body from infection or disease. This virus is called HIV (Human Immunodeficiency Virus). However, one must do something to become infected with the virus—AIDS can be avoided. You don't have to get it. At the present time there is no cure or vaccine for AIDS; however, research for an AIDS vaccine to prevent the disease is being explored.

How One Becomes Infected

HIV is a very difficult virus to acquire. A person may become infected with HIV any time the virus enters the bloodstream. It can only be passed from one person to another through the blood, semen, vaginal secretions, or mother's breast milk of an infected person. The direct exchange of these infected fluids causes one to be infected with HIV. The HIV virus is not spread from any form of casual contact (handshakes, touch-ing, hugging, holding hands, or even casual kissing). In addition, the virus is not spread by sweat, tears, urine or saliva. There also have been no known cases of AIDS from sharing kitchens, bathrooms, laundries, eating utensils, or living space. There are three main methods of transmission: sexual activity, contaminated blood, and from mother to child. Before blood screening was performed, many hemophiliacs also became infected with HIV.

It is possible that some people infected with the virus will remain healthy for many years before symptoms of AIDS appear. It may take up to fifteen years for the symptoms to appear in some people.

There has been a dramatic increase of reported cases in the heterosexual population, but the risk is greatest among gay men and intravenous drug users. In 1991, it was estimated that in college-age students, one in 100 males and one in 600 females were HIV positive.

It is possible that some people infected with the virus will remain healthy for many years before symptoms of AIDS appear. It may take ten years or more for the symptoms to appear in some people. Eventually HIV causes the body's immune system to weaken. Once it is weakened, a person infected with HIV can develop many health problems. Extreme weight loss, severe pneumonia, cancers, and damage to the central nervous system signal the onset of AIDS.

Reducing Your Risk of Contracting AIDS

There is no vaccine to protect one from getting AIDS—you must protect yourself. As former U.S. Surgeon General Dr. C. Everett Koop states, the best protection against sexual transmission of HIV is to abstain from sex or to have one uninfected

185

partner who is faithful to you. The more sexual partners a person has, the greater the risk of infection. While proper use of a latex condom during sex can greatly reduce the risk of infection with HIV, they are not 100% safe. Therefore, there is no such thing as completely safe sex with an infected person.

The U.S. Public Health Service recommends a number of precautions to reduce your risk of contracting AIDS. Some of these recommendations are:

- Know your sexual partners.
- Use a condom during sexual activity.
- Avoid intravenous drug use.
- Avoid having unprotected sexual contact with anyone who has AIDS symptoms or is in an AIDS high-risk group.
- Contact your local public health office for more information or use one of the toll-free hotlines:

  National AIDS Hotline: 1-800-342-AIDS (English)

  National AIDS Hotline: 1-800-342-SIDA (Spanish)

LOW BACK PAIN

Back trouble is a common ailment—about 80% of all Americans will have at least one backache during their lifetime. It is so common because being erect puts extra pressure on the vertebrae of the lower back, or lumbar region, where the back curves most and where pain most often occurs. Most backaches develop as we get older (between 30-50 years of age) as the disks in the back lose water and elasticity and thus their ability to absorb shock. In addition, many people tend to become less active and their muscles supporting the back (abdominal and lower back) lose their strength and flexibility. One of the primary causes of lower back pain is an imbalance between muscle groups associated with the back. In particular, one may find that the abdominal muscles are weak, that the hamstring muscles are inflexible, or that the erector muscles are inflexible. Participation in an exercise program to improve these areas of weakness is important in avoiding lower back problems.

Backaches can be caused by a variety of factors such as sudden movement, poor posture, swayback, sideways curvature, improper sitting or lifting, or imbalance between muscle groups. It can range from mild discomfort to excruciating pain. It may be necessary to call a doctor if you have any of the following symptoms: radiating pain, numbness, tingling in an arm or leg, back pain that doesn't improve after two days of rest, or vomiting or fever associated with back pain. For minor soreness and pain in the back, avoiding physically demanding activity may be sufficient. It may help to lie down in order to relieve the pain. As soon as you can comfortably get up, you should gradually resume activity. Aspirin or ibuprofen will help reduce the intensity of pain and inhibit inflammation.

The question of whether to use heat or ice on your back depends on several factors. Icing is recommended immediately after a sudden, wrenching back injury that causes pain in a localized portion of the back. Cold can relax the spasm and minimize the swelling. Ice is recommended for 10-20 minutes several times a day during the first 48 hours. For chronic back discomfort, hot baths or heating pad may be soothing and promote healing. You may need to experiment and find out which treatment is best for you.

A major factor in preventing and rehabilitating lower back problems is performing exercises to stretch and strengthen the back and abdominal muscles. The exercises which follow are recommended to prevent lower back pain.

Exercises for the Lower Back

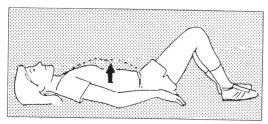

Pelvic Tilt. Lie on your back with knees bent, feet flat on the floor, and arms at your sides. Tighten your stomach muscles and flatten the small of your back against the floor, without pushing down with the legs. Hold for five seconds, then slowly relax.

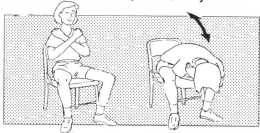

Trunk Flexion, seated. Sitting near the edge of a chair, spread legs apart and cross arms over your chest. Be sure the chair will not slip backward or tip. Tuck your chin and slowly curl your trunk downward. Relax. Uncurl slowly into an upright position, raising your head last.

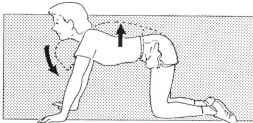

Cat and Camel. On your hands and knees, relax your abdomen and let your back sag. Then tighten your stomach muscles and arch your back.

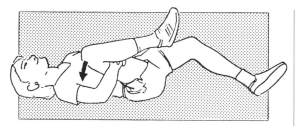

Lying Knee to Chest (One Knee). Assume a lying position with both knees bent. Bring just one knee to your chest and hold onto that knee with your hands. Pull downward until your knee is firmly against your abdomen. Now pull your knee toward your head. Hold for 15-20 seconds. Repeat 2-3 times for each leg.

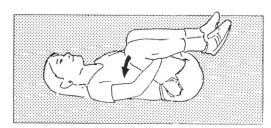

Lying Knee to Chest (Both Knees). Assume a lying position with both knees bent. Bring your knees to your chest one at a time until both knees are near the chest. Place your hands either on top of the knees or directly under your knees (with your forearms resting on the back of your thighs). Pull your knees toward your chest until they are against your abdomen firmly. Now pull your knees toward your head. Hold for 15-20 seconds. Repeat 3-5 times.

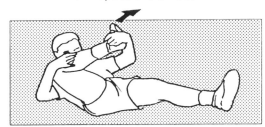

Leg Cradle. Lie on your back. Bend the right knee and cradle the leg at the knee and ankle. Keep the left leg straight. Slowly pull the leg toward the chest while lifting

187

your head off the mat. A pull in the opposite direction (toward the left) will increase the stretch of the right hip. Repeat 15 times on each side.

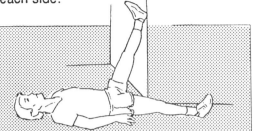

Lying Hamstring Stretch. Start this exercise by elevating your left leg on a portion of the wall that is near a doorway or hall. This allows the right leg to extend beyond the wall into the doorway or hall. Keep the left leg straight; to do so, you may need to place your buttocks several inches away from the wall. Do not arch your lower back but keep if flat and relaxed. Hold for 20-30 seconds. Repeat 2-3 times on each side. You can intensify the stretch by placing your buttocks closer to the wall.

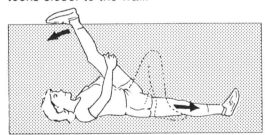

Lying Straight Leg Stretch: Lie on your back; place your hands behind your left thigh near your knee and lace the fingers firmly. Do not extend your lower leg yet; it should still be bent with your heel near your buttocks. Keep your arms extended as you hold your leg. Now attempt to straight out your knee. You should feel a good stretch behind your knee and in the back of your thigh. Hold for 20-30 seconds. Repeat 2-3 times with each leg.

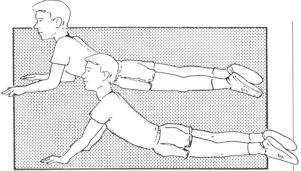

Extension in Lying. Adopt the prone position, press the top half of your body up by straightening your arms, *while the bottom half, from the pelvis down is allowed to move with gravity.* The top half of the body is then lowered. Repeat five times. (Each time exercise is performed you should try to achieve more elevation.)

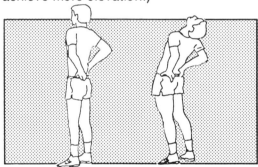

Extension in Standing. Stand with feet apart and place hands (fingers pointing backwards) in the small of your back across the belt line. Lean backwards as far as possible, using the hands as a fulcrum, and then return to neutral position. Repeat two times. Hold position for ten minutes.

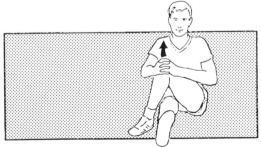

Sitting Stretch. Sit with the right leg straight in front of your left knee, bent and crossed over the right. Pull the left knee across your body toward the opposite shoulder until a stretch is felt on the side of the hip. Hold for a count of 5. Repeat 15 times on each side.

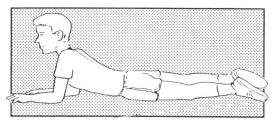

Lying Prone in Extension. Adopt the prone lying position. Place elbow under shoulders and raise the top half of your body. *Keep pelvis and thighs on the mat.* Maintain position for three minutes.

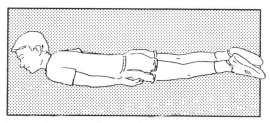

Lying Prone. Adopt the prone lying position with arms along side of trunk, relax buttocks and low back. Maintain position for two minutes.

QUESTIONS AND ANSWERS

There are many authorities arguing that people should take more calcium in their diet as a means of combating osteoporosis. What are the limits?

Dr. Kenneth Cooper writes, "Studies have shown that women can take up to 2000 milligrams of calcium daily and not be at risk of absorbing too much of the mineral." Although the current RDA is 800 mg, this figure is being reevaluated. The Institute of Aerobic Research recommends that women up to age 50 maintain a daily intake of 1,200 mg of calcium and that women over 50 maintain a daily intake of 1,500 mg.

What kinds of people are most apt to develop osteoporosis in later life?

In his book *Preventing Osteoporosis,* Cooper says all men and women over the age of 65 are susceptible. However, particularly high-risk people are heavy drinkers, smokers, female runners who run extensively, people who are allergic to dairy products, fair and slim women, teenagers who subsist on junk foods, postmenopausal women, and users of steroids.

Is exercise during pregnancy unsafe?

Most physicians indicate that if women were exercising before pregnancy, there is no reason they cannot continue during pregnancy. Of course, it is advisable to consult with your doctor to determine the exact exercise program for you. It may be necessary to make certain adjustments in your program from time to time.

If I hurt should I take a "pill" before exercising?

Drug dependency can arise from the regular use of any drug taken for the purpose of killing pain or mood altering. The most commonly used drugs are tobacco, alcohol, caffeine, sedatives, amphetamines, marijuana, cocaine, and hallucinogens.

Each of these substances affects the individual physically and psychologically. Serious damage to the body can occur from most of them when they are taken in large amounts or over an extended period of time. Repeated use also causes the body to develop a tolerance for certain drugs which leads to requiring larger or more frequent doses for the same effect.

As pain killers, drugs mask body signals that are saying some part of your body is hurting and needs a rest for healing purposes. It is quite possible that recovery time will take longer and an injury increased by taking even a simple pain killing drug such as aspirin.

189

What causes the "stitch in the side"?

A "stitch," or sudden, sharp pain in the side or upper part of the abdomen, is a form of muscle cramp. Physicians now believe that a cramp occurs in the diaphragm muscle due to the blood supply being cut off by the pressure from the lungs above and the abdomen below during exercise. The muscle goes into a spasm when it is unable to get enough oxygen. You can help prevent a "stitch" by strengthening your diaphragm and abdominal muscles. To relieve the pain, slow down and push your fingers deep into the site of the pain, just below the last rib on the upper right part of the abdomen. Then bend forward and exhale, puckering your lips. When the pain disappears, you can continue exercising.

What about reducing suits?

By all means, *avoid* rubberized suits. This type of clothing can be dangerous in hot, humid weather. The attire does not aid in weight reduction, only in water loss which is temporary. The best clothing is that which is loose, comfortable, absorbent, and (in hot climates) reflects the sun.

I have heard there are many injuries related to aerobic dance. Is there any truth to the statement?

According to Dr. Kenneth Cooper, aerobic dance injuries have been greatly exaggerated. When one stops to consider that basketball players have been practicing from two to three hours per day on hardwood floors for years with a negligible injury rate, it does not seem logical to think that aerobic dance should be more dangerous. Of course, there aren't many fat basketball players.

What you heard or read may have alluded to research done by Douglas, Kelso, and Bellvei in 1985. They found that approximately 75% of aerobic dance instructors and 43% of students reported injuries due to aerobic dancing.

While the authors in no way question the authenticity of the researchers' statistics, there are a number of variables which must be examined. For example, when participants increased their number of sessions from 3.3 classes per week to 4.7 classes there was a significant increase in injuries.

Another interesting fact was that a soft shock-absorbing floor did not produce a corresponding decrease in injuries. As an example, wood over air is one of the safest of floors, but when the wood is covered with a carpet it assumes one of the highest injury rates. Douglas also stated that when a concrete floor is covered with a carpet it produced an injury rate of 50%.

Douglas also found that barefoot participants had a 65% injury rate as compared to a 49% rate for participants wearing shoes. Vetter et al. found that the two most common sites of injury were the heel and the inner portion of the shins (shin splints.)

In summary, the following factors must be considered in any discussion of dangers or injury risk pertaining to aerobic movement.

- Number of classes participated in per week
- Type of floor and/or covering
- Training techniques (no stretching before and after or progressing too quickly)
- Footwear

Are ankle weights or hand weights safe to use and do they help?

Most experts agree that ankle or shoe weights *increase* chances for injury. The problem is that normally the opposing leg muscles are in balance; i.e., the quadriceps raise the knee while the hamstrings lower it. Running with weights can strengthen the quadriceps out of proportion and possibly damage the hamstrings.

The supposed purpose of carrying such weights while running or walking is to increase or speed up the metabolic cost of running or walking. The research however does not substantiate most claims. One group of researchers studied cardiac patients using the treadmill at speeds of 2.0, 3.0, and 3.5 miles per hour. Patients walked for 5 minutes at each speed with no weights, 1 pound weights, and 3 pound weights. Oxygen uptake and heart rate were monitored. Their conclusion after extensive testing was that the metabolic cost of walking with hand weights was only slightly greater than walking alone. Minimal increases in walking speed would accomplish the same thing but more easily.

Is it true that taking "No Doz" tablets and certain diet pills before exercising could trigger a case of heatstroke?

"No Doz" tablets and many diet pills are basically caffeine, and when ingested by a susceptible person, operating in high temperature, can elevate body temperature to a critical level.

Does jogging produce or contribute to varicose veins?

There are few runners who have varicose veins. What is not known is whether running has a beneficial effect or whether people who have varicose veins do not run. We do know that muscular action plays a significant role in the blood change process in the leg. Running enhances the return flow of blood from the legs.

While exercising last week, I acquired a pain in the center of my chest. Is this normal?

No, it is not. Pain should always be regarded as a red light in any exercise program.

I have heard that most runners who are prone to "stress fractures" have a peculiar style. Is this so?

There are a number of contributing factors involved in stress fractures. These vary from amount and shape of bone mass to structural imbalance and the body's use of calcium. However, many of these runners do display a strong "pavement pounding" running style, i.e., fists clenched, knees high, bending the toes and foot upward just before contact, almost like stamping the heel into the ground.

What is the cause of breast soreness from exercise?

It is generally believed that damage to the underlying muscle and connective tissue due to improperly supported breasts is the major cause of breast soreness during exercise. Properly constructed sport bras can be useful in controlling breast motion and thereby reduce the possibility of injury and discomfort. Other factors in selecting an exercise bra include one without underwires, padding or lace and one that has sufficient lateral support.

Does running cause bone and joint problems?

Two studies as published in the March 7, 1987 issue of the *Journal of the American Medical Association* concluded the following:

- No increased evidence of osteoarthritis could be shown in the runners evaluated.
- Both male and female runners had approximately 40% more bone mineral than a control group.
- Using x-ray examination, no increased prevalence of osteoarthritis could be determined.
- High mileage running in men need not be associated with premature arthritis or degenerative joint disease in the lower extremities.

191

As a female jogger, I am concerned with the problem of developing amenorrhea. What can you tell me about it?

Amenorrhea is the absence or abnormal stoppage of the menstrual cycle. The cause is not known; however, the incidence seems to be more prevalent among those women who train daily for many hours and who have low levels of body fat or weight. If a woman misses her monthly period, however, this does not necessarily mean that she has not ovulated and that she cannot become pregnant.

Can exercise help relieve menstrual cramps?

Exercise can be one of the best remedies to relieve cramps because it helps improve blood circulation in the uterus. It is also believed that exercise produces a release of endorphins, natural opiate-like substances that are produced in the brain and relieve pain just as narcotics do.

How does alcohol affect my fitness?

According to the American College of Sports Medicine, ingestion of alcohol can exert a harmful effect upon a wide variety of psychomotor skills such as reaction time, hand-eye coordination, accuracy, balance, and complex coordination. It also may decrease strength, power, local muscular endurance, speed, and cardiovascular endurance.

The effects of alcohol intake can be rapid because 20% of the alcohol ingested is absorbed directly and immediately into the bloodstream through the stomach walls. The blood then carries it to the brain. In the brain, the thought processes are slowed as alcohol numbs the brain cells. The higher the alcohol concentration, the greater the number of affected cells. The body can metabolize one drink per hour or hour and a half, and nothing can be done to speed up the process.

Additional problems in regard to nutrition are that alcohol contains about seven calories per gram and several of the B vitamins and other nutrients are depleted in meeting the need to metabolize the alcohol. And finally, a serious disease, cirrhosis of the liver, is associated with long-term intake of excessive amounts of alcohol.

Can drinking alcoholic beverages have an effect on my blood pressure?

Yes. Research shows that up to 80% of all patients with high blood pressure who undergo alcoholic rehabilitation programs end up with normal blood pressure 30-60 days after they have quit drinking.

I have heard that females are more susceptible to the effects of alcoholism. True or not?

You have heard right. Two diseases associated with alcoholism, cirrhosis of the liver and hepatitis, seem to develop more rapidly with females, the diseases are more severe, and they develop more rapidly with less alcohol.

How can I tell if I have developed a drug dependency?

Drug dependency can arise from the regular use of any drug taken for the purpose of mood altering. The most commonly used drugs are tobacco, alcohol, caffeine, sedatives, amphetamines, marijuana, cocaine, and hallucinogens.

Each of these substances affects the individual physically and psychologically. Serious damage to the body can occur from most of them when taken in large amounts or over an extended period of time. Repeated use also causes the body to develop a tolerance for certain drugs which leads to requiring larger or more frequent doses for the same effect.

Why do we hear so much about the steroid problem?

One of the reasons we hear so much about steroids is because the *Journal of the American Medical Association* (December 1988) published the results of a study revealing that 6.6% of male high school seniors have used steroids to improve appearance and performance.

The steroid problem arose more than thirty years ago when the Communist countries, most notably Russia, were winning so many Olympic events. Their athletes were being given so much of the male hormone testosterone that many of their male athletes had to be catheterized (that's running a tube up the penis) just to urinate. Their women athletes began to appear so much like men that chromosome tests were mandated by Olympic officials to prove they were really females before they were allowed to compete. Over the years so many horror stories, ranging from cancer to irreversible body changes from the use of steroids have been brought to light, that most intelligent people now gain their strength and muscle the old-fashioned and smart way—they do it by hard work.

What about the dangers of the sun's rays to the eyes?

The sun's rays pose a special danger to the eyes. The UV (ultraviolet) light can be transmitted directly to the retina and cause cataracts as well as macular degeneration. It is estimated that up to 100,000 cataracts that are removed each year may be sun-related and thus preventable. A key to protecting against these rays is the regular use of high-quality sunglasses. Eye specialists recommend wearing UV absorbing sunglasses all year long whenever you are in the sun.

Many people think that the darkest sunglasses must be the best ones. This is not true. You should use the following guidelines when selecting your sunglasses:

- Know how much UV radiation is blocked by the glasses and get those that block up to 400 nanometers. Glasses that conform to the ANSI standard (American National Standard Institute) have "Z-80.3" printed on the frame.
- Violet/blue light rays can be particularly dangerous to the retina of the eye and the best glasses will block most rays.
- Lenses should also block between 75% to 90% of the visible light. The label should state the transmission factor, and it should not exceed 25%. If this information is not on the label, try the glasses on and look in a mirror. Those that are dark enough will not allow you to see your eyes.
- The lenses should be large enough to protect against light that comes in from the top, bottom, and sides of the frames. Wrap-around sunglasses are a good choice.
- Make certain the glasses fit and do not slip down your nose. When glasses slip they can allow more UV rays to enter your eyes.
- Don't just go by how glasses look when you try them on—make certain you are getting the eye protection you need!

REFERENCES

1. Douglas, Jr., R., Kelso, S., and Bellvei, P., *Aerobic Dance Injuries*: A retrospective study of instructors and participants, Physical Sports Medicine 13, (2); 130-144, 1985.
2. Vetter, W., Helfet, D., Spear, B. A. and Matthews, L., *Aerobic Dance Injuries*, Physician and Sports Medicine 13 (2), 1985.

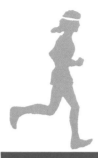

Consumer Beware!

Objectives

- List some of the "tests" to use in determining the validity of information or products.
- Discuss some of the more common techniques employed by "quacks" and dishonest business enterprises.
- Discuss points to consider when joining a fitness club or spa.

Key Words

- Better Business Bureau
- FDA (Food and Drug Administration)
- Quackery
- Testimonial

Fitness, nutrition, and exercise seem to be on everybody's mind these days. Unfortunately, this increased concern has caused the market to be filled with a variety of products claiming to help improve your health. In recent years Americans have been spending billions of dollars on products that not only do nothing for them but may even harm them.

Another problem associated with these fraudulent products is that they keep people from seeking the professional help they really need. Since obviously not all advertisements are false, how does one identify the quack? Health fraud or quackery is the promotion of a medical remedy that doesn't work or hasn't been proven to work.

One of the main agencies responsible for regulating the safety of foods, cosmetics, drugs, and medical devices is the Food and Drug Administration (FDA), which is part of the United States Department of Health and Human Services. Products which are sold with a medical claim must be approved by the FDA before they are marketed. However, many companies carefully avoid making a medical claim even though to the average consumer it may appear they are. Therefore, it is important that each consumer learn to evaluate such advertisements and claims in order to avoid the purchase of worthless and potentially dangerous products.

FACTORS TO CONSIDER

One root of the problem is that people want to believe in miracles, the quick-fix, the easy cure. We are constantly searching for the simple solution and the shortcuts to health and fitness. The wise consumer, on the other hand, will apply the following principles when evaluating a product:

Look out for the "it sounds too good to be true" claim. These claims are characterized by statements such as:
— "a quick and painless cure"
— "a scientific breakthrough"
— "a miracle product"
— "a special, secret, or foreign formula"
— "available only through the mail"
— "a product that cures a variety of ailments"
— "testimonials from satisfied users"
— "a promise to save you money or time"

Watch for certain signals that the product is a fraud such as:
— Claims it is endorsed by the FDA. It is against the law to say that the government endorses any non-prescription drug or medical device.
— Non-prescription drugs that claim to cure cancer or arthritis.
— Claims that a vitamin or mineral supplement will cure a variety of illnesses.
— Products that claim to be endorsed by *Consumer Reports*—this magazine does not allow the use of its name in the marketing of a product.
— Advertisements that describe a health problem (tired, run-down, etc.) and try to sell you a cure.
— Products advertised to "tone your body," "remove fat," or "take off a pound a day" are useless and can be dangerous. There really is no substitute for exercising and proper diet.

Take time to investigate a questionable product or treatment. Good sources of information include:
— your doctor, pharmacist, or other health professional
— your local consumer protection office

— the Better Business Bureau
— your nearest office of the Food and Drug Administration
— if it is a mail order, your local postmaster or the Postal Inspector Service.

Remember there is no federal, state, or local government agency that approves or verifies claims in advertisements before they are printed. Authorities can take action only after the ads appear and this applies to claims of "money back guarantees." Quacks have no intention of responding to refund demands.

EVALUATING INFORMATION

With the numerous articles in magazines and newspapers and the growing list of books on the market which also offer the consumer advice, how does the consumer know what to believe—especially when many claims appear to be contradictory? The following guidelines may be helpful in this evaluation:

— The author's statements should be supported by scientifically valid evidence (watch out for testimonials).
— The article or book should avoid vague medical terms and unsupported promises.
— The author should not be trying to "sell" a particular product.
— Consider who sponsored the study. Did the Dairy Council, Tobacco Industry, or other group with a vested monetary interest back the research and select the researchers?
— Identify the source of the study. Was it conducted by an objective, non-biased group or by those with a special interest in the outcome?

— What technique was used in securing the evidence? Was the study performed according to good research design?
— Are the claims justified according to the evidence collected or are they extended beyond the actual results?
— What are the credentials and background of the individuals conducting the study?
— Does the report conflict with information you previously received from a knowledgeable source? If so, have you resolved the areas of differences and accepted one as being more factual or current?
— Is the magazine or newspaper in which the article appears known for its accuracy and selection of factual material?

FITNESS CLUBS AND SPAS

A special area of interest to many who are anxious to do something about their fitness is that of selecting a fitness or health club. For many who lack the discipline to exercise on their own the fitness club has been the answer. However, in recent years many of these clubs and spas have faced financial ruin.

There is no way to guarantee that a club will not go out of business while you are a member, but the following tips may provide some protection against financial loss due to that possibility:

• Don't buy pre-construction memberships. The club may never open and you may lose your fee.
• Ask for a copy of the membership contract and review it thoroughly. It should contain costs, terms of what you are paying to use the club, a cancel clause,

information about financing agreements. It should contain a provision which allows you to stop paying if you become physically disabled. It should allow you to stop paying if the club closes a branch and does not offer a similar facility within five miles.

- Visit the club and ask for a tour. Meet the instructors and participate in a sample class or two. Plan your visit during the busiest hours and the hours you will most likely be attending. Is it too crowded? Is all the equipment working? Is the club clean? Does it include opportunities for developing cardiovascular fitness (swimming, stationary bicycle, etc.) as well as strength-building devices?

- Make certain that the club meets your state's requirements before signing a contract.

- Realize that if the club closes you will probably not get your membership fee back.

- Be certain you understand the terms of the financing agreement if you are paying for your membership in installments. The club, in most cases, sells these credit agreements to financing companies. If the club closes, you may still be responsible for continuing to make payments to the finance company.

- Get all agreements in writing. Sales people will promise you anything but unless you have it in writing, they may not honor it later.

- If possible, seek a monthly pay-as-you-go plan. The less you pay in advance, the less you will lose if the club goes out of business.

- There is no such thing as a lifetime membership. The contract cannot be longer than three years.

Guidelines for Purchasing Specialized Exercise Equipment

- Purchase from businesses that are reputable—a check with the Better Business Bureau or Chamber of Commerce would be wise.

- Seek the advice of experts or check consumer reports. Your local colleges or universities or YMCAs usually have knowledgeable professionals willing to give you information.

- Make certain you will continue to use the equipment. Many people purchase expensive exercise equipment that ends up gathering dust.

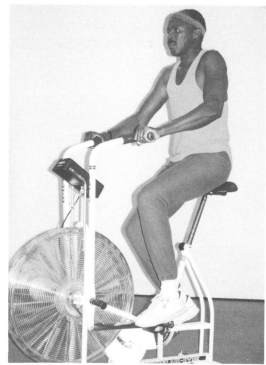

Research the product before buying specialized exercise equipment.

- Avoid impulse buying after seeing a television commercial or receiving a sales pitch. Give yourself a few days to think it over before buying.

- Be certain you know what the equipment can and cannot do, how it works, and how to care for it.

PRODUCTS TO AVOID

The following is just a sample of products that the consumer should avoid because there is no evidence to prove their effectiveness.

- Electrical muscle stimulators which are sold as body toning devices. They are not effective in body toning and can even be dangerous.
- Quick weight loss products can affect your health and harm you. Remember there are no medicines or devices that will let you lose weight effortlessly.
- Cancer cure claims which promote one device or remedy capable of diagnosing or treating all types of cancers are fraudulent.
- The results from tests of hair analysis have not been verified.

QUESTIONS AND ANSWERS

What about tanning salons?

Just one word—don't! The horror stories are too many to count and range from second degree burns to serious eye damage. Excessive ultraviolet light in any form is damaging to the human body. So be smart!

Is massage an effective means of developing fitness and losing weight?

Massage, whether by machine or masseur, will help to increase circulation and may promote relaxation, but has no value in removing fatty tissue or in developing physical fitness.

Are there any "special" foods for building strength?

None that we know of, but there are many quacks convincing a lot of people that they have the "perfect" food. Of course, they want a heavy price.

Do special belts and girdles cause spot reductions?

There is absolutely no evidence to substantiate that the wearing of such clothing causes a loss of weight or spot reductions of adipose tissue. Such clothing may promote sweating and therefore temporary loss of fluids, but it is the exercise that is beneficial. In addition, vibration machines and steam cabinets do not contribute to loss of body fat.

What are continuous passive motion (CPM) tables?

This is the latest in a long line of "machines" that are being touted to eliminate fat, lose inches, and tone muscles—all while lying down! What these high-powered hucksters are pushing are motorized tables that move a person's arms, legs, abdomen, and back. They are most frequently found in high-priced spas and may include as many as six different varieties supposedly to change the entire body.

The reduction of fat in specific areas of the body by vigorous exercise, either by machine or self, does not happen. To lose inches, you must lose weight. And to lose weight demands that you use more calories than you take in. When you do this, your body will utilize energy stored as fat, and the inches will come off, but proportionately.

An additional false claim is that CPM tables decrease blood pressure and enhance circulation. All experts agree there is only one way to increase circulation and that is by active muscle contraction.

SUGGESTED LAB: 31.

GLOSSARY

Glossary

Aerobics - Activities in which the oxygen supply is sufficient to meet the body's demand.

Aerobic metabolism - When adequate oxygen is supplied to the cells during an activity.

Agility - The capacity to change direction of the body quickly and effectively.

AIDS - Acquired Immune Deficiency Syndrome. A disease of the body's immune system.

Alveoli - The tiny air sacs which are part of the lungs.

All or none principle - When a muscle contracts, it contracts maximally.

Amenorrhea - The absence or abnormal cessation of menstruation.

Amino acids - The main structural component of proteins.

Anabolic steroids - Synthetic versions of the male hormone testosterone.

Anaerobic metabolism - When the work demand is greater than the body's capacity.

Anaerobic threshold - A level of work that leads to the accumulation of lactic acid in the muscles and body fluids.

Arteries - Blood vessels that carry blood away from the heart.

Atherosclerosis - The narrowing of arteries due to deposits in the inside arterial walls.

Atherosclerotic disease - An accumulation of fatty plaque and a narrowing of the coronary arteries of the heart.

Balance - A kind of coordination involving vision, reflexes, and the skeletal muscular system which provides the maintenance of equilibrium.

Blood pressure - The pressure that the blood exerts against the internal walls of the arteries.

Body composition - The relative distribution of lean and fat body tissue.

CPM - Continuous passive motion. CPM tables or machines claim to do many things for you. They may relax you, but that is about all.

Calorie - A measure of heat energy. A small calorie represents the amount of heat needed to raise one gram of water one degree Celsius.

Capillaries - The smallest blood vessels that serve as bridges between arteries and veins.

Carbohydrates - One of the key food sources primarily responsible for providing energy. Typical carbohydrates are starches, celluloses, and sugars.

Cardiovascular endurance - The ability of the body to persist in strenuous tasks over a prolonged period of time.

Cartilage - A tough, elastic tissue that acts as a buffer between bones.

Cholesterol - A fatty substance transported in the blood. It is found in all animal fats.

Cirrhosis - A disease in which liver cells are destroyed and liver function is impaired. The disease is frequently associated with excessive consumption of alcohol.

Clonic cramp - A type of muscle cramp characterized by repeated contractions and relaxations of the muscle.

Complete protein - A protein containing all the essential amino acids necessary for growth and repair of tissue.

Concentric contraction - The gradual releasing of a contraction. Example: lifting a weight over one's head.

Constipation - The inability or difficulty in having a bowel movement. A symptom of stress.

Cool down - The period following an exercise session which is designed to slowly decelerate the heart rate, aid the return of blood to the heart (to prevent pooling in the extremities), and reduce the possibility of muscle soreness.

Coordination - The ability to integrate the senses with the muscles so as to produce accurate, smooth, and harmonious body movement.

Cross training - The use of one or more exercise programs to train for fitness.

Diastole - The relaxed phase of a muscular contraction of the heart.

Diastolic - The pressure in the arteries when the heart is relaxing between beats.

Disaccharides - A sugar compound containing two monosaccharides such as sucrose.

Distress - A body response to negative stressors accompanied by a deterioration in performance and health.

Eccentric contraction - The gradual releasing of a contraction. Example: lowering the same weight.

Electrical impedance - A unit used to measure body fat by measuring the electrical resistance of the body tissue.

Electrolyte - Ions that are essential for muscle contraction (sodium, calcium, potassium) because they are capable of carrying an electrical current.

Endorphins - Morphine-like substances secreted by the body which act as pain killers, and is sometimes associated with the feeling of euphoria that frequently occurs during and after exercise.

Ergometer - A device for measuring the work performed by a group of muscles (i.e., stationary bicycle, treadmill).

Eustress - A body response to positive stressors, which usually results in improved performance and health.

External respiration - The exchange of gases between the blood and tissue fluids.

F.D.A. - Food and Drug Administration, a federal agency regulating the safety of foods, drugs, cosmetics, and medical devices.

Fast twitch fiber - A thick strong muscle fiber that responds very quickly.

Fat soluble vitamins - One of two general classes of vitamins that are soluble in fat. They are stored to a greater degree in the body and include Vitamin A, D, E, and K.

Fiber - The indigestible portion of plant food.

Fibrin - Tiny threadlike substances that assist the blood in clotting.

Flexibility - The functional capacity of a joint to move through a normal range of motion.

Frequency - The number of times per day or week that an exercise is performed.

Heat exhaustion - A body response to excessive heat. Caused by lack of fluids resulting in pale, and cool skin, profuse perspiration, weakness, and feeling of weakness.

Heat stroke - A body response to excessive heat resulting in high body temperature, hot dry skin, and frequent unconsciousness. This is a life-threatening problem.

HIV - Human Immunodeficiency Virus associated with AIDS victims.

High density lipoprotein (HDL) - A type of cholesterol containing a high proportion of protein that is transported in the blood. HDL protects against plaque formation.

Hemoglobin - The part of the blood that transports oxygen from the lungs to the capillaries, and returns to the lungs with waste carbon dioxide.

Homeostasis - A state of physical balance; the body constantly attempts to maintain homeostasis.

Hydrogenated fat - Fats or oils that have been treated by a process that adds hydrogen to some of the unfilled bonds, thus hardening the fat or oil. This process makes the fat more saturated.

Hypertension - A blood pressure reading that is consistently higher then the recommended level (high blood pressure).

Imagery - A process of relaxation involving deep breathing, closing the eyes and imagining beautiful or peaceful scenery.

Incomplete protein - A protein lacking one or more of the essential amino acids.

Interval training - Alternating periods of high intensity work with periods of rest or recovery.

Insomnia - Inability or difficulty in falling asleep.

Isokinetic contraction - A muscular contraction executed at a constant speed and with maximal tension in the muscle throughout the full range of motion.

Isometric contraction - A muscular contraction in which there is tension but no noticeable movement at the joints. This is often called a static contraction and the muscle length remains constant.

Isotonic contraction - A muscular contraction in which the muscle shortens or lengthens as it moves a constant weight. This is often called a dynamic contraction with the shortening called concentric contraction and the lengthening called eccentric contraction.

Ligament - Connective tissue that binds bones together.

Low density lipoprotein (LDL) - A type of cholesterol containing a higher proportion of cholesterol to protein than HDL. LDL is a lightweight molecule which is transported in the blood and promotes the formation of plaque on the walls of the arteries.

Maximum oxygen uptake (VO$_2$) - The maximum rate at which oxygen can be taken in and utilized per minute during exercise.

METS - A measurement unit for energy expenditure.

Minerals - Inorganic compounds that are essential for normal body function.

Monosaccharides - The simple sugars such as glucose, fructose, and galactose.

Monounsaturated fat - Fat capable of absorbing two or more hydrogen ions. They are usually liquid and derived from plant sources.

Muscle - A band of contractile fibers held together by a sheath of connective tissues.

Muscle recruitment - The ability of the body to call upon additional muscle units to perform a task.

Muscular endurance - The ability to continue selected muscle group movements for prolonged periods of time.

Muscular strength - The ability of a muscle group to contract against a resistance.

Myofibrils - The contractile units of muscle fibers. They shorten or lengthen the muscle.

Myoglobin - Facilitates the absorption of oxygen from the blood into the muscle cells.

Obesity - An excessive accumulation of body fat. It usually refers to those who are 20-30% or greater above the average weight for their size.

Osteoporosis - A condition in which the bones are weakened by a deficiency in calcium.

Overload - Any type of physical activity which exercises a muscle or group of muscles beyond that which it normally encounters.

Oxygen debt - The volume of oxygen consumed during the recovery.

PNF stretch (proprioceptive neuromuscular facilitation) - A group of stretching techniques which involve alternating contractions and relaxations of the opposing muscle groups.

Polyunsaturated fat - Fat capable of absorbing four or more hydrogen ions. They are usually liquid and derived from plant sources.

Power - The speed of muscle contraction which, when combined with strength, provides an explosive type of movement.

Progression - The process in which the amount of work done is periodically increased as the body adapts to the current workload.

Proteins - One of the key food sources which provides the basic building components for the cells. Proteins are formed by various combinations of amino acids.

RDA (Recommended Dietary Allowances) - The levels of intake of essential nutrients considered to be adequate to meet the known nutritional needs of practically all healthy people.

Reaction time - The time required to respond or initiate a movement as a result of a given stimulus.

Resting heart rate - The number of times the heart beats per minute when at rest.

Retrogression - A period during training in which performance seems to decrease or reach a temporary plateau.

Residual volume - The air remaining in the lungs after a complete exhalation.

Sarcolemma - The cell membrane of the muscle cell.

Sarcoplasm - The fluid part of the muscle cell.

Saturated fat - Fat that has all chemical bonds filled with hydrogen. They are usually solid and derived mainly from animal sources.

Set point - The weight you normally maintain when you are not consciously attempting to control it.

Shin splints - A condition caused by tearing or inflammation of the muscles and tendons of the lower leg.

Skinfold caliper - A device used to measure the amount of fat between two layers of skin.

Specificity - The principle of training which states that the improvements made are specific to the type of training program which is used.

Speed - The ability to move one's body from one point to another.

Sphygmomanometer - A device for measuring blood pressure.

Spirometer - A device used to measure the vital lung capacity.

Spot reducing - The idea that exercising a specific body part will facilitate the loss of body fat from that spot. Studies show this does not happen.

Sprain - An injury to ligaments or the capsule-like sac that surrounds a joint.

Static contraction - When muscles which are antagonistic to each other contract with equal strength, or when the muscle is held in a partial or complete contraction against another immovable force.

Steady state - When a balance between supply and demand of oxygen is reached.

Stress - A non-specific response of the body to any demand made upon it.

Stressor - A stimulus that initiates the stress response; may be phsyiological, psychological, or social.

Stroke - Occurs when the blood supply is cut off to part of the brain.

Systole - the heart's normal contraction, squeezing blood from its chambers.

Systolic - The pressure produced in the artery each time the blood is forcibly pushed from the heart into the large blood vessels.

Target heart rate - The optimal rate at which the heart should be beating during exercise in order to receive a training benefit (i.e., cardiovascular improvement).

Tonic cramp - A continuous and steady contraction of a muscle, characterized by extreme pain.

Trachea - The windpipe.

Training - An exercise program designed to improve the physical functioning of an individual.

Triglycerides - The storage medium for fatty acids in the body. The fatty acids are packaged in threes with glycerol to make triglycerides.

Unsaturated fat - Fat that can absorb more hydrogen. They are usually liquid and derived from plant sources.

Use and disuse - If you train, there will be improvement or maintenance; if not physical performance will decline.

VLDL - The lightest fat-protein molecule in the blood stream which carries the largest amount of triglycerides.

Veins - Blood vessels carrying blood back to the heart.

Vital lung capacity - The maximum volume of air which can be forcefully expelled from the lungs after a maximum inhalation.

Vitamins - Organic compounds essential for the normal metabolic functioning of the body.

Warmup - The preparation phase of an exercise session in which the body is prepared for the stress which will be placed upon it.

Water soluble vitamins - One of the two general classes of vitamins that soluble in water. They include the B vitamins and vitamin C.

White blood cells - Smaller in number than red cells, these cells are primarily responsible for defending the body against infection.

APPENDICES

APPENDIX A

Fitness Assessments

Test		Page
A-1	Rockport Fitness Walking Test (1 mile walk)	208
A-2	Bicycle Ergometer	209
A-3	Harvard Step Test	213
A-4	One-Minute Step Test	215
A-5	Vital Lung Capacity Assessment	216
A-6	Body Fat Analysis with Skinfold Calipers	217
A-7	Flexibility Assessments	220
A-8	Muscular Strength and Endurance Assessments	222
A-9	Blood Pressure	227

A-1

ROCKPORT FITNESS WALKING TEST™

(One Mile Walk)

Preliminary Procedure

1. Wear appropriate exercise clothes—especially comfortable exercise shoes (i.e., walking or jogging shoes).

2. Check your pulse rate. (See Chapter Two for directions.)

3. Stretch for 5-10 minutes to warmup for the test.

Action

1. Walk a mile as fast as comfortably possible trying to maintain a steady pace.

2. As soon as you complete the mile, check your pulse for 15 seconds (multiply by four to get a one-minute count). Record this number.

3. Record your time for completing the mile.

4. Stretch for 5-10 minutes to cool down.

Valuation

1. Refer to the charts in Appendix B-2 to determine your relative fitness level based on age and sex.

2. The fitness level determined by the test can be used as a guideline for beginning your fitness program.

A-2

BICYCLE ERGOMETER

Preliminary Procedure

1. One should not exercise before the test and should refrain from eating two hours before and smoking three hours before the test.
2. Set the seat of the bicycle so that the arch of the foot is in the middle of the pedal and the leg is in full extension. Make note of the number on the shaft of the seat so that you can adjust the seat accordingly in the future.
3. Set the RPM (revolutions per minute) at 120 and "free wheel" for 1-2 minutes warmup.
4. Set the RPM at 60 and the work load at 450 KPM* for women and 600 KPM for men. After initial practice on the bike these work loads may need to be adjusted so that the load is great enough to allow you to reach but not exceed your target heart rate zone.

Action

1. On signal, begin pedaling and maintain a constant rate of work at designated level.
2. After 45 seconds, a partner using a stethoscope will check your pulse or heart rate for 15 seconds and multiply by four to get your BPM (beats per minute).
3. This procedure is continued for each minute of the test until a "steady state" is achieved. The test may be terminated if after the sixth minute the difference between the BPM for the fifth and sixth minutes does not vary more than five beats. If the difference is greater than five beats, the test is continued until the difference between the last two scores is less than five.
4. If stabilization does not occur within the first ten minutes, the test should be discontinued and repeated on another day.
5. Extreme care must be taken as the upper limit of the individual's target rate is being reached. The instructor should be alerted at once.
6. After stabilization occurs, reset the RPM to 120 and cool down by "free wheeling" for 1-2 minutes.

Incorrect Procedure or Inadequate Performance

1. Failing to maintain appropriate workload throughout the test.
2. Stopping test before stabilization is achieved.

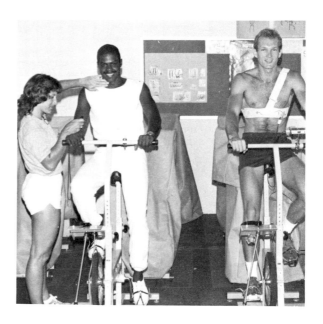

Valuation

Using the accompanying tables (Tables 1, 2 and 3):
1. Calculate the liters per minute of work based on heart rate achieved for that workload (Table 1).
2. Correct this value of age, using the correction factor in Table 2. Multiply the correction factor times liters per minute.
3. Next determine oxygen consumption (Ml/Kg/Min*) using the chart which makes the adjustment for body size (Table 3).
4. Record the fitness rating based on sex and age for level of oxygen consumption (Appendix B-2).

* KPM represents Kilipond Meters per Minute which indicates a unit of work on the bicycle. On the bicycle test, this number indicates the workload at which the individual performs the test.

**Ml/Kg/Min represents your maximum oxygen uptake divided by body weight in kilograms. This adjustment is necessary because the amount of oxygen needed for any task is a function of size. Oxygen uptake values can only be compared if weight is equalized among individuals.

TABLE 1
PREDICTION OF MAXIMAL OXYGEN UPTAKE FROM HEART RATE AND WORKLOAD ON A BICYCLE ERGOMETER*

Part A - Men

Maximal oxygen uptake, liters min^{-1}

Heart rate	300 kpm/min 50W	600 kpm/min 100W	900 kpm/min 150W	1200 kpm/min 200W	1500 kpm/min 250W
120	2.2	3.5	4.8		
121	2.2	3.4	4.7		
122	2.2	3.4	4.6		
123	2.1	3.4	4.6		
124	2.1	3.3	4.5	6.0	
125	2.0	3.2	4.4	5.9	
126	2.0	3.2	4.4	5.8	
127	2.0	3.1	4.3	5.7	
128	2.0	3.1	4.2	5.6	
129	1.9	3.0	4.2	5.6	
130	1.9	3.0	4.1	5.5	
131	1.9	2.9	4.0	5.4	
132	1.8	2.9	4.0	5.3	
133	1.8	2.8	3.9	5.3	
134	1.8	2.8	3.9	5.2	
135	1.7	2.8	3.8	5.1	
136	1.7	2.7	3.8	5.0	
137	1.7	2.7	3.7	5.0	
138	1.6	2.7	3.7	4.9	
139	1.6	2.6	3.6	4.8	
140	1.6	2.6	3.6	4.8	6.0
141		2.6	3.5	4.7	5.9
142		2.5	3.5	4.6	5.8
143		2.5	3.4	4.6	5.7
144		2.5	3.4	4.5	5.7
145		2.4	3.4	4.5	5.6
146		2.4	3.3	4.4	5.6
147		2.4	3.3	4.4	5.5
148		2.4	3.2	4.3	5.4
149		2.3	3.2	4.3	5.4
150		2.3	3.2	4.2	5.3
151		2.3	3.1	4.2	5.2
152		2.3	3.1	4.1	5.2
153		2.2	3.0	4.1	5.1
154		2.2	3.0	4.0	5.1
155		2.2	3.0	4.0	5.0
156		2.2	2.9	4.0	5.0
157		2.1	2.9	3.9	4.9
158		2.1	2.9	3.9	4.9
159		2.1	2.8	3.8	4.8
160		2.1	2.8	3.8	4.8
161		2.0	2.8	3.7	4.7
162		2.0	2.8	3.7	4.6
163		2.0	2.8	3.7	4.6
164		2.0	2.7	3.6	4.5
165		2.0	2.7	3.6	4.5
166		1.9	2.7	3.6	4.5
167		1.9	2.6	3.5	4.4
168		1.9	2.6	3.5	4.4
169		1.9	2.6	3.5	4.3
170		1.8	2.6	3.4	4.3

Part B - Women

Maximal oxygen uptake, liters min^{-1}

Heart rate	300 kpm/min 50W	450 kpm/min 75W	600 kpm/min 100W	750 kpm/min 125W	900 kpm/min 150W
120	2.6	3.4	4.1	4.8	
121	2.5	3.3	4.0	4.8	
122	2.5	3.2	3.9	4.7	
123	2.4	3.1	3.9	4.6	
124	2.4	3.1	3.8	4.5	
125	2.3	3.0	3.7	4.4	
126	2.3	3.0	3.6	4.3	
127	2.2	2.9	3.5	4.2	
128	2.2	2.8	3.5	4.2	4.8
129	2.2	2.8	3.4	4.1	4.8
130	2.1	2.7	3.4	4.0	4.7
131	2.1	2.7	3.4	4.0	4.6
132	2.0	2.7	3.3	3.9	4.5
133	2.0	2.6	3.2	3.8	4.4
134	2.0	2.6	3.2	3.8	4.4
135	2.0	2.6	3.1	3.7	4.3
136	1.9	2.5	3.1	3.6	4.2
137	1.9	2.5	3.0	3.6	4.2
138	1.8	2.4	3.0	3.5	4.1
139	1.8	2.4	2.9	3.5	4.0
140	1.8	2.4	2.8	3.4	4.0
141	1.8	2.3	2.8	3.4	3.9
142	1.7	2.3	2.8	3.3	3.9
143	1.7	2.2	2.7	3.3	3.8
144	1.7	2.2	2.7	3.2	3.8
145	1.6	2.2	2.7	3.2	3.7
146	1.6	2.2	2.6	3.2	3.7
147	1.6	2.1	2.6	3.1	3.6
148	1.6	2.1	2.6	3.1	3.6
149		2.1	2.6	3.0	3.5
150		2.0	2.5	3.0	3.5
151		2.0	2.5	3.0	3.4
152		2.0	2.5	2.9	3.4
153		2.0	2.4	2.9	3.3
154		2.0	2.4	2.8	3.3
155		1.9	2.4	2.8	3.2
156		1.9	2.3	2.8	3.2
157		1.9	2.3	2.7	3.2
158		1.8	2.3	2.7	3.1
159		1.8	2.2	2.7	3.1
160		1.8	2.2	2.6	3.0
161		1.8	2.2	2.6	3.0
162		1.8	2.2	2.6	3.0
163		1.7	2.2	2.6	2.9
164		1.7	2.1	2.5	2.9
165		1.7	2.1	2.5	2.9
166		1.7	2.1	2.5	2.8
167		1.6	2.1	2.4	2.8
168		1.6	2.0	2.4	2.8
169		1.6	2.0	2.4	2.8
170		1.6	2.0	2.4	2.7

TABLE 2

AGE CORRECTION FACTORS FOR ESTIMATING MAXIMAL OXYGEN UPTAKE

AGE	FACTOR
15	1.10
25	1.00
35	0.87
40	0.83
45	0.78
50	0.75
55	0.71
60	0.68
65	0.65

* The value should be corrected for age according to Table 2

Source: Astrand, P.O., *Ergometry Test of Physical Fitness,* Varberg, Sweden: Monark-Crescent AB.

TABLE 3

CALCULATION OF MAXIMUM OXYGEN UPTAKE - ML/KG X MIN

Body Weight pound	kg	Maximum Oxygen Uptake - litres/min. 1.5	1.6	1.7	1.8	1.9	2.0	2.1	2.2	2.3	2.4	2.5	2.6	2.7	2.8	2.9	3.0	3.1	3.2	3.3	3.4	3.5	3.6	3.7
96		33	35	37	39	41	43	45	47	49	51	53	55	57	59	61	63	65	67	69	71	73	75	77
99		32	34	36	38	40	42	44	46	48	50	52	54	56	58	60	62	64	66	68	70	72	74	76
101		32	34	36	38	40	42	44	46	48	50	52	54	56	58	60	62	64	66	68	70	72	74	76
103		31	33	35	37	39	41	43	45	47	49	51	53	55	57	59	61	63	65	67	69	71	73	75
106		31	33	35	37	39	41	43	45	47	49	51	53	55	57	59	61	63	65	67	69	71	73	75
108		30	32	34	36	38	40	42	44	46	48	50	52	54	56	58	60	62	64	66	68	70	72	74
110	50	30	32	34	36	38	40	42	44	46	48	50	52	54	56	58	60	62	64	66	68	70	72	74
112	51	29	31	33	35	37	39	41	43	45	47	49	51	53	55	57	59	61	63	65	67	69	71	73
115	52	29	31	33	35	37	38	40	42	44	46	48	50	52	54	56	58	60	62	63	65	67	69	71
117	53	28	30	32	34	36	38	40	42	43	45	47	49	51	53	55	57	58	60	62	64	66	68	70
119	54	28	30	31	33	35	37	39	41	43	44	46	48	50	52	54	56	57	59	61	63	65	67	69
121	55	27	29	31	33	35	36	38	40	42	44	45	47	49	51	53	55	56	58	60	62	64	65	67
123	56	27	29	30	32	34	36	38	39	41	43	45	46	48	50	52	54	55	57	59	61	63	64	66
126	57	26	28	30	32	33	35	37	39	40	42	44	46	47	49	51	53	54	56	58	60	61	63	65
128	58	26	28	29	31	33	34	36	38	40	41	43	45	47	48	50	52	53	55	57	59	60	62	64
130	59	25	27	29	31	32	34	36	37	39	41	42	44	46	47	49	51	53	54	56	58	59	61	63
132	60	25	27	28	30	32	33	35	37	38	40	42	43	45	47	48	50	52	53	55	57	58	60	62
134	61	25	26	28	30	31	33	34	36	38	39	41	43	44	46	48	49	51	52	54	56	57	59	61
137	62	24	26	27	29	31	32	34	35	37	39	40	42	44	45	47	48	50	52	53	55	56	58	60
139	63	24	25	27	29	30	32	33	35	37	38	40	41	43	44	46	48	49	51	52	54	56	57	59
141	64	23	25	27	28	30	31	33	34	36	38	39	41	42	44	45	47	48	50	52	53	55	56	58
143	65	23	25	26	28	29	31	32	34	35	37	38	40	42	43	45	46	48	49	51	52	54	55	57
146	66	23	24	26	27	29	30	32	33	35	36	38	39	41	42	44	45	47	48	50	52	53	55	56
148	67	22	24	25	27	28	30	31	33	34	36	37	39	40	42	43	45	46	48	49	51	52	54	55
150	68	22	24	25	26	28	29	31	32	34	35	37	38	40	41	43	44	46	47	49	50	51	53	54
152	69	22	23	25	26	28	29	30	32	33	35	36	38	39	41	42	43	45	46	48	49	51	52	54
154	70	21	23	24	26	27	29	30	31	33	34	36	37	39	40	41	43	44	46	47	49	50	51	53
157	71	21	23	24	25	27	28	30	31	32	34	35	37	38	39	41	42	44	45	46	48	49	51	52
159	72	21	22	24	25	26	28	29	31	32	33	35	36	38	39	40	42	43	44	46	47	49	50	51
161	73	21	22	23	25	26	27	29	30	32	33	34	36	37	38	40	41	42	44	45	47	48	49	51
163	74	20	22	23	24	26	27	28	30	31	32	34	35	36	38	39	41	42	43	45	46	47	49	50
165	75	20	21	23	24	25	27	28	29	31	32	33	35	36	37	39	40	41	43	44	45	47	48	49
168	76	20	21	22	24	25	26	28	29	30	32	33	34	36	37	38	39	41	42	43	45	46	47	49
170	77	19	21	22	23	25	26	27	29	30	31	32	34	35	36	38	39	40	42	43	44	45	47	48
172	78	19	21	22	23	24	26	27	28	29	31	32	33	35	36	37	38	40	41	42	44	45	46	47
174	79	19	20	22	23	24	25	27	28	29	30	32	33	34	35	37	38	39	41	42	43	44	46	47
176	80	19	20	21	23	24	25	26	28	29	30	31	33	34	35	36	38	39	40	41	43	44	45	46
179	81	19	20	21	22	23	25	26	27	28	30	31	32	33	35	36	37	38	40	41	42	43	44	46
181	82	18	20	21	22	23	24	26	27	28	29	30	32	33	34	35	37	38	39	40	41	43	44	45
183	83	18	19	20	22	23	24	25	27	28	29	30	31	33	34	35	36	37	39	40	41	42	43	45
185	84	18	19	20	21	23	24	25	26	27	29	30	31	32	33	35	36	37	38	39	40	42	43	44
187	85	18	19	20	21	22	24	25	26	27	28	29	31	32	33	34	35	36	38	39	40	41	42	44
190	86	17	19	20	21	22	23	24	26	27	28	29	30	31	33	34	35	36	37	38	40	41	42	43
192	87	17	18	20	21	22	23	24	25	26	28	29	30	31	32	33	34	36	37	38	39	40	41	43
194	88	17	18	19	20	22	23	24	25	26	27	28	30	31	32	33	34	35	36	38	39	40	41	42
196	89	17	18	19	20	21	22	24	25	26	27	28	29	30	31	33	34	35	36	37	38	39	40	42
198	90	17	18	19	20	21	22	23	24	26	27	28	29	30	31	32	33	34	36	37	38	39	40	41
201	91	16	18	19	20	21	22	23	24	25	26	27	29	30	31	32	33	34	35	36	37	38	40	41
203	92	16	17	18	20	21	22	23	24	25	26	27	28	29	30	32	33	34	35	36	37	38	39	40
205	93	16	17	18	19	20	22	23	24	25	26	27	28	29	30	31	32	33	34	35	37	38	39	40
207	94	16	17	18	19	20	21	22	23	24	26	27	28	29	30	31	32	33	34	35	36	37	38	39
209	95	16	17	18	19	20	21	22	23	24	25	26	27	28	29	31	32	33	34	35	36	37	38	39
212	96	16	17	18	19	20	21	22	23	24	25	26	27	28	29	30	31	32	33	34	35	36	38	39
214	97	15	16	18	19	20	21	22	23	24	25	26	27	28	29	30	31	32	33	34	35	36	37	38
216	98	15	16	17	18	19	20	21	22	23	24	26	27	28	29	30	31	32	33	34	35	36	37	38
218	99	15	16	17	18	19	20	21	22	23	24	25	26	27	28	29	30	31	32	33	34	35	36	37
220	100	15	16	17	18	19	20	21	22	23	24	25	26	27	28	29	30	31	32	33	34	35	36	37

TABLE 3

CALCULATION OF MAXIMUM OXYGEN UPTAKE, *Continued*

Body Weight pound		Maximum Oxygen Uptake - litres/min. 3.8	3.9	4.0	4.1	4.2	4.3	4.4	4.5	4.6	4.7	4.8	4.9	5.0	5.1	5.2	5.3	5.4	5.5	5.6	5.7	5.8	5.9	6.0
96		79	81	83	85	87	89	91	93	95	97	99	101	103	105	107	109	111	113	115	117	119	121	123
99		78	80	82	84	86	88	90	92	94	96	98	100	102	104	106	108	110	112	114	116	118	120	122
101		78	80	82	84	86	88	90	92	94	96	98	100	102	104	106	108	110	112	114	116	118	120	122
103		77	79	81	83	85	87	89	91	93	95	97	99	101	103	105	107	109	111	113	115	117	119	121
106		77	79	81	83	85	87	89	91	93	95	97	99	101	103	105	107	109	111	113	115	117	119	121
108		76	78	80	82	84	86	88	90	92	94	96	98	100	102	104	106	108	110	112	114	116	118	120
110	50	76	78	80	82	84	86	88	90	92	94	96	98	100	102	104	106	108	110	112	114	116	118	120
112	51	75	76	78	80	82	84	86	88	90	92	94	96	98	100	102	104	106	108	110	112	114	116	118
115	52	73	75	77	79	81	83	85	87	88	90	92	94	96	98	100	102	104	106	108	110	112	113	115
117	53	72	74	75	77	79	81	83	85	87	89	91	92	94	96	98	100	102	104	106	108	109	111	113
119	54	70	72	74	76	78	80	81	83	85	87	89	91	93	94	96	98	100	102	104	106	107	109	111
121	55	69	71	73	75	76	78	80	82	84	85	87	89	91	93	95	96	98	100	102	104	105	107	109
123	56	68	70	71	73	75	77	79	80	82	84	86	88	89	91	93	95	96	98	100	102	104	105	107
126	57	67	68	70	72	74	75	77	79	81	82	84	86	88	89	91	93	95	96	98	100	102	104	105
128	58	66	67	69	71	72	74	76	78	79	81	83	84	86	88	90	91	93	95	97	98	100	102	103
130	59	64	66	68	69	71	73	75	76	78	80	81	83	85	86	88	90	92	93	95	97	98	100	102
132	60	63	65	67	68	70	72	73	75	77	78	80	82	83	85	87	88	90	92	93	95	97	98	100
134	61	62	64	66	67	69	70	72	74	75	77	79	80	82	84	85	87	89	90	92	93	95	97	98
137	62	61	63	65	66	68	69	71	73	74	76	77	79	81	82	84	85	87	89	90	92	94	95	97
139	63	60	62	63	65	67	68	70	71	73	75	76	78	79	81	83	84	86	87	89	90	92	94	95
141	64	59	61	63	64	66	67	69	70	72	73	75	77	78	80	81	83	84	86	88	89	91	92	94
143	65	58	60	62	63	65	66	68	69	71	72	74	75	77	78	80	82	83	85	86	88	89	91	92
146	66	58	59	61	62	64	65	67	68	70	71	73	74	76	77	79	80	82	83	85	86	88	89	91
148	67	57	58	60	61	63	64	66	67	69	70	72	73	75	76	78	79	81	82	84	85	87	88	90
150	68	56	57	59	60	62	63	65	66	68	69	71	72	74	75	76	78	79	81	82	84	85	87	88
152	69	55	57	58	59	61	62	64	65	66	67	69	71	71	73	74	76	77	79	80	81	83	84	86
154	70	54	56	57	59	60	61	63	64	66	67	69	70	70	72	73	75	76	77	79	80	82	83	85
157	71	54	55	56	58	59	61	62	63	65	66	68	69	70	72	73	75	76	77	79	80	82	83	85
159	72	53	54	56	57	58	60	61	63	64	65	67	68	69	71	72	74	75	76	78	79	81	82	83
161	73	52	53	55	56	58	59	60	62	63	64	66	67	68	70	71	73	74	75	77	78	79	80	81
163	74	51	53	54	55	57	58	59	61	62	64	65	66	68	69	70	72	73	74	76	77	78	80	81
165	75	51	52	53	55	56	57	59	60	61	63	64	65	67	68	69	71	72	73	75	76	77	79	80
168	76	50	51	53	54	55	57	58	59	61	62	63	64	66	67	68	70	71	72	74	75	76	78	79
170	77	49	51	52	53	55	56	57	58	60	61	62	64	65	66	68	69	70	71	73	74	75	77	78
172	78	49	50	51	53	54	55	56	58	59	60	62	63	64	65	67	68	69	71	72	73	74	76	77
174	79	48	49	51	52	53	54	56	57	58	59	61	62	63	65	66	67	68	70	71	72	73	75	76
176	80	48	49	50	51	53	54	55	56	58	59	60	61	63	64	65	66	68	69	70	71	72	74	75
179	81	47	48	49	51	52	53	54	56	57	58	59	60	62	63	64	65	67	68	69	70	72	73	74
181	82	46	48	49	50	51	52	54	55	56	57	59	60	61	62	63	65	66	67	68	70	71	72	73
183	83	46	47	48	49	51	52	53	54	55	57	58	59	60	61	63	64	65	66	67	69	70	71	72
185	84	45	46	48	49	50	51	52	54	55	56	57	58	60	61	62	63	64	65	67	68	69	70	71
187	85	45	46	47	48	49	51	52	53	54	55	56	58	59	60	61	62	64	65	66	67	68	69	71
190	86	44	45	47	48	49	50	51	52	53	55	56	57	58	59	60	62	63	64	65	66	67	69	70
192	87	44	45	46	47	48	49	51	52	53	54	55	56	57	59	60	61	62	63	64	66	67	68	69
194	88	43	44	45	47	48	49	50	51	52	53	55	56	57	58	59	60	61	63	64	65	66	67	68
196	89	43	44	45	46	47	48	49	51	52	53	54	55	56	57	58	60	61	62	63	64	65	66	67
198	90	42	43	44	46	47	48	49	50	51	52	53	54	56	57	58	59	60	61	62	63	64	66	67
201	91	42	43	44	45	46	47	48	49	51	52	53	54	55	56	57	58	59	60	62	63	64	65	66
203	92	41	42	43	45	46	47	48	49	50	51	52	53	54	55	57	58	59	60	61	62	63	64	65
205	93	41	42	43	44	45	46	47	48	49	51	52	53	54	55	56	57	58	59	60	61	62	63	65
207	94	40	41	43	44	45	46	47	48	49	50	51	52	53	54	55	56	57	59	60	61	62	63	64
209	95	40	41	42	43	44	45	46	47	48	49	51	52	53	54	55	56	57	58	59	60	61	62	63
212	96	40	41	42	43	44	45	46	47	48	49	50	51	52	53	54	55	56	57	58	59	60	61	63
214	97	39	40	41	42	43	44	45	46	47	48	49	51	52	53	54	55	56	57	58	59	60	61	62
216	98	39	40	41	42	43	44	45	46	47	48	49	50	51	52	53	54	55	56	57	58	59	60	61
218	99	38	39	40	41	42	43	44	45	46	47	48	49	51	52	53	54	55	56	57	58	59	60	61
220	100	38	39	40	41	42	43	44	45	46	47	48	49	50	51	52	53	54	55	56	57	58	59	60

A-3

HARVARD STEP TEST

The Harvard Step Test was developed in 1943 at the Harvard University Fatigue Laboratories in Cambridge, Massachusetts, by Lucien Brouha and associates, as a relatively simple, easily administered measure of cardiovascular endurance.

The test is based upon the premise that for a given work task, the person with a higher level of cardiovascular fitness will have a smaller increase in heart rate and, that following the task, heart rate will return to normal much faster than for a person who has a lower level of cardiovascular fitness.

Purpose
To measure cardiovascular fitness

Objectives
1. To provide for self-evaluation.
2. To provide motivation for self-improvement
3. To provide a laboratory experience for a better understanding of the relationship between heart rate and cardiovascular endurance.

Validity
The original evidence of validity was based upon endurance in treadmill running, heart rate, and blood lactate level.

Description of the Test
The test consists of stepping up and down on a bench or box, 20 inches high for males and 16 inches high for females, at the rate of 30 times per minute for a period of five minutes, or until unable to continue the exercise at the prescribed rate.

Scoring
Two forms are in general use—the long form (also known as the slow form) and the short form (also known as the rapid form). In both forms, scoring is based upon recovery pulse rate and no reference is made to resting or pretest pulse rate.

Long Form Scoring. Recovery pulse rate is counted three times for 30 seconds each time, at 1, 2, and 3 minutes following cessation of the exercise. The sum of these three pulse rates is used in calculating test results.

Short Form Scoring. At one minute following cessation of the exercise, a 30-second pulse count is made, and this one pulse count is used in

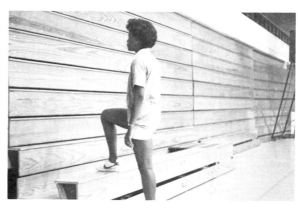

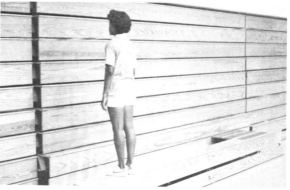

calculating test results.

Pulse counts in both the long form and the short form developed as simplifications of the original method of counting pulse beats for ten minutes following cessation of the exercise.

Scoring Formulae and Classification of Scores:
1. **Long form**

$$\text{Index of Fitness} = \frac{\text{Time of Stepping in Seconds X 100}}{2 \text{ (Sum of 3 Pulse Counts)}}$$

Classification Scores:

Below 55	Poor
55-64	Low Average
65-79	High Average
80-90	Good
Above 90	Excellent

Note: T scores for the Harvard Step Test were developed from the above scale which represents approximately 8,000 college freshmen.

2. Short form

$$\text{Index of Fitness} = \frac{\text{Time of Stepping X 100}}{5.5 \text{ X Pulse Count}}$$

Scoring: Refer to the classifications above.

TEST INSTRUCTIONS

Preparatory Procedure

1. Assistant counts and records resting or pre-test pulse rate for 30 seconds. Palpate radial artery (hollow of wrist just above thumb) or carotid artery (in the neck alongside the wind-pipe).

2. Starting position: Stand erect facing side of box at a comfortable stepping distance.

Action (Begin on Starting Signal)

1. Step up onto the box with first one foot and then the other, assuming a momentary straight stand.

2. Immediately step down to the starting position.

3. Repeat continuously until the signal to stop is given.

4. Either foot may precede the other in any combination of stepping throughout the exercise.

5. Rate of stepping: Thirty times per minute, i.e., one complete sequence every two seconds.

6. Duration of action: five minutes.

Incorrect Procedure or Inadequate Performance

1. Failure to maintain proper rate of action.

2. Failure to come to a straight stance on the box; i.e., straight knees, straight body.

3. Failure to continue for the full five minutes.

Valuation

1. Immediately sit down on the box and rest.

2. Assistant locates the pulse.

3. One minute after cessation of exercise, assistant counts the pulse beat for thirty seconds and records.

4. Two minutes after cessation of exercise, assistant counts the pulse beat for 30 seconds and records.

5. Three minutes after cessation of exercise, assistant counts the pulse beat for 30 seconds and records.

6. Record the sum of the above three pulse counts.

7. The scoring table is contained in Appendix B-2 for those able to complete five minutes of stepping.

A-4
ONE-MINUTE STEP TEST

1. Secure a bench, bleacher or chair between 16 and 20 inches high.

2. Work with a partner.

3. Sit quietly and allow the pulse to settle.

4. Determine starting heart rate by counting the pulse for ten seconds.

Action
1. Begin stepping up and down on the bench in a 4-count movement at a rate of two complete up and down movements every five seconds (24 per minute).

2. Continue the test for one minute.

3. One minute after completing the test, partner takes a ten second standing pulse count to determine your heart recovery rate.

Incorrect Procedure or
Inadequate Performance
1. Failure to maintain the proper rate of action.

2. Failure to come to a straight stand on the bench; i.e., straight knees and straight body.

3. Failure to continue for the full minute.

Scoring Procedure
1. Note the difference between the starting pulse rate and the recovery heart rate.

2. Obtain rating from the chart in Appendix B-2.

A-5

VITAL LUNG CAPACITY

Purpose
1. To measure lung capacity

2. To provide for self-evaluation

Objectives
1. To provide motivation for improvement

2. To provide for a better understanding of the components of fitness

VITAL CAPACITY (DRY SPIROMETER)

Preliminary Procedure
1. Set the index to zero by rotating the outer ring until the pointer is even with the red 0 mark.

2. Attach a clear disposable mouthpiece.

Action
1. Stand erect, take several forced inspirations and exhale completely following each inspiration.

2. Following the hyperventilation exercise, take another deep breath and then exhale forcibly into the mouthpiece connected to the instrument. The forced expiration should be regular and even. It is not necessary to blow hard.

Incorrect Procedure or
Inadequate Performance
1. Successive exhalations

2. Uneven or incomplete expiration

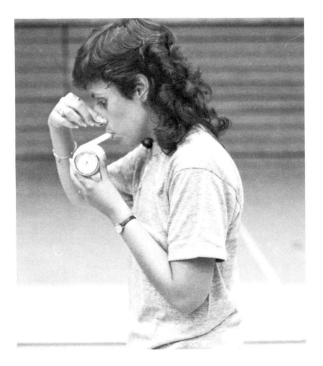

Valuation
1. Note the position of the pointer and read the vital capacity from the dial.

2. Additional trials are permitted when necessary.

3. Scoring tables for Vital Capacity Assessment are contained in Appendix B-1.

A-6

BODY FAT ANALYSIS WITH SKIN-FOLD CALIPERS

Purpose
1. To assess percentage of body fat

2. To become aware of differences between overweight and obesity

Objectives
1. To provide for self-assessment

2. To provide motivation for improvement

Preliminary Procedure
Stand with right side next to the person taking measurements.

Action
1. Measurements are taken for the following areas of the body:

   Triceps (women and men) — midpoint between the shoulder and elbow on the posterior (back) of the arm.

   Subscapula (women and men) — below the shoulder blade

   Suprailiac (women) — above the crest of the hip.

   Abdomen (men) — vertically beside the navel.

   Chest (men) — between the armpit and nipple.

   Thigh (women and men) — between the hip and knee.

2. Measurement is made by pinching a fold of skin between the thumb and forefinger, pulling the fold away from the underlying muscle, and applying the caliper to the fold.

3. The thickness of the fold reflects the amount of body fat. The calipers must be placed one-half inch from the thumb and index finger and allowed to close completely before the measurement is recorded.

4. At least three measurements of each area should be taken to assure accuracy.

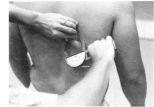
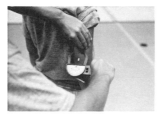

| Triceps | Subscapula |

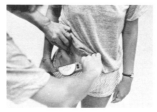
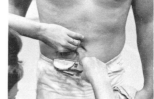

| Suprailiac | Abdomen |

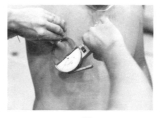
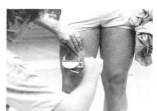

| Chest | Thigh |

Incorrect Procedure or Inadequate Performance
1. Including muscle tissue in the measurement.

2. Incorrect positioning of the calipers.

3. Failure to allow adequate time for the calipers to close.

Valuation
1. Record the measurement to the nearest millimeter using the mean of the two closest readings.

2. Additional measurements may be necessary.

Scoring Procedure
Use Table 4 to determine percentage of body fat based on the sum of three skinfolds.

TABLE 4: PART I
PERCENTAGE OF BODY FAT — WOMEN
(Sum of Triceps, Iliac, and Thigh Skinfolds)

Sum of Skinfolds (mm)	AGE TO THE LAST YEAR								
	Under 22	23 to 27	28 to 32	33 to 37	38 to 42	43 to 47	48 to 52	53 to 57	Over 58
23-25	9.7	9.9	10.2	10.4	10.7	10.9	11.2	11.4	11.7
26-28	11.0	11.2	11.5	11.7	12.0	12.3	12.5	12.7	13.0
29-31	12.3	12.5	12.8	13.0	13.3	13.5	13.8	14.0	14.3
32-34	13.6	13.8	14.0	14.3	14.5	14.8	15.0	15.3	15.5
35-37	14.8	15.0	15.3	15.5	15.8	16.0	16.3	16.5	16.8
38-40	16.0	16.3	16.5	16.7	17.0	17.2	17.5	17.7	18.0
41-43	17.2	17.4	17.7	17.9	18.2	18.4	18.7	18.9	19.2
44-46	18.3	18.6	18.8	19.1	19.3	19.6	19.8	20.1	20.3
47-49	19.5	19.7	20.0	20.2	20.5	20.7	21.0	21.2	21.5
50-52	20.6	20.8	21.1	21.3	21.6	21.8	22.1	22.3	22.6
53-55	21.7	21.9	22.1	22.4	22.6	22.9	23.1	23.4	23.6
56-58	22.7	23.0	23.2	23.4	23.7	23.9	24.2	24.4	24.7
59-61	23.7	24.0	24.2	24.5	24.7	25.0	25.2	25.5	25.7
62-64	24.7	25.0	25.2	25.5	25.7	26.0	26.7	26.4	26.7
65-67	25.7	25.9	26.2	26.4	26.7	26.9	27.2	27.4	27.7
68-70	26.6	26.9	27.1	27.4	27.6	27.9	28.1	28.4	28.6
71-73	27.5	27.8	28.0	28.3	28.5	28.8	28.0	29.3	29.5
74-76	28.4	28.7	28.9	29.2	29.4	29.7	29.9	30.2	30.4
77-79	29.3	29.5	29.8	30.0	30.3	30.5	30.8	31.0	31.3
80-82	30.1	30.4	30.6	30.9	31.1	31.4	31.6	31.9	32.1
83-85	30.9	31.2	31.4	31.7	31.9	32.2	32.4	32.7	32.9
86-88	31.7	32.0	32.2	32.5	32.7	32.9	33.2	33.4	33.7
89-91	32.5	32.7	33.0	33.2	33.5	33.7	33.9	34.2	34.4
92-94	33.2	33.4	33.7	33.9	34.2	34.4	34.7	34.9	35.2
95-97	33.9	34.1	34.4	34.6	34.9	35.1	35.4	35.6	35.9
98-100	34.6	34.8	35.1	35.3	35.5	35.8	36.0	36.3	36.5
101-103	35.3	35.4	35.7	35.9	36.2	36.4	36.7	36.9	37.2
104-106	35.8	36.1	36.3	36.6	36.8	37.1	37.3	37.5	37.8
107-109	36.4	36.7	36.9	37.1	37.4	37.6	37.9	38.1	38.4
110-112	37.0	37.2	37.5	37.7	38.0	38.2	38.5	38.7	38.9
113-115	37.5	37.8	38.0	38.2	38.5	38.7	39.0	39.2	39.5
116-118	38.0	38.3	38.5	38.8	39.0	39.3	39.5	39.7	40.0
119-121	38.5	38.7	39.0	39.2	39.5	39.7	40.0	40.2	40.5
122-124	39.0	39.2	39.4	39.7	39.9	40.2	40.4	40.7	40.9
125-127	39.4	39.6	39.9	40.1	40.4	40.6	40.9	41.1	41.4
128-130	39.8	40.0	40.3	40.5	40.8	41.0	41.3	41.5	41.8

Source: Pollock, M.L., Schmidt, D.H., and Jackson, A.S.: Measurement of Cardiorespiratory Fitness and Body Composition in the Clinical Setting, *Comprehensive Therapy,* Vol. 6, No. 9, pp. 12-27, 1980.

TABLE 4: PART II
PERCENTAGE OF BODY FAT — MEN
(Sum of Chest, Abdominal, and Thigh Skinfolds)

Sum of Skinfolds (mm)	AGE TO THE LAST YEAR								
	Under 22	23 to 27	28 to 32	33 to 37	38 to 42	43 to 47	48 to 52	53 to 57	Over 58
8-10	1.3	1.8	2.3	2.9	3.4	3.9	4.5	5.0	5.5
11-13	2.2	2.8	3.3	3.9	4.4	4.9	5.5	6.0	6.5
14-16	3.2	3.8	4.3	4.8	5.4	5.9	6.4	7.0	7.5
17-19	4.2	4.7	5.3	5.8	6.3	6.9	7.4	8.0	8.5
20-22	5.1	5.7	6.2	6.8	7.3	7.9	8.4	8.9	9.5
23-25	6.1	6.6	7.2	7.7	8.3	8.8	9.4	9.9	10.5
26-28	7.0	7.6	8.1	8.7	9.2	9.8	10.3	10.9	11.4
29-31	8.0	8.5	9.1	9.6	10.2	10.7	11.3	11.8	12.4
32-34	8.9	9.4	10.0	10.5	11.1	11.6	12.2	12.8	13.3
35-37	9.8	10.4	10.9	11.5	12.0	12.6	13.1	13.7	14.3
38-40	10.7	11.3	11.8	12.4	12.9	13.5	14.1	14.6	15.2
41-43	11.6	12.2	12.7	13.3	13.8	14.4	15.0	15.5	16.1
44-46	12.5	13.1	13.6	14.2	14.7	15.3	15.9	16.4	17.0
47-49	13.4	13.9	14.5	15.1	15.6	16.2	16.8	17.3	17.9
50-52	14.3	14.0	15.4	15.9	16.5	17.1	17.6	18.2	18.8
53-55	15.1	15.7	16.2	16.8	17.4	17.9	18.5	18.1	19.7
56-58	16.0	16.5	17.1	17.7	18.2	18.8	19.4	20.0	20.5
59-61	16.9	17.4	17.9	18.5	19.1	19.7	20.2	20.8	21.4
62-64	17.6	18.2	18.8	19.4	19.9	20.5	21.1	21.7	22.2
65-67	18.5	19.0	19.6	20.2	20.8	21.3	21.9	22.5	23.1
68-70	19.3	19.9	20.4	21.0	21.6	22.2	22.7	23.3	23.9
71-73	20.1	20.7	21.2	21.8	22.4	23.0	23.6	24.1	24.7
74-76	20.9	21.5	22.0	22.6	23.2	23.8	24.4	25.0	25.5
77-79	21.7	22.2	22.8	23.4	24.0	24.6	25.2	25.8	26.3
80-82	22.4	23.0	23.6	24.2	24.8	25.4	25.9	26.5	27.1
83-85	23.2	23.8	24.4	25.0	25.5	26.1	26.7	27.3	27.9
86-88	24.0	24.5	25.1	25.7	26.3	26.9	27.5	28.1	28.7
89-91	24.7	25.3	25.9	25.5	27.1	27.6	28.2	28.8	29.4
92-94	25.4	26.0	26.6	27.2	27.8	28.4	29.0	29.6	30.2
92-97	26.1	16.7	27.3	27.9	28.5	29.1	29.7	30.3	30.9
98-100	26.9	27.4	28.0	28.6	29.2	29.8	30.4	31.0	31.6
101-103	27.5	28.1	28.7	29.3	29.9	30.5	31.1	31.7	32.3
104-106	28.2	28.8	29.4	30.0	30.6	31.2	31.8	32.4	33.0
107-109	28.9	29.5	30.1	30.7	31.3	31.9	32.5	33.1	33.7
110-112	29.6	30.2	30.8	31.4	32.0	32.6	33.2	33.8	34.4
113-115	30.2	30.8	31.4	32.0	32.6	33.2	33.8	34.5	35.1
116-118	30.9	31.5	32.1	32.7	33.3	33.9	34.5	35.1	35.7
119-121	31.5	32.1	32.7	33.3	33.9	34.5	35.1	35.7	36.4
122-124	32.1	32.7	33.3	33.9	34.5	35.1	35.8	36.4	37.0
125-127	32.7	33.3	33.9	34.5	35.1	35.8	36.4	37.0	37.6

219

A-7

FLEXIBILITY ASSESSMENTS

Flexibility is the ability to move the body parts through their full range of motion at their joints. Your muscle system, including ligaments, the bones, and the joints, is critical to the degree of flexibility you possess.

There are two areas of flexibility, static and dynamic. *Static* flexibility is the ability to move or stretch the body, or some part of it, freely in various directions. Dynamic flexibility is the ability to perform repeated flexing or stretching exercises or the ability to move a joint through various ranges of motion at varying speeds.

Flexibility is specific to a joint or a combination of joints and, for that reason, it is possible to have adequate back flexibility without having arm and shoulder joint flexibility.

Purpose
1. To measure general flexibility

2. To measure specific flexibility

Objectives
1. To provide for self-evaluation

2. To provide motivation for improvement

3. To provide for a better understanding of flexibility

SIT AND REACH HIP FLEXIBILITY

Starting Position
Sit on the floor with your back straight; knees are together and feet are flat against the box.

Action
1. As an assistant holds your knees straight, reach forward with your arms fully extended, palms down, fingers straight and one hand on top of the other.

2. Hold this position for at least three seconds.

3. Measure the distance the fingertips reach on the box to the nearest one-quarter inch.

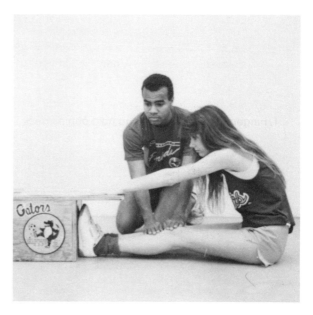

Incorrect Procedure or Inadequate Performance
1. Bouncing

2. Knees not straight

3. Feet not held against the box

4. Reach position not held for at least 3 seconds

Valuation
1. Two trials are allowed with the best being scored.

2. Score to the nearest one-quarter inch.

3. Incorrect procedure invalidates the measurement.

PRONE-TRUNK EXTENSION

Starting Procedure
1. Lie prone on the floor with an assistant sitting astride and holding your buttocks and legs down.

2. Interlock your fingers behind your neck with your elbows outward.

Action
1. Raise your chest and head off the floor as high as possible.

2. Keep your pelvis and legs in contact with the floor.

3. Measure the distance to the nearest quarter-inch from the floor to the bottom of your chin.

Incorrect Procedure or
Inadequate Performance
1. Fingers not interlocked and held behind neck

2. Buttocks and legs not held down

Valuation
1. Two trials are allowed, with the better being scored.

2. Measure to the nearest quarter-inch.

3. Incorrect procedure invalidates results.

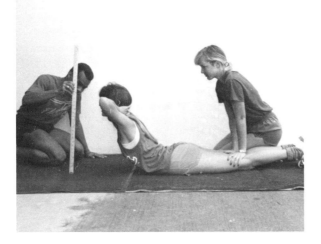

SHOULDER LIFT

Starting Procedure
1. Lie prone on the floor with the chin touching the floor and extend the arms forward directly in front of the shoulders.

2. Hold a stick horizontally with both hands, keeping elbows straight, hands 6" apart, wrists straight.

Action
1. Raise the arms upward as far as possible with chin still touching the floor.

2. Keep legs and feet on the floor.

3. Hold upraised arms for a three second count.

4. Measure the distance to the nearest quarter-inch from the bottom of the stick to the floor.

Incorrect Procedure or
Inadequate Performance
1. Lifting chin off floor.

2. Lifting legs and feet off floor.

3. Hyperextending wrists.

Valuation
1. Two trials are allowed, with the better being scored.

2. Incorrect procedure invalidates results.

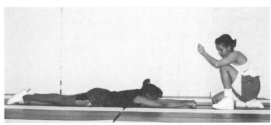

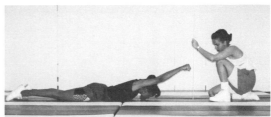

SCORING TABLES FOR FLEXIBILITY ASSESSMENTS ARE CONTAINED IN APPENDIX B-4.

A-8

MUSCULAR STRENGTH AND ENDURANCE ASSESSMENTS

Purpose
1. To measure muscular strength
2. To measure muscular endurance

Objectives
1. To provide for self-evaluation
2. To provide motivation for improvement
3. To provide for a better understanding of the components of fitness

CRUNCHES
Measure of Abdominal Muscular Endurance

Preliminary Procedure
1. Lie on your back, knees bent and feet flat on floor, with heels approximately 12" from buttocks.
2. Place your hands with palms facing down on the tops of your thighs.

Action
1. Raise your head and shoulders, exhaling as you extend your arms so that your fingers touch the center of your kneecaps.

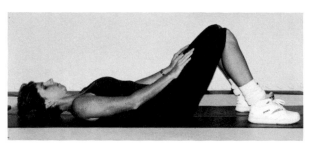

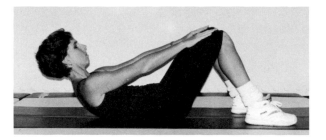

2. Lower your shoulders to the floor. It is not necessary to return head to the floor each time.
3. Complete as many as you can in 60 seconds.

Incorrect Procedure or Inadequate Performance
1. Using hands to pull up body.
2. Failing to lift shoulders off floor.
3. Lifting upper body off floor beyond a 45 degree angle (hip flexors are used).

PUSH-UPS
Measure of Arm-Shoulder Strength and Endurance

Preliminary Procedure
1. Assume a front-leaning position on the floor with the hands on the floor next to the shoulder.
2. Partner places fist under chin or chest as marker.

Action
1. Keep the body straight while lowering, until the chin or chest touches the partner's fist.
2. Only the hands and toes should touch the floor as the body is lowered.
3. Return to the starting position by pushing up until the arms are straight.
4. Repeat continuously as many times as possible without stopping.

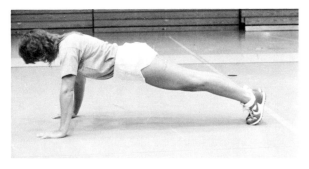

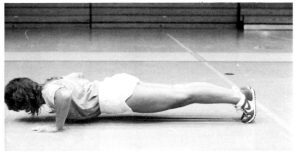

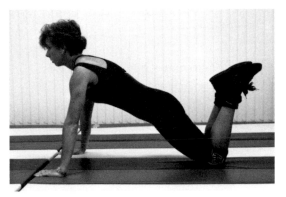

Static Push-up
Start in the standard push-up position with arms completely extended. Then lower the body until the elbows are flexed at a 90 degree angle or less. The score is the number of seconds this position can be held.

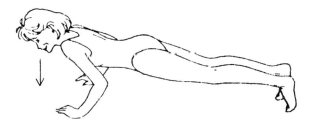

Incorrect Procedure or Inadequate Performance
1. Allowing the thigh, chest or other parts of the body to touch the floor

2. Failing to lower all the way to the partner's hand or extend until the arms are straight on the return

3. Failing to lower and raise the body in a straight line

Counting
1. Count one for each correctly performed push-up.

2. Do not count any exercises that are performed with incorrect procedure.

3. Stop counting when reasonably continuous action cannot be maintained.

Modified Push-Up
Start in the standard push-up position with the weight supported on the hands and knees—feet are off the floor.

PULL-UPS (Males)
Measure of Arm and Shoulder Girdle Strength and Muscular Endurance

Preliminary Procedure
1. Straight arm, extended body hang, on horizontal bar

2. Overhand grip (palms forward), thumbs around bar

Action
1. Pull up so that the chin is well above the bar.

2. Lower to the starting position.

3. Repeat continuously as many times as possible.

223

**Incorrect Procedure or
Inadequate Performance**
1. Use of incorrect grip

2. Failure to rise high enough

3. Failure to lower to full extension

4. Bending hips or knees

5. Swinging, kicking, thrusting, or "kipping" action

6. Tilting head backward (hyperextension of neck) to raise chin above the bar

Counting
1. Count one for each correctly performed pull-up.

2. Count "zero" if exercise is performed with incorrect procedure.

3. Terminate the exercise when reasonably continuous action cannot be maintained.

BACK LIFT (Male and Female)
Measure of Muscular Strength

Safety Note: Students with a history of lower back trouble should be advised to omit this item

Preliminary Procedure
1. Chalk hands. Use carbonate of magnesia.

2. Stand on dynamometer base:
   a. Feet parallel and six inches apart
   b. Ankle joints alongside base hook
   c. Back straight, head erect
   d. Arms straight, fingers extended downward along front of thighs

3. Assistant hold the bar even with your fingertips and connects the lower end of the chain to the basehook.

4. Bend slightly forward with the knees straight and grasp the bar with a mixed grip (one palm forward and one palm toward the body).

Action
1. Lift straight up with steady, even extension of the back only.

2. Maintain steady effort until you feel maximum exertion has been applied.

**Incorrect Procedure or
Inadequate Performance**
1. Bending knees

2. Bending arms

3. Any sudden jerking action

4. Allowing chain to slacken prior to the lift

Valuation
1. Read scale in pounds as indicated.

2. Incorrect procedure invalidates results.

3. Additional trials are permitted when necessary.

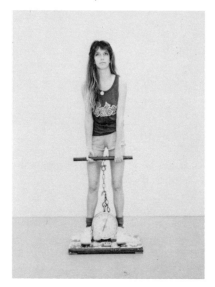

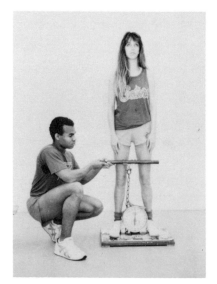

LEG LIFT (Male and Female)
Measure of Muscular Strength

Safety Note: Students with a history or predisposition to rupture should be advised to omit this item.

Preliminary Procedure
1. Check maximum indicator hand on dynamometer for correct setting.

2. Stand on dynamometer base:
   a. Feet parallel and six inches apart
   b. Ankle joints alongside base hook
   c. Back straight and head erect

3. Hold the center of the bar, palm down, at the level of the pubic bone.

4. Assistant attaches lifting belt as follows:
   a. Slip the belt loop over the right hand end of bar.
   b. Pass the belt around subject's hips and over the top of the left hand end of the bar.
   c. Reach down between subject's body and the bar and pull the free end of the belt up between the body and the bar.
   d. Pull the belt snug and fold the free end over and around the standing part of the belt so as to form a timber hitch.

5. Squat slightly so that the knees are bent at an angle of 115 to 125 degrees between the back of the thighs and the calf of the leg.

6. Assistant connects the lower end of the chain to the base hook.

Action
1. Lift straight up with steady, even extension of knees only.

2. Maintain steady effort until you feel maximum exertion has been reached.

Incorrect Procedure or Inadequate Performance
1. Lifting with the back

2. Any sudden jerking action

3. Allowing chain to slacken prior to the lift

Valuation
1. Read scale in pounds as indicated.

2. Incorrect procedure invalidates the results.

3. Additional trials are permitted when necessary.

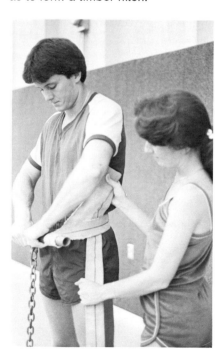

GRIP (Dominant and Non-Dominant Hand, Male and Female)

Measurement of Grip Strength

Preliminary Procedure
1. Check dynamometer for zero setting.

2. Chalk hands. Use carbonate of magnesia.

3. Grasp the dynamometer so that hand and fingers do not interfere with the dial.

Action
1. Dominant hand: Exert maximum gripping force upon the dynamometer.

2. Non-dominant hand (reset instrument): Exert maximum gripping force on dynamometer.

3. Almost any movement is permitted. However, the most common procedure is to crouch slightly forward and execute an uppercut or hook-like punch as in boxing, while applying maximum gripping force on the dynamometer.

Incorrect Procedure or Inadequate Performance
1. Placing fist (knuckles) against body or other object and pushing

2. Striking closed fist against the palm of the other hand or other object in a punching movement.

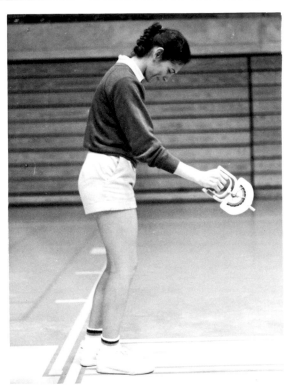

Valuation
1. Read the scale in kilograms as recorded.

2. Incorrect procedure invalidates the results.

3. Three trials are allowed, with the best being measured.

SCORING TABLES FOR STRENGTH ASSESSMENT ARE CONTAINED IN APPENDIX B-4.

A-9

BLOOD PRESSURE

Preliminary Procedure

1. Sit comfortably with your arm slightly flexed and the forearm supported at heart level.

2. Fasten the arm band snugly around your arm just above the elbow. Be certain there are no unnecessary folds in the arm band.

3. Locate the brachial artery in the forearm just below the elbow.

Action

1. Inflate the arm band until the pressure is about 100 mm mercury - just above the diastolic pressure and below the systolic pressure.

2. Place the stethoscope over the artery and become familiar with the sounds of blood spurting through the arteries. Do not leave the artery occluded for more than three minutes.

3. With the stethoscope in place, raise the pressure approximately 30 mm above the usual systolic reading and release it at a rate of two to three mm Hg per second. Faster or slower deflation will cause systematic errors.

4. When the first sound of arterial blood flow becomes audible, record the level of mm Hg - this is the systolic blood pressure.

5. When the point is reached that the sound disappears, record the level of mm Hg - this is the diastolic blood pressure.

Incorrect Procedure or
Inadequate Performance

1. Improper placement of the inflatable cuff

2. Incorrect release of cuff pressure

3. Inability to distinguish accurately the systolic and diastolic periods

Valuation

1. Additional trials should be utilized if necessary.

2. Record results with the systolic pressure over the diastolic: $\frac{120}{80}$

Refer to Chapter 2 for further explanation of the results.

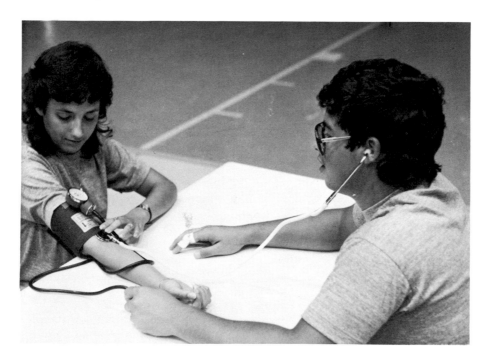

Fitness Evaluation

Fitness Area   **Page**

B-1 Health Screening Tests 230
      Resting Blood Pressure 230
      Resting Heart Rate 231
      Lung Capacity 232

B-2 Cardiovascular Tests 235

B-3 Body Fat Assessment 242

B-4 Muscular Fitness Tests 243
      Strength...243
      Muscular Endurance 244
      Flexibility 247

B-1
HEALTH SCREENING TESTS

One method of evaluating your results of the various fitness assessments is by noting the fitness category as designated by qualitative terms such as Superior, Excellent, Good, etc. Such categories have been determined by compiling data from many subjects and comparing results achieved by those with varying degrees of fitness.

Also taken into consideration for some assessments is age. The charts which follow are examples of this method of evaluating test results.

RESTING BLOOD PRESSURE				
FEMALES				
FITNESS CATEGORY	Under Age 30 Systolic-Diastolic	30-39 Systolic-Diastolic	40-49 Systolic-Diastolic	50-59 Systolic-Diastolic	60-Plus Systolic-Diastolic
Very Low	90-100 56-67	90-103 60-70	90-104 58-70	90-110 58-70	109-120 66-74
Low	101-110 68-74	104-110 71-75	105-114 71-78	111-120 71-79	121-130 75-79
Moderate	111-118 75-78	111-119 76-80	115-120 79-80	121-130 80-84	131-139 80-81
High	119-122 79-80	120-124 81-85	121-131 81-86	131-142 85-90	140-150 82-90
Very High	123-141 81-90	125-160 86-110	132-164 87-110	143-172 91-110	151-168 92-100

RESTING BLOOD PRESSURE				
MALES				
FITNESS CATEGORY	Under Age 30	30-39	40-49	50-59	60-Plus
	Systolic-Diastolic	Systolic-Diastolic	Systolic-Diastolic	Systolic-Diastolic	Systolic-Diastolic
Very Low	94-112 60-72	96-110 60-74	96-110 60-76	98-116 60-78	98-119 59-76
Low	113-120 73-80	111-120 75-80	112-120 77-80	117-125 79-80	120-130 77-180
Moderate	121-130 80-83	121-126 81-84	121-130 81-85	126-132 81-88	131-140 81-86
High	131-140 84-90	127-138 85-90	131-140 86-92	133-144 89-95	141-152 87-94
Very High	141-158 91-109	139-168 91-110	141-166 93-110	145-180 96-114	153-184 95-118

RESTING HEART RATES					
FEMALES Beats Per Minute - Age in Years					
FITNESS CATEGORY	Under 30	30-39	40-49	50-59	60 plus
Superior	<47	<47	<47	<47	<47
Excellent	47-59	47-59	47-60	47-60	47-57
Good	58-64	60-65	61-65	61-65	58-64
Moderate	65-70	67-72	66-72	66-71	65-71
High	71-79	73-80	73-80	72-79	72-78
Very High	>84	>81	>81	>80	>79

RESTING HEART RATES					
MALES Beats Per Minute - Age in Years					
FITNESS CATEGORY	**Under 30**	**30-39**	**40-49**	**50-59**	**60 Plus**
Superior	< 39	< 39	< 42	< 42	< 46
Excellent	39-54	39-55	42-54	42-55	47-55
Good	55-61	56-62	55-61	56-62	56-61
Moderate	62-68	63-67	62-67	63-67	62-67
High	69-79	68-79	68-82	68-82	68-82
Very High	> 80	> 80	> 83	> 83	> 83

LUNG CAPACITY ASSESSMENT SCORES		
FITNESS CATEGORY	MALE	FEMALE
Excellent	> 5500	> 4000
Good	4700-5400	3600-3900
Average	3900-4600	2800-3500
Poor	3100-3800	2100-2700
Very Poor	< 3000	< 2000

Note: See charts on next page for Lung Capacity Rating based on height and age.

LUNG CAPACITY
MALES

Ht. in Inches	20					30					40				
	Excell.	Good	Average	Fair	Poor	Excell.	Good	Average	Fair	Poor	Excell.	Good	Average	Fair	Poor
60	5439	4662	3885	3108	2331	5131	4398	3665	2932	2199	4823	4134	3445	2756	2067
62	5815	4984	4154	3323	2492	5495	4710	3925	3140	2355	5187	4446	3705	2964	2223
64	6174	5292	4410	3528	2646	5866	5028	4190	3352	2514	5558	4764	3970	3176	2382
66	6545	5610	4675	3740	2805	6237	5346	4455	3564	2673	5929	5082	4235	3388	2541
68	6916	5928	4940	3952	2964	6608	5664	4720	3776	2832	6300	5400	4500	3600	2700
70	7288	6247	5206	4164	3123	6980	5983	4986	3988	2991	6672	5719	4766	3812	2859
72	7659	6565	5471	4376	3282	7351	6301	5251	4200	3150	7043	6037	5031	4024	3018
74	8030	6883	5736	4588	3441	7722	6619	5516	4412	3309	7414	6355	5296	4236	3177

Ht. in Inches	50					60					70				
	Excell.	Good	Average	Fair	Poor	Excell.	Good	Average	Fair	Poor	Excell.	Good	Average	Fair	Poor
60	4515	3870	3225	2580	1935	4207	3606	3005	2404	1803	3899	3342	2785	2228	1671
62	4879	4182	3485	2788	2091	4571	3918	3235	2612	1959	4263	3654	3045	2436	1461
64	5250	4500	3750	3000	2250	4952	4236	3530	2824	2118	4634	3972	3310	2648	1986
66	5621	4818	4015	3212	2409	5313	4554	3795	3036	2277	5005	4290	3575	2860	2145
68	5992	5136	4280	3424	2568	5684	4872	4060	3248	2436	5376	4608	3840	3072	2304
70	6364	5455	4546	3636	2727	6056	5191	4326	3460	2625	5748	4927	4106	3284	2463
72	6735	5773	4811	3848	2886	6427	5509	4591	3672	2754	6119	5245	4371	3496	2622
74	7106	6091	5076	4060	3045	6798	5827	4856	3884	2913	6490	5563	4636	3708	2781

LUNG CAPACITY
FEMALES

Ht. in Inches	20					30					40				
	Excell.	Good	Aver.	Fair	Poor	Excell.	Good	Aver.	Fair	Poor	Excell.	Good	Aver.	Fair	Poor
58	4184	3586	2989	2391	1793	3932	3370	2809	2247	1685	3680	3154	2629	2103	1577
60	4477	3837	3198	2558	1918	4225	3621	3018	2414	1810	3973	3405	2838	2270	1702
62	4764	4083	3403	2722	2041	4512	3867	3223	2578	1933	2860	2451	2043	1634	1225
64	5056	4334	3612	2889	2167	3404	2918	2432	1945	1459	4552	3902	3252	2601	1951
66	5350	4586	3822	3057	2293	5098	4370	3642	2913	2185	4856	4154	3462	2769	2077
68	5643	4837	4031	3224	2418	5391	4621	3851	3080	2310	5139	4405	3671	2936	2202
70	5978	5124	4270	3416	2562	5726	4908	4090	3272	2454	5474	4692	3910	3128	2346
72	6228	5338	4449	3559	2669	5976	5122	4269	3415	2561	5724	4906	4089	3271	2453

Ht. in Inches	50					60					70				
	Excell.	Good	Aver.	Fair	Poor	Excell.	Good	Aver.	Fair	Poor	Excell.	Good	Aver.	Fair	Poor
58	3428	2938	2449	1959	1469	3176	2722	2269	1815	1361	2924	2506	2089	1671	1253
60	3721	3189	2658	2126	1594	3469	2973	2478	1982	1486	3217	2757	2298	1838	1378
62	4008	3435	2863	2290	1717	3756	3219	2683	2146	1609	3504	3003	2503	2002	1501
64	4300	3686	3072	2457	1843	4048	3470	2892	2313	1735	3794	3252	2710	2168	1626
66	4594	3938	3282	2625	1969	4342	3722	3102	2481	1861	4090	3506	2922	2337	1753
68	4887	4189	3491	2792	2094	4635	3973	3311	2648	1986	4383	3757	3131	2504	1878
70	5222	4476	3730	2984	2238	4970	4260	3550	2840	2130	4718	4044	3370	2696	2022
72	5472	4690	3909	3127	2345	5220	4474	3729	2983	2237	4968	4258	3549	2839	2129

B-2
CARDIOVASCULAR TESTS

PREDICTED MAXIMUM OXYGEN UPTAKE (Bicycle Ergometer)									
FITNESS CATEGORY	MALES (BY AGE)					FEMALES (BY AGE)			
	20-29	30-39	40-49	50-65	66-69	20-29	30-39	40-49	50-65
Very High	> 57	> 52	> 48	> 44	> 40	> 49	> 48	> 46	< 42
High	52-56	48-51	44-47	40-43	36-39	44-48	42-47	41-45	37-41
Average	44-51	40-47	36-43	32-39	27-35	35-43	34-41	32-40	29-36
Somewhat Low	39-43	35-39	31-35	26-31	22-26	29-34	28-33	26-31	22-28
Low	< 38	< 34	< 30	< 25	< 21	< 28	<27	< 25	< 21

ONE MINUTE STEP TEST	
FITNESS CATEGORY male & females	Score Related to Starting Heart Rate
Excellent	Same or less
Good	1-2 beats
Fair	3-4 beats
Poor	5-6 beats
Very Poor	7+ beats

235

B-2 CARDIOVASCULAR TESTS, Continued

ONE MILE RUN TEST						
	MALES (BY AGE)					
FITNESS CATEGORY	13-19	20-29	30-39	40-49	50-59	> 60
Excellent	< 6:00	< 6:30	< 7:00	< 7:30	< 8:00	< 8:30
Good	6:01-6:30	6:31-7:00	7:01-7:30	7:31-8:00	8:01-8:30	8:31-9:00
Fair	6:31-7:30	7:01-8:00	7:31-8:30	8:01-9:00	8:31-9:30	9:01-10:00
Poor	7:31-8:30	8:01-9:00	8:31-9:30	9:01-10:00	9:31-10:30	10:01-11:00
Very Poor	> 8:30	> 9:00	> 9:30	> 10:00	> 10:30	> 11:00

ONE MILE RUN TEST						
	FEMALES (BY AGE)					
FITNESS CATEGORY	13-19	20-29	30-39	40-49	50-59	> 60
Excellent	< 7:00	< 7:30	< 8:00	< 8:30	< 9:00	< 9:30
Good	7:01-7:30	7:31-8:00	8:01-8:30	8:31-9:00	9:01-9:30	9:31-10:00
Fair	7:31-8:30	8:01-9:00	8:31-9:30	9:01-10:00	9:31-10:30	10:01-11:00
Poor	8:31-9:30	9:01-10:00	9:31-10:30	10:01-11:00	10:31-11:30	11:01-12:00
Very Poor	> 9:30	> 10:00	> 10:30	> 11:00	> 11:30	> 12:00

B-2 CARDIOVASCULAR TESTS, Continued

1.5 MILE RUN						
FITNESS CATEGORY	MALES (BY AGE)					
	13-19	**20-29**	**30-39**	**40-49**	**50-59**	**60+**
Superior	< 8:37	< 9:45	< 10:00	< 10:30	< 11:00	< 11:15
Excellent	8:37-9:40	9:45-10:45	10:00-11:00	10:30-11:30	11:00-12:30	11:15-13:59
Good	9:41-10:48	10:46-12:00	11:01-12:30	11:31-13:00	12:31-14:30	14:00-16:15
Fair	10:49-12:10	12:01-14:00	12:31-14:45	13:01-15:35	14:31-17:00	16:16-19:00
Poor	12:11-15:30	14:01-16:00	14:46-16:30	15:36-17:30	17:01-19:00	19:01-20:00
Very Poor	> 15:31	> 16:10	> 17:31	> 17:31	> 19:01	> 20:01

1.5 MILE RUN						
FITNESS CATEGORY	FEMALES (BY AGE)					
	13-19	**20-29**	**30-39**	**40-49**	**50-59**	**60+**
Superior	> 11:50	> 12:30	> 13:00	> 13:45	> 14:30	> 16:30
Excellent	11:50-12:29	12:30-13:30	13:00-14:30	13:45-15:55	14:30-16:30	16:30-17:30
Good	12:30-14:30	13:31-15:54	14:31-16:30	15:56-17:30	16:31-19:00	17:31-19:30
Fair	14:31-16:54	15:55-18:30	16:31-19:00	17:31-19:30	19:01-20:00	19:31-20:30
Poor	16:55-18:30	18:31-19:00	19:01-19:30	19:31-20:00	20:01-20:30	20:31-21:00
Very Poor	< 18:31	< 19:01	< 19:31	< 20:01	< 20:31	< 21:01

B-2 CARDIOVASCULAR TESTS, Continued

12 MINUTE RUN						
	FEMALES (BY AGE)					
FITNESS CATEGORY	13-19	20-29	30-39	40-49	50-59	60+
Superior	> 1.52	> 1.46	> 1.40	> 1.35	> 1.31	> 1.19
Excellent	1.44-1.51	1.35-1.45	1.30-1.39	1.25-1.34	1.19-1.30	1.10-1.18
Good	1.30-1.43	1.23-1.34	1.19-1.29	1.12-1.24	1.06-1.18	.99-1.09
Fair	1.19-1.29	1.12-1.22	1.06-1.18	.99-1.11	.94-1.05	.87-.98
Poor	1.00-1.18	.96-1.11	.95-1.05	.88-.93	.84-.93	.78-.86
Very Poor	< 1.00	< .96	< .95	< .88	< .84	< .78

12 MINUTE RUN						
	MALES (BY AGE)					
FITNESS CATEGORY	13-19	20-29	30-39	40-49	50-59	60+
Superior	> 1.87	> 1.77	> 1.70	> 1.66	> 1.59	> 1.56
Excellent	1.73-1.86	1.65-1.76	1.57-1.69	1.54-1.65	1.45-1.58	1.33-1.55
Good	1.57-1.72	1.50-1.64	1.46-1.56	1.40-1.53	1.31-1.44	1.21-1.32
Fair	1.38-1.56	1.32-1.49	1.31-1.45	1.25-1.39	1.17-1.30	1.03-1.20
Poor	1.30-1.37	1.22-1.31	1.18-1.30	1.14-1.24	1.03-1.16	.87-1.02
Very Poor	< 1.30	< 1.22	< 1.18	< 1.14	< 1.03	< .87

B-2 CARDIOVASCULAR TESTS, Continued

12 MINUTE RUN

Scoring Value

2-.50	4-1.0	6-1.50
2 1/8-.53	4 1/8-1.03	6 1/8-1.53
2 2/8-.56	4 2/8-1.06	6 2/8-1.56
2 3/8-.59	4 3/8-1.09	6 3/8-1.59
2 4/8-.62	4 4/8-1.12	6 4/8-1.62
2 5/8-.65	4 5/8-1.15	6 5/8-1.65
2 6/8-.68	4 6/8-1.18	6 6/8-1.68
2 7/8-.71	4 7/8-1.21	6 7/8-1.71
3-.75	5-1.25	7-1.75
3 1/8-.78	5 1/8-1.28	7 1/8-1.78
3 2/8-.81	5 2/8-1.31	7 2/8-1.81
3 3/8-.84	5 3/8-1.34	7 3/8-1.84
3 4/8-.87	5 4/8-1.37	7 4/8-1.87
3 5/8-.90	5 5/8-1.40	7 5/8-1.90
3 6/8-.93	5 6/8-1.43	7 6/8-1.93
3 7/8-.96	5 7/8-1.46	7 7/8-1.96
		8.2.0

B-2 CARDIOVASCULAR TESTS, continued

Rockport Fitness Walking Test™ Results

Note: The charts below are reprinted by permission of the Rockport Walking Institute. Copyright 1989 by the Rockport Company. All rights reserved.

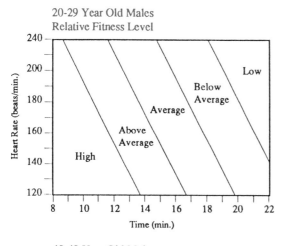

20-29 Year Old Males
Relative Fitness Level

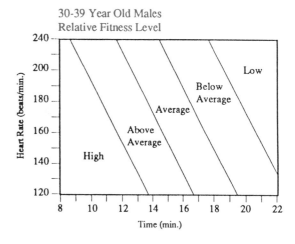

30-39 Year Old Males
Relative Fitness Level

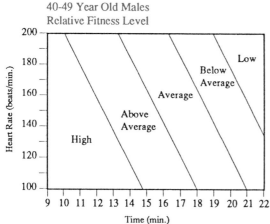

40-49 Year Old Males
Relative Fitness Level

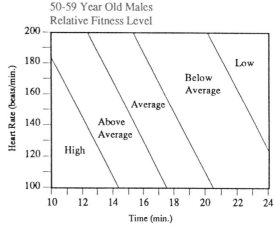

50-59 Year Old Males
Relative Fitness Level

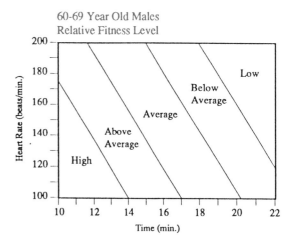

60-69 Year Old Males
Relative Fitness Level

Exercise Level:
Low = Introductory level
Below Average = Beginner
Average = Advanced Beginner
Above Average = Intermediate
High = High Intermediate to Advanced

B-2 CARDIOVASCULAR TESTS, continued

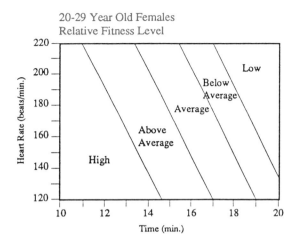

20-29 Year Old Females
Relative Fitness Level

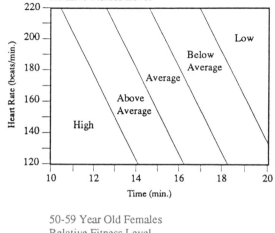

30-39 Year Old Females
Relative Fitness Level

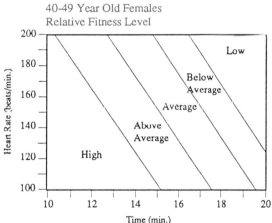

40-49 Year Old Females
Relative Fitness Level

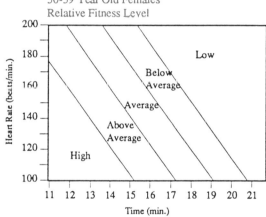

50-59 Year Old Females
Relative Fitness Level

Exercise Level:
Low = Introductory level
Below Average = Beginner
Average = Advanced Beginner
Above Average = Intermediate
High = High Intermediate to Advanced

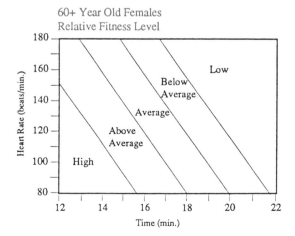

60+ Year Old Females
Relative Fitness Level

241

B-3
BODY FAT ASSESSMENT

PERCENTAGE BODY FAT					
FITNESS CATEGORY	MALES (BY AGE)				
	< 30	**30-39**	**40-49**	**50-59**	**> 60**
Excellent	< 9.7	< 13.4	< 15.6	< 17.6	< 17.2
Good	9.8-14.0	13.5-17.0	15.7-19.1	17.7-21.1	17.3-21.2
Fair	14.1-17.5	17.1-20.0	19.2-22.1	21.2-23.9	21.3-24.6
Poor	17.6-22.0	20.1-23.7	22.2-25.8	24.0-27.3	24.7-28.4
Very Poor	> 22.1	> 23.8	> 25.9	> 27.4	> 28.5

PERCENTAGE BODY FAT					
FITNESS CATEGORY	FEMALES (BY AGE)				
	< 30	**30-39**	**40-49**	**50-59**	**> 60**
Excellent	< 14.8	< 16.7	< 20.1	< 23.3	< 24.6
Good	14.9-18.9	16.8-20.6	20.2-24.1	23.4-27.4	24.7-29.0
Fair	19.0-22.8	20.7-24.0	24.2-27.2	27.5-30.9	29.1-31.2
Poor	22.9-27.1	24.1-28.6	27.3-31.4	31.0-35.0	31.3-36.1
Very Poor	> 27.2	> 28.7	> 31.5	> 35.1	> 45.9

B-4
MUSCULAR FITNESS TESTS

	GRIP STRENGTH			
	MALES		FEMALES	
FITNESS CATEGORY	Kg. Dominant	Kg. Non-Dominant	KG. Dominant	KG. Non-Dominant
Superior	99-65	99-60	99-40	99-35
Excellent	64-60	59-55	39-36	34-31
Good	59-55	54-50	35-32	30-27
Average	54-48	49-43	31-29	26-23
Fair	47-38	42-33	28-21	22-16
Poor	37-0	32-0	20-0	15-0

STRENGTH TESTS		
	MALES	FEMALES
Leg Strength		
Excellent	1100 lbs.	670 lbs.
Good	870-1099	500-669
Average	630-869	330-499
Fair	390-629	160-329
Poor	Below 390	Below 160
Back Strength		
Excellent	430 lbs.	255 lbs.
Good	350-429	205-254
Average	280-349	150-204
Fair	200-279	100-149
Poor	Below 200	Below 100
Dips		
Excellent	23	
Good	15-22	
Average	8-14	
Fair	3-7	
Poor	Below 4	

243

B-4 MUSCULAR FITNESS TESTS, continued

	SIT UPS									
	MALES					FEMALES				
AGE	Excellent	Good	Average	Fair	Poor	Excellent	Good	Average	Fair	Poor
20-29	48-above	43-47	37-42	33-36	0-32	44-above	39-43	33-38	29-32	0-28
30-39	40-above	35-39	29-34	25-28	0-24	36-above	31-35	25-30	21-24	0-20
40-49	35-above	30-34	24-29	20-23	0-19	31-above	26-30	19-25	16-18	0-15
50-59	30-above	25-29	19-24	15-18	0-14	26-above	21-25	15-20	11-14	0-10
60-69	25-above	20-24	14-19	10-13	0-9	21-above	16-20	10-15	6-9	0-5

INCLINED PULL-UP (Females)	
Excellent	21
Good	12-20
Average	8-12
Fair	3-7
Poor	Below 3

PULL-UPS (Males)	
Excellent	15
Good	11-14
Average	6-10
Fair	2-5
Poor	1

B-4 MUSCULAR FITNESS TESTS, continued

PUSH-UPS					
	MALES				
AGE	Excellent	Good	Average	Fair	Poor
20-29	55-above	45-54	35-44	20-34	0-19
30-39	45-above	35-44	25-34	15-24	0-14
40-49	40-above	30-39	20-29	12-19	0-11
50-59	35-above	25-34	15-24	8-14	0-7
60-69	30-above	20-29	10-19	5-9	0-4

PUSH-UPS					
	FEMALES				
AGE	Excellent	Good	Average	Fair	Poor
20-29	25+	20-24	14-19	9-13	0-8
30-39	23+	18-22	12-17	7-11	0-6
40-49	18+	14-17	9-13	5-8	0-4
50-59	14+	10-13	6-9	3-5	0-2

B-4 MUSCULAR FITNESS TESTS, continued

STATIC PUSH-UP RATINGS			
MALES		FEMALES	
Rating	Total Time Held	Rating	Total Time Held
Excellent	111 sec. - above	Excellent	35 sec. - above
Good	102-110 sec.	Good	30-34 sec.
Average	97-101 sec.	Average	26-29 sec.
Fair	88-96 sec.	Fair	20-25 sec.
Poor	0-87 sec.	Poor	0-19 sec.

MODIFIED PUSH-UP				
Excellent	Good	Average	Fair	Poor
49-above	34-48	17-33	6-16	0-5
40-above	25-39	12-24	4-11	0-3
35-above	20-34	8-19	3-7	0-2
30-above	15-29	6-14	2-5	0-1
20-above	5-19	3-4	1-2	0

Reprinted with the permission of Macmillan Publishing Company from HEALTH AND FITNESS THROUGH PHYSICAL ACTIVITY by Pollock, Wilmore and Fox. Copyright © 1978 by Macmillan Publishing Company.

B-4 MUSCULAR FITNESS TESTS, continued

FLEXIBILITY			
FITNESS CATEGORY	MALES		
	Shoulder Lift	**Trunk Ext.**	**Sit & Reach**
Superior	> 28	> 24	> 8
Excellent	26-27	22-23	6-7
Good	24-25	20-21	4-5
Average	22-23	18-19	2-3
Fair	20-21	16-17	0-1
Poor	< 19	< 16	< 0

FLEXIBILITY			
FITNESS CATEGORY	FEMALES		
	Shoulder Lift	**Trunk Ext.**	**Sit & Reach**
Superior	> 27	> 22	> 8
Excellent	25-26	20-21	6-7
Good	22-24	17-19	4-5
Average	19-21	15-16	2-3
Fair	17-18	13-14	0-1
Poor	< 17	< 13	< 0

Nutritive Values of Foods

Food Analysis

Which of the following contains the most sugar?
1. Heinz Tomato Ketchup — Sealtest Ice Cream
2. Wishbone Russian Dressing — Coca Cola
3. Coffee-mate Non-Dairy Creamer — Hershey's Milk Chocolate

Here's how they shape up:
1. Ketchup, 29% sugar; 21% for the ice cream
2. Dressing, 30% sugar; Coca Cola, 8.8%
3. Coffee-mate, 65% sugar; Hershey bar, 51%

Sugar content of some other foods:

4.	Shake-n-Bake, barbecue style	51%
5.	Quaker 100% Natural Cereal	24%
6.	Ritz Crackers	12%
7.	Fruits and vegetables	3.7%
8.	Cremora	56.9%
9.	Delmonte Whole Kernel Corn	10.7%
10.	Libby's Peaches	17.9%
11.	Dannon Lowfat Yogurt	13.7%
12.	Wyler's Beef Bouillon Cubes	14.8%
13.	Skippy Peanut Butter	9.2%
14.	Post Raisin Bran	55.0%

We get about 24% of our calories from sugar — "empty calories" — and only 3% from natural sugars (fruits and vegetables).

15.	Hamburger Helper	23.0%
16.	Ragu Spaghetti Sauce	6.2%
17.	Cool Whip	21.0%
18.	Wishbone Italian Dressing	7.3%
19.	Wishbone Russian Dressing	30.2%
20.	Wishbone French Dressing	23.0%
21.	Cherry Jello	82.6%
22.	Sara Lee Chocolate Cake	35.9%
23.	Shake-n-Bake Chicken	14.7%

The sugar content is based on all sources of sugar as they occur in the products. The analysis of these products was carried out by Consumer's Union.

NUTRITIVE VALUES OF FOODS

	Amount	Grams (g)	Calories	Protein (g)	Fat (g)	Carbohydrates (g)	Calcium (mg)	Phosphorus (mg)	Iron (mg)	Potassium (mg)	Vitamin A (I. Units)	Thiamine (mg)	Riboflavin (mg)	Niacin (mg)	Ascorbic acid (mg)
DAIRY PRODUCTS															
Butter (see Fats)															
Cheese:															
Blue	1 oz.	28	100	6	8	1	150	110	0.1	73	200	0.01	0.11	0.3	0
Cheddar	1 oz.	28	115	7	9	Tr	204	145	.2	28	300	.01	.11	Tr	0
Cottage Cheese:															
(large curd)	1 cup	225	235	28	10	6	135	297	.3	190	370	.05	.37	.3	Tr
(small curd)	1 cup	210	220	26	9	6	126	277	.3	177	340	.04	.34	.3	Tr
Cream	1 oz.	28	100	2	10	1	23	30	.3	34	400	Tr	.06	Tr	0
Mozzarella															
(skim milk)	1 oz.	28	80	8	5	1	207	149	.1	27	180	.01	.10	Tr	0
Parmesan, grated:	1 tbsp	5	25	2	2	Tr	69	40	Tr	5	40	Tr	.02	Tr	0
Provolone	1 oz.	28	100	7	8	1	214	141	.1	39	230	.01	.09	Tr	0
Ricotta (skim milk)	1 cup	246	340	28	19	13	669	449	1.1	308	1060	.05	.46	.2	0
Romano	1 oz.	28	110	9	8	1	302	215			160		.11	Tr	0
Swiss	1 oz.	28	105	8	8	1	272	171	Tr	31	240	.01	.10	Tr	0
Cream, sweet:															
Half and Half	1 tbsp	15	20	Tr	2	1	16	14	Tr	19	20	.01	.02	Tr	Tr
Cream, sour	1 tbsp	12	25	Tr	3	1	14	10	Tr	17	90	Tr	.02	Tr	Tr
Whipped Topping	1 tbsp	4	15	Tr	1	1	Tr	Tr	Tr	1	30	0	0	0	0
	1 cup	75	240	1	19	17	5	6	.1	14	650	0	0	0	0
Milk:															
Whole	1 cup	244	150	8	8	11	291	228	.1	370	310	.09	.40	.2	2
Lowfat (2%)	1 cup	244	120	8	5	12	297	232	.1	377	500	.10	.40	.2	2
Nonfat (skim)	1 cup	245	85	8	Tr	12	302	247	.1	406	500	.09	.37	.2	2
Buttermilk	1 cup	245	100	8	2	12	285	219	.1	371	80	.08	.38	.1	2
Canned:															
Evaporated:															
Whole milk	1 cup	252	340	17	19	25	657	510	.5	764	610	.12	.80	.5	5
Sweet condensed	1 cup	306	980	24	27	166	868	775	.6	1136	1000	.28	1.27	.6	8
Dried:															
Nonfat Instant	1 cup	68	245	24	Tr	35	837	670	.2	1160	1610	.28	1.19	.6	4
Milk Beverages:															
Chocolate milk	1 cup	250	210	8	8	26	280	251	.6	417	300	.09	.41	.3	2
(Lowfat 2%)	1 cup	250	180	8	5	26	284	254	.6	422	500	.10	.42	.3	2
Eggnog	1 cup	254	340	10	19	34	330	278	.5	420	890	.09	.48	.3	4
Shakes:															
Chocolate	10.6 oz	300	355	9	8	63	396	378	.9	672	260	.14	.67	.4	0
Vanilla	11 oz	313	350	12	9	56	457	361	.3	572	360	.09	.61	.5	0

	Amount	Grams (g)	Calories	Protein (g)	Fat (g)	Carbohydrates (g)	Calcium (mg)	Phosphorus (mg)	Iron (mg)	Potassium (mg)	Vitamin A (I. Units)	Thiamine (mg)	Riboflavin (mg)	Niacin (mg)	Ascorbic acid (mg)
Dairy Products, continued															
Milk Desserts (Frozen):															
Ice cream	1 cup	133	270	5	14	32	176	134	.1	257	540	.05	.33	.1	1
Ice milk, soft	1 cup	175	225	8	5	38	274	202	0.3	412	180	0.12	0.54	0.2	1
Sherbet	1 cup	193	270	2	4	59	103	74	.3	198	190	.03	.09	.1	4
Milk Desserts (Other):															
Custard, baked	1 cup	265	305	14	15	29	297	310	1.1	387	930	.11	.50	.3	1
Puddings:															
Home recipe: Vanilla	1 cup	255	285	9	10	41	298	232	Tr	352	410	.08	.41	.3	2
Home recipe:Choc.	1 cup	260	385	8	12	67	250	255	1.3	445	390	.05	.36	.3	1
From instant mix	1 cup	260	325	8	7	63	374	237	1.3	335	340	.08	.39	.3	2
Regular mix	1 cup	260	320	9	8	59	265	247	.8	354	340	.05	.39	.3	2
Tapioca	1 cup	165	220	8	8	28	173	180	.7	223	480	.07	.30	.2	2
Yogurt:															
Fruit-flavored	8 oz	227	230	10	3	42	343	269	.2	439	120	.08	.40	.2	1
Plain	8 oz	227	145	12	4	16	415	326	.2	531	150	.10	.49	.3	2
Eggs:															
Fried in butter	1	46	85	5	6	1	26	80	.9	58	290	.03	.13	Tr	0
Scrambled	1	64	95	6	7	1	47	97	.9	85	310	.04	.16	Tr	0
Boiled	1	50	80	6	6	1	28	90	1.0	65	260	.04	.13	Tr	0
Poached	1	50	80	6	6	1	28	90	1.0	65	260	.04	.13	Tr	0

BUTTER, FATS, OILS, AND RELATED PRODUCTS

	Amount	Grams (g)	Calories	Protein (g)	Fat (g)	Carbohydrates (g)	Calcium (mg)	Phosphorus (mg)	Iron (mg)	Potassium (mg)	Vitamin A (I. Units)	Thiamine (mg)	Riboflavin (mg)	Niacin (mg)	Ascorbic acid (mg)
Butter	1 tbsp	14	100	Tr	12	Tr	3	3	Tr	4	430	Tr	Tr	Tr	0
Butter Pat (1 in.)	1	5	35	Tr	4	Tr	1	1	Tr	1	150	Tr	Tr	Tr	0
Butter, Whipped	1 tbsp	9	65	Tr	8	Tr	2	2	Tr	2	290	Tr	Tr	Tr	0
Margarine	1 tbsp	14	100	Tr	12	Tr	3	3	Tr	4	470	Tr	Tr	Tr	0
Margarine Pat (1 in)	1	5	35	Tr	4	Tr	1	1	Tr	1	170	Tr	Tr	Tr	0
Margarine, Whipped	1 tbsp	9	70	Tr	8	Tr	2	2	Tr	2	310	Tr	Tr	Tr	0
Oils, salad or cooking:															
Corn oil	1 tbsp	14	120	0	14	0	0	0	0	0	--	0	0	0	0
Olive	1 tbsp	14	120	0	14	0	0	0	0	0	--	0	0	0	0
Peanut	1 tbsp	14	120	0	14	0	0	0	0	0	--	0	0	0	0
Safflower	1 tbsp	14	120	0	14	0	0	0	0	0	--	0	0	0	0
Salad dressings:															
Blue cheese: regular	1 tbsp	15	75	1	8	1	12	11	Tr	6	30	Tr	.02	Tr	Tr
Low-calorie	1 tbsp	16	10	Tr	1	1	10	8	Tr	5	30	Tr	.01	Tr	Tr
French: regular	1 tbsp	16	65	Tr	6	3	2	2	.1	13	--	--	--	--	--
Low-calorie	1 tbsp	16	15	Tr	1	2	2	2	.1	13	--	--	--	--	--
Italian: regular	1 tbsp	15	85	Tr	9	1	2	1	Tr	2	Tr	Tr	Tr	Tr	--
Low-calorie	1 tbsp	15	10	Tr	1	Tr	Tr	1	Tr	2	Tr	Tr	Tr	Tr	--
Thousand Island: reg	1 tbsp	1680	Tr	8	2	2	3		.1	18	50	Tr	Tr	Tr	Tr
Low-calorie	1 tbsp	15	25	Tr	2	2	2	3	.1	17	50	Tr	Tr	Tr	Tr
Mayonnaise: regular	1 tbsp	14	100	Tr	11	Tr	3	4	.1	5	40	Tr	.01	Tr	--
Low-calorie	1 tbsp	16	20	Tr	2	2	3	4	Tr	1	40	Tr	Tr	Tr	--
Tartar Sauce	1 tbsp	14	75	Tr	8	1	3	4	.1	11	30	Tr	Tr	Tr	Tr

252

FISH, SHELLFISH, MEAT, POULTRY, AND RELATED PRODUCTS

	Amount	Grams (g)	Calories	Protein (g)	Fat (g)	Carbohydrates (g)	Calcium (mg)	Phosphorus (mg)	Iron (mg)	Potassium (mg)	Vitamin A (I. Units)	Thiamine (mg)	Riboflavin (mg)	Niacin (mg)	Ascorbic acid (mg)
Fish:															
Bluefish, baked	3 oz	85	135	22	4	0	25	244	0.6	--	40	0.09	0.08	1.6	--
Haddock, fried	3 oz	85	140	17	5	5	34	210	1.0	296	--	.03	.06	2.7	2
Perch Filet, fried	1	85	195	16	11	6	28	192	1.1	242	--	.10	.10	1.6	--
Salmon, canned	3 oz	85	120	17	5	0	167	243	.7	307	60	.03	.16	6.8	--
Sardine, canned in oil	3 oz	85	175	20	9	0	372	424	2.5	502	190	.02	.17	4.6	--
Tuna, canned in oil	3 oz	85	170	24	7	0	7	199	1.6	--	70	.04	.10	10.1	--
Tuna salad	1 cup	205	350	30	22	7	41	291	2.7	--	590	.08	.23	10.3	2
Shellfish:															
Clams, raw, canned	3 oz	85	65	11	1	2	59	138	5.2	154	90	.08	.15	1.1	8
Clams, canned	3 oz	85	45	7	1	2	47	116	3.5	119	--	.01	.09	.9	--
Crab, canned	1 cup	135	135	24	3	1	61	246	1.1	149	--	.11	.11	2.6	--
Oysters, raw	1 cup	240	160	20	4	8	226	343	13.2	290	740	.34	.43	6.0	--
Scallop, breaded	6	90	175	16	8	9	--	--	--	--	--	--	--	--	--
Shrimp, canned	3 oz	85	100	21	1	1	98	224	2.6	104	50	.01	.03	1.5	--
Shrimp, fried	3 oz	85	190	17	9	9	61	162	1.7	195	--	.03	.07	2.3	--
Meat and Meat Products:															
Bacon, fried	2 slices	15	85	4	8	Tr	2	34	.5	35	0	.08	.05	.8	--
Beef, Pot Roast	3 oz	85	245	23	16	0	10	114	2.9	184	30	.04	.18	3.6	--
Ground	2.9 oz	82	235	20	17	0	9	159	2.6	221	30	.07	.17	4.4	--
Roast	3 oz	85	375	17	33	0	8	158	2.2	189	70	.05	.13	3.1	--
Steak, sirloin	3 oz	85	330	20	27	0	9	162	2.5	220	50	.05	.15	4.0	--
Steak, round	3 oz	85	220	24	13	0	10	213	3.0	272	20	.07	.19	4.8	--
Beef Products:															
Corned beef	3 oz	85	185	22	10	0	17	90	3.7	--	--	.01	.20	2.9	--
Corned beef hash	1 cup	220	400	19	25	24	29	147	4.4	440	--	.02	.20	4.6	--
Dried chip beef	2.5 oz	71	145	24	4	0	14	287	3.6	142	--	.05	.23	2.7	0
Beef/veg. stew	1 cup	245	220	16	11	15	29	184	2.9	613	2400	.15	.17	4.7	17
Beef pot pie	1 slice	210	515	21	30	39	29	149	3.8	334	1720	.30	.30	5.5	6
Chili Con Carne/Beans	1 cup	255	340	19	16	31	82	321	4.3	594	150	.08	.18	3.3	--
Lamb Shoulder Roast	3 oz.	85	285	18	23	0	9	146	1.0	206	--	.11	.20	4.0	--
Beef Liver	3 oz.	85	195	22	9	5	9	405	7.5	323	45390	.22	3.56	14.0	23
Ham, cured	3 oz.	85	245	18	19	0	8	146	2.2	199	0	.40	.15	3.1	--
Luncheon Meat:															
Canned Ham	1 slice	60	175	9	15	1	5	65	1.3	133	0	.19	.13	1.8	--
Bologna	1 slice	28	85	3	8	Tr	2	36	.5	65	--	.05	.06	.7	--
Braunschweiger	1 slice	28	90	4	8	1	3	69	1.7	--	1850	.05	.41	2.3	--
Pork Chop	2.7 oz.	78	305	19	25	0	9	209	2.7	216	0	0.75	0.22	4.5	--
Brown 'n Serve Sausage	1 link	1770	3	6	Tr	--	--	--	--	--	--	--	--	--	--
Deviled Ham, Canned	1 tbsp	13	45	2	4	0	1	12	.3	--	0	.02	.01	.2	--
Frankfurter	1	56	170	7	15	1	3	57	.8	--	--	.08	.11	1.4	--
Potted Meat,canned (Beef,chicken,turkey)	1 tbsp	13	30	2	2	0	--	--	--	--	--	Tr	.03	.2	--
Salami,cooked	1 slice	28	90	5	7	Tr	3	57	.7	--	--	.07	.07	1.2	--
Vienna Sausage	1	16	40	2	3	Tr	1	24	.3	--	--	.01	.02	.4	--
Veal cutlet	3 oz.	85	185	23	9	0	9	196	2.7	258	--	.06	.21	4.6	--

	Amount	Grams (g)	Calories	Protein (g)	Fat (g)	Carbohydrates (g)	Calcium (mg)	Phosphorus (mg)	Iron (mg)	Potassium (mg)	Vitamin A (I. Units)	Thiamine (mg)	Riboflavin (mg)	Niacin (mg)	Ascorbic acid (mg)

Fish, Shellfish, Meat, Poultry and Related Products (continued)

Chicken:

	Amount	Grams	Cal	Prot	Fat	Carb	Ca	P	Fe	K	Vit A	Thia	Ribo	Niac	Asc
Fried Breast	2.8 oz.	79	160	26	5	1	9	218	1.3	--	70	.04	.17	11.6	--
Drum Stick	1.3 oz.	38	90	12	4	Tr	6	89	.9	--	50	.03	.15	2.7	--
Canned Chicken	3 oz.	85	170	13	10	0	18	210	1.3	117	200	.03	.11	3.7	3
Chicken a la King	1 cup	245	470	27	34	12	127	358	2.5	404	1130	.10	.42	5.4	12
Chicken n Noodles	1 cup	240	365	22	18	26	26	247	2.2	149	430	.05	.17	4.3	Tr
Chicken Chow Mein (canned)	1 cup	250	95	7	Tr	18	45	85	1.3	418	150	0.05	0.10	1.0	13
Chicken Pot Pie	1 piece	232	545	23	31	42	70	232	3.0	343	3090	.34	.31	5.5	5

Turkey:

	Amount	Grams	Cal	Prot	Fat	Carb	Ca	P	Fe	K	Vit A	Thia	Ribo	Niac	Asc
Dark roasted	4 pieces	85	175	26	7	0	--	--	2.0	338	--	.03	.20	3.6	--
Light roasted	2 pieces	85	150	28	3	0	--	--	1.0	349	--	.04	.12	9.4	--
Chopped/Diced (light & dark)	1 cup	140	265	44	9	0	11	351	2.5	514	--	.07	.25	10.8	--

Fruits and Fruit Products

	Amount	Grams	Cal	Prot	Fat	Carb	Ca	P	Fe	K	Vit A	Thia	Ribo	Niac	Asc
Apples, raw	2.75"	138	80	Tr	1	20	10	14	.4	152	120	.04	.03	.1	6
	3.25"	212	125	Tr	1	31	15	21	.6	233	190	.06	.04	.2	8
Apple Juice	1 cup	248	120	Tr	Tr	30	15	22	1.5	250	--	.02	.05	.2	2
Apple Sauce, sweet	1 cup	255	230	1	Tr	61	10	13	1.3	166	100	.05	.03	.1	3
Apple Sauce,unsweet	1 cup	244	100	Tr	Tr	26	10	12	1.2	190	100	.05	.02	.1	2
Apricots, raw	3	107	55	1	Tr	14	18	25	.5	301	2890	.03	.04	.6	11
(canned, syrup)	1 cup	258	220	2	Tr	57	28	39	.8	604	4490	.05	.05	1.0	10
(dried)	1 cup	130	340	7	1	86	87	140	7.2	1273	14170	.01	.21	4.3	16
Avocado, raw	1	216	370	5	37	13	22	91	1.3	1303	630	.24	.43	3.5	30
Banana	1	119	100	1	Tr	26	10	31	.8	440	230	.06	.07	.8	12
Blackberries	1 cup	144	85	2	1	19	46	27	1.3	245	290	0.04	0.06	0.6	30
Blueberries	1 cup	145	90	1	1	22	22	19	1.5	117	150	.04	.09	.7	20
Cantaloupe, raw	1 half	477	80	2	Tr	20	38	44	1.1	682	9240	.11	.08	1.6	90
Cherries, tart canned	1 cup	244	105	2	Tr	26	37	32	.7	317	1660	.07	.05	.5	12
Cherries, sweet	10	68	45	1	Tr	12	15	13	.3	129	70	.03	.04	.3	7
Cranberry Juice,sweet	1 cup	253	165	Tr	Tr	42	13	8	.8	25	Tr	.03	.03	.1	81
Cranberry Sauce	1 cup	277	405	Tr	1	104	17	11	.6	83	60	.03	.03	.1	6
Dates, pitted	10	80	220	2	Tr	58	47	50	2.4	518	40	.07	.08	1.8	0
Dates, chopped	1 cup	178	490	4	1	130	105	112	5.3	1153	90	.16	.18	3.9	0
Fruit Cocktail,canned	1 cup	255	195	1	Tr	50	23	31	1.0	411	360	.05	.03	1.0	5
Grapefruit, pink	1 half	241	50	1	Tr	13	20	20	.5	166	540	.05	.02	.2	44
Grapefruit, white	1 half	241	45	1	Tr	12	19	19	.5	159	10	.05	.02	.2	44
Grapefruit, canned	1 cup	254	180	2	Tr	45	33	36	.8	343	30	.08	.05	.5	76
Grapefruit Juice	1 cup	246	95	1	Tr	23	22	37	.5	399	.10	.05	.5	93	
Grapes, raw	10	50	35	Tr	Tr	9	6	10	.2	87	50	.03	.02	.2	2
Grape Juice	1 cup	253	165	1	Tr	42	28	30	.8	293	--	.10	.05	.5	Tr
Frozen Grape Juice	1 cup	250	135	1	Tr	33	8	10	.3	85	10	.05	.08	.5	10
Grape Drink, canned	1 cup	250	135	Tr	Tr	35	8	10	.3	88	--	.03	.03	.3	--

	Amount	Grams (g)	Calories	Protein (g)	Fat (g)	Carbohydrates (g)	Calcium (mg)	Phosphorus (mg)	Iron (mg)	Potassium (mg)	Vitamin A (I. Units)	Thiamine (mg)	Riboflavin (mg)	Niacin (mg)	Ascorbic acid (mg)
Fruits and Fruit Products (continued)															
Lemon	1	74	20	1	Tr	6	19	12	.4	102	10	.03	.01	.1	39
Lemonade	1 cup	248	105	Tr	Tr	28	2	3	.1	40	10	.01	.02	.2	17
Limeade	1 cup	247	100	Tr	Tr	27	3	3	Tr	32	Tr	Tr	Tr	Tr	6
Honey Dew Melon	1/10	226	50	1	Tr	11	21	24	.6	374	60	.06	.04	.9	34
Orange	2 5/8"	131	65	1	Tr	16	54	26	.5	263	260	.13	.05	.5	66
Orange Juice,fresh	1 cup	248	110	2	Tr	26	27	42	.5	496	500	.22	.07	1.0	124
Orange juice,unsweet	1 cup	249	120	2	Tr	28	25	45	1.0	496	500	.17	.05	.7	100
Frozen Orange Juice	1 cup	249	120	2	Tr	29	25	42	.2	503	540	.23	.03	.9	120
Papayas,raw cubes	1 cup	140	55	1	Tr	14	28	22	.4	328	2450	.06	.06	.4	78
Peaches	2 1/2"	100	40	1	Tr	10	9	19	.5	202	1330	.02	.05	1.0	7
Sliced Peaches	1 cup	170	65	1	Tr	16	15	32	.9	343	2260	.03	.09	1.7	12
Peaches, canned (syrup)	1 cup	256	200	1	Tr	51	10	31	.8	333	1100	.03	.05	1.5	8
Pears, Bartlett	2 1/2"	164	100	1	1	25	13	18	.5	213	30	.03	.07	.2	7
Pineapple,raw diced	1 cup	155	80	1	Tr	21	26	12	.8	226	110	.14	.05	.3	26
Pineapple, canned (syrup)	1 cup	255	190	1	Tr	49	28	13	.8	245	130	.20	.05	.5	18
Pineapple Slices	1 slice	105	80	Tr	Tr	20	12	5	.3	101	50	.08	.02	.2	7
Pineapple Juice (unsweetened)	1 cup	250	140	1	Tr	34	38	23	.8	373	130	.13	.05	.5	80
Plums	2 1/8"	66	30	Tr	Tr	8	8	12	.3	112	160	.02	.02	.3	4
"	1 1/2""	28	20	Tr	Tr	6	3	5	.1	48	80	.01	.01	.1	1
Prunes, uncooked	4 lg.	49	110	1	Tr	29	22	34	1.7	298	690	.04	.07	.7	1
Prunes Juice	1 cup	256	195	1	Tr	49	36	51	1.8	602	--	.03	.03	1.0	5
Raisins, packet	1	14	40	Tr	Tr	11	9	14	.5	107	Tr	.02	.01	.1	Tr
Raspberries	1 cup	123	70	1	1	17	27	27	1.1	207	160	.04	.11	1.1	31
Raspberries, Frozen	10 oz.	284	280	2	1	70	37	48	1.7	284	200	.06	.17	1.7	60
Rhubarb, cooked	1 cup	270	380	1	Tr	97	211	41	1.6	548	220	.05	.14	.8	16
Strawberries	1 cup	149	55	1	1	13	31	31	1.5	244	90	0.04	0.10	0.9	88
Tangerine	2 3/8"	86	40	1	Tr	10	34	15	.3	108	360	.05	.02	.1	27
Watermelon 4x8	1 wedge	926	110	2	1	27	30	43	2.1	426	2510	.13	.13	.9	30
Grain Products:															
Bagel, egg	1	55	165	6	2	28	9	43	1.2	41	30	.14	.10	1.2	0
Bagel, water	1	55	165	6	1	30	8	41	1.2	42	0	.15	.11	1.4	0
Biscuit, home 2"	1	28	105	2	5	13	34	49	.4	33	Tr	.08	.08	.7	Tr
Biscuit, mix	1	28	90	2	3	15	19	65	.6	32	Tr	.09	.08	.8	Tr
Breads:															
Brown Bread	1 slice	45	95	2	1	21	41	72	.9	131	0	.06	.04	.7	0
Cracked Wheat	1 slice	25	65	2	1	13	22	32	.5	34	Tr	.08	.06	.8	Tr
French	1 slice	35	100	3	1	19	15	30	.8	32	Tr	.14	.08	1.2	Tr
Vienna	1 slice	25	75	2	1	14	11	21	.6	23	Tr	.10	.06	.8	Tr
Italian	1 slice	30	85	3	Tr	17	5	23	.7	22	0	.12	.07	1.0	0
Raisin	1 slice	25	65	2	1	13	18	22	.6	58	Tr	.09	.06	.6	Tr
Rye	1 slice	25	60	2	Tr	13	19	37	.5	36	0	.07	.05	.7	0
Pumpernickel	1 slice	32	80	3	Tr	17	27	73	.8	145	0	.09	.07	.6	0
White	1 slice	25	70	2	1	13	21	24	.6	26	Tr	.10	.06	.8	Tr
Whole Wheat	1 slice	28	65	3	1	14	24	71	.8	72	Tr	.09	.03	.8	Tr

Grain Products (continued)

	Amount	Grams (g)	Calories	Protein (g)	Fat (g)	Carbohydrates (g)	Calcium (mg)	Phosphorus (mg)	Iron (mg)	Potassium (mg)	Vitamin A (I. Units)	Thiamine (mg)	Riboflavin (mg)	Niacin (mg)	Ascorbic acid (mg)
Breakfast Cereals:															
Corn (hominy, grits) enriched	1 cup	245	125	3	Tr	27	2	25	.7	27	Tr	.10	.07	1.0	0
Oatmeal, rolled oats	1 cup	240	130	5	2	23	22	137	1.4	146	0	.19	.05	.2	0
Bran Flakes,sweet	1 cup	35	105	4	1	28	19	125	15.6	137	1650	.41	.49	4.1	12
w/raisins	1 cup	50	145	4	1	40	28	146	16.9	154	2350	.58	.71	5.8	18
Corn Flakes,plain	1 cup	25	95	2	Tr	21	--	9	0.6	30	1180	0.29	0.35	2.9	9
(sugar coated)	1 cup	40	155	2	Tr	37	1	10	1.0	27	1880	.46	.56	4.6	14
Puffed Corn	1 cup	20	80	2	1	16	4	18	2.3	--	940	.23	.28	2.3	7
Corn Shredded,sweet	1 cup	25	95	2	Tr	22	1	10	.6	--	0	.11	.05	.5	0
Puffed Oats, sweet	1 cup	25	100	3	1	19	44	102	2.9	--	1180	.29	.35	2.9	9
Puffed Rice, plain	1 cup	15	60	1	Tr	13	3	14	.3	15	0	.07	.01	.7	0
sweetened	1 cup	28	115	1	0	26	3	14	1.1	43	1250	.38	.43	5.0	15
Wheat Flakes, sweet	1 cup	30	105	3	Tr	24	12	83		81	1410	.35	.42	3.5	11
Plain Puffed Wheat	1 cup	15	55	2	Tr	12	4	48	.6	51	0	.08	.03	1.2	0
Sweetened	1 cup	38	140	3	Tr	33	7	52	1.6	63	1680	.50	.57	6.7	20
Shredded Wheat, plain	1/2 cup	25	90	2	1	20	11	97	.9	87	0	.06	.03	1.1	0
Wheat Germ	1 tbsp	6	25	2	1	3	3	70	.5	57	10	.11	.05	.3	1
Cakes:															
Angel Food	1 slice	53	135	3	Tr	32	50	63	.2	32	0	.03	.08	.3	0
Coffee Cake	1 slice	72	230	5	7	38	44	125	1.2	78	120	.14	.15	1.3	Tr
Cupcakes, no icing	1	25	90	1	3	14	40	59	.3	21	40	.05	.05	.4	Tr
w/Chocolate icing	1	36	130	2	5	21	47	71	.4	42	60	.05	.06	.4	Tr
Devils Food Cake	1 slice	69	235	3	8	40	41	72	1.0	90	100	.07	.10	.6	Tr
Gingerbread	1 slice	63	175	2	4	32	57	63	.9	173	Tr	.09	.11	.8	Tr
White w/chocolate icing	1 slice	69	235	3	8	40	63	126	.8	75	100	.08	.10	.7	Tr
Boston Cream Pie	1 slice	69	210	3	6	34	46	70	.7	61	140	.09	.11	.8	Tr
Fruit Cake	1 slice	15	55	1	2	9	11	17	.4	74	20	.02	.02	.2	Tr
Pound Cake	1 slice	33	160	2	10	16	6	24	.5	20	80	.05	.06	.4	0
Sponge Cake	1 slice	66	195	5	4	36	20	74	1.1	57	300	.09	.14	.6	Tr
Cookies:															
Brownie with nuts	1	20	95	1	6	10	8	30	.4	38	40	.04	.03	.2	Tr
Chocolate Chip (commercial) 2.25"	4	42	200	2	9	29	16	48	1.0	56	50	.10	.17	.9	Tr
Gingersnaps 2"	4	28	90	2	2	22	20	13	.7	129	20	.08	.06	.7	0
Oatmeal with raisins	4	52	235	3	8	38	11	53	1.4	192	30	.15	.10	1.0	Tr
Vanilla Wafers 1 3/4"	10	40	185	2	6	30	16	25	.6	29	50	.10	.09	.8	0

	Amount	Grams (g)	Calories	Protein (g)	Fat (g)	Carbohydrates (g)	Calcium (mg)	Phosphorus (mg)	Iron (mg)	Potassium (mg)	Vitamin A (I. Units)	Thiamine (mg)	Riboflavin (mg)	Niacin (mg)	Ascorbic acid (mg)
Grain Products (continued)															
Crackers:															
Graham, plain 2 /12"	2	14	55	1	1	10	6	21	.5	55	0	.02	.08	.5	0
Saltines	4	11	50	1	1	8	2	10	.5	13	0	.05	.05	.4	0
Danish Pastry, plain	4 1/4"	65	275	5	15	30	33	71	1.2	73	200	.18	.19	1.7	Tr
Doughnuts, plain	1	25	100	1	5	13	10	48	.4	23	20	.05	.05	.4	Tr
" Yeast, Glazed	1	50	205	3	11	22	16	33	.6	34	25	.10	.10	.8	0
Macaroni and Cheese															
Canned	1 cup	240	230	9	10	26	199	182	1.0	139	260	.12	.24	1.0	Tr
Home recipe	1 cup	200	430	17	22	40	362	322	1.8	240	860	.20	.40	1.8	Tr
Muffins:															
Blueberry	1	40	110	3	4	17	34	53	.6	46	90	.09	.10	.7	Tr
Bran	1	40	105	3	4	17	57	162	1.5	172	90	.07	.10	1.7	Tr
Corn	1	40	125	3	4	19	42	68	.7	54	120	.10	.10	.7	Tr
Plain	1	40	120	3	4	17	42	60	0.6	50	40	0.09	0.12	0.9	Tr
Pancakes: 4" dia.															
Buckwheat	1	27	55	2	2	6	59	91	.4	66	60	.04	.05	.2	Tr
Plain	1	27	60	2	2	9	27	38	.4	33	30	.06	.07	.5	Tr
Pies(9") 1 slice= 1/7															
Apple	1 slice	135	345	3	15	51	11	30	.9	108	40	.15	.11	1.3	2
Banana Cream	1 slice	130	285	6	12	40	86	107	1.0	264	330	.11	.22	1.0	1
Blueberry	1 slice	135	325	3	15	47	15	31	1.4	88	40	.15	.11	1.4	4
Cherry	1 slice	135	350	4	15	52	19	34	.9	142	590	.16	.12	1.4	Tr
Custard	1 slice	130	285	8	14	30	125	147	1.2	178	300	.11	.27	.8	0
Lemon Meringue	1 slice	120	305	4	12	45	17	59	1.0	60	200	.09	.12	.7	4
Mince	1 slice	135	365	3	16	56	38	51	1.9	240	Tr	.14	.12	1.4	1
Peach	1 slice	135	345	3	14	52	14	39	1.2	201	990	.15	.14	2.0	4
Pecan	1 slice	118	495	6	27	61	55	122	3.7	145	190	.26	.14	1.0	Tr
Pumpkin	1 slice	130	275	5	15	32	66	90	1.0	208	3210	.11	.18	1.0	Tr
Pizza															
Cheese,4 3/4"	1 slice	60	145	6	4	22	86	89	1.1	67	230	0.16	0.18	1.6	4
Popcorn, plain	1 cup	6	25	1	Tr	5	1	17	.2	--	--	--	.01	.1	0
(oil, salt)	1 cup	9	40	1	2	5	1	19	.2	--	--	--	.01	.2	0
Pretzels:															
Dutch	1	16	60	2	1	12	4	21	.2	21	0	.05	.04	.7	0
Thin Twisted	10	60	235	6	3	46	13	79	.9	78	0	.20	.15	2.5	0
Stick 2 1/4"	10	3	10	Tr	Tr	2	1	4	Tr	4	0	.01	.01	.1	0
Instant White Rice	1 cup	165	180	4	Tr	40	5	31	1.3	--	0	.21		1.7	0
Long Grain Rice	1 cup	205	225	4	Tr	50	21	57	1.8	57	0	.23	.02	2.1	0
Par Boiled Rice	1 cup	175	185	4	Tr	41	33	100	1.4	75	0	.19	.02	2.1	0
Brown n Serve Rolls	1	26	85	2	2	14	20	23	.5	25	Tr	.10	.06	.9	Tr
Frankfurter/Hamburger:															
Buns	1	40	120	3	2	21	30	34	.8	38	Tr	.16	.10	1.3	Tr
Hard Rolls	1	50	155	5	2	30	24	46	1.2	49	Tr	.20	.12	1.7	Tr

257

	Amount	Grams (g)	Calories	Protein (g)	Fat (g)	Carbohydrates (g)	Calcium (mg)	Phosphorus (mg)	Iron (mg)	Potassium (mg)	Vitamin A (I. Units)	Thiamine (mg)	Riboflavin (mg)	Niacin (mg)	Ascorbic acid (mg)
Grain Products (continued)															
Hoagie	1	135	390	12	4	75	58	115	3.0	122	Tr	.54	.32	4.5	Tr
Spaghetti	1 cup	140	155	5	1	32	11	70	1.3	85	0	.20	.11	1.5	0
Spagehtti Sauce															
w/cheese, home	1 cup	250	260	9	9	37	80	135	2.3	408	1080	.25	.18	2.3	13
canned	1 cup	250	190	6	2	39	40	88	2.8	303	930	.35	.28	4.5	10
Spaghetti & meat sauce:															
Home	1 cup	248	330	19	12	39	124	236	3.7	665	1590	.25	.30	4.0	22
Canned	1 cup	250	260	12	10	29	53	113	3.3	245	1000	.15	.18	2.3	5
Toaster Pastries	1	50	200	3	6	36	54	67	1.9	74	500	.16	.17	2.1	
Waffles:															
Home 7"	1	75	210	7	7	28	85	130	1.3	109	250	.17	.23	1.4	Tr
Mix	1	75	205	7	8	27	179	257	1.0	146	170	.14	.22	.9	Tr

Legumes, Nuts, Seeds and Related Products

	Amount	Grams (g)	Calories	Protein (g)	Fat (g)	Carbohydrates (g)	Calcium (mg)	Phosphorus (mg)	Iron (mg)	Potassium (mg)	Vitamin A (I. Units)	Thiamine (mg)	Riboflavin (mg)	Niacin (mg)	Ascorbic acid (mg)
Chopped Almonds	1 cup	130	775	24	70	25	304	655	6.1	1005	0	.31	1.20	4.6	Tr
Almond Slivers	1 cup	115	690	21	62	22	269	580	5.4	889	0	.28	1.06	4.0	Tr
Brazil Nuts	1 oz.	28	185	4	19	3	53	196	1.0	203	Tr	.27	.03	.5	--
Cashew Nuts, Roasted	1 cup	140	785	24	64	41	53	522	5.3	650	140	.60	.35	2.5	--
Filberts/ Hazel Nuts	1 cup	115	730	14	72	19	240	388	3.9	810	--	.53	--	1.0	Tr
Peanuts,roasted/salted	1 cup	144	840	37	72	27	107	577	3.0	971	--	.46	.19	24.8	0
Peanut Butter	1 tbsp	16	95	4	8	3	9	61	.3	100	--	.02	.02	2.4	0
Pecans	1 cup	118	810	11	84	17	86	341	2.8	712	150	1.01	.15	1.1	2
Black Walnuts	1 cup	125	785	26	74	19	Tr	713	7.5	575	380	.28	.14	.9	--
English Walnuts	1 cup	120	780	18	77	19	119	456	3.7	540	40	.40	.16	1.1	2
Coconut Meat	1 piece	45	155	2	16	4	6	43	.8	115	0	.02	.01	.2	1
Lentils	1 cup	200	210	16	Tr	39	50	238	4.2	498	40	.14	.12	1.2	0
Pumpkin Seeds	1 cup	140	775	41	65	21	71	1602	15.7	1386	100	.34	.27	3.4	--
Sunflower Seeds	1 cup	145	810	35	69	29	174	1214	10.3	1334	70	2.84	.33	7.8	--

Sugars and Sweets

	Amount	Grams (g)	Calories	Protein (g)	Fat (g)	Carbohydrates (g)	Calcium (mg)	Phosphorus (mg)	Iron (mg)	Potassium (mg)	Vitamin A (I. Units)	Thiamine (mg)	Riboflavin (mg)	Niacin (mg)	Ascorbic acid (mg)
Cake Icing-White	1 cup	94	295	1	0	75	2	2	Tr	17	0	Tr	0.03	Tr	0
White w/coconut	1 cup	166	605	3	13	124	10	50	0.8	277	0	0.02	.07	0.3	0
Cake Icing-Chocolate	1 cup	275	1035	9	38	185	165	305	3.3	536	580	.06	.28	.6	1
Fudge Icing/mix	1 cup	245	830	7	16	183	96	218	2.7	238	Tr	.05	.20	.7	Tr
Candy:															
Caramel	1 oz.	28	115	1	3	22	42	35	.4	54	Tr	.01	.05	.1	Tr
Milk Chocolate	1 oz.	28	145	2	9	16	65	65	.3	109	80	.02	.10	.1	Tr
Semi-Sweet	1 cup	170	860	7	61	97	51	255	4.4	553	30	.02	.14	.9	0
Chocolate Peanuts	1 oz.	28	160	5	12	11	33	84	.4	143	Tr	.10	.05	2.1	Tr
Chocolate Fudge	1 oz.	28	115	1	3	21	22	24	.3	42	Tr	.01	.03	.1	Tr
Gum Drops	1 oz.	28	100	Tr	Tr	25	2	Tr	.1	1	0	0	Tr	Tr	0
Hard Candy	1 oz.	28	110	0	Tr	28	6	2	.5	1	0	0	0	0	0
Marshmallows	1 oz.	28	90	1	Tr	23	5	2	.5	2	0	0	Tr	Tr	0
Chocolate powder:															
Non fat dry milk	1 oz.	28	100	5	1	20	167	155	.5	227	10	.04	.21	.2	1
Without milk	1 oz.	28	100	1	1	25	9	48	.6	142	--	.01	.03	.1	0
Honey	1 tbsp	21	65	Tr	0	17	1	1	.1	11	0	Tr	.01	.1	Tr

	Amount	Grams (g)	Calories	Protein (g)	Fat (g)	Carbohydrates (g)	Calcium (mg)	Phosphorus (mg)	Iron (mg)	Potassium (mg)	Vitamin A (I. Units)	Thiamine (mg)	Riboflavin (mg)	Niacin (mg)	Ascorbic acid (mg)
Legumes, Nuts, Seeds and Related Products (continued)															
Jams/Preserves	1 tbsp.	20	55	Tr	Tr	14	4	2	.2	18	Tr	Tr	.01	Tr	Tr
Jelly	1 tbsp.	18	50	Tr	Tr	13	4	1	.3	14	Tr	Tr	.01	Tr	1
Syrups:															
Chocolate topping	2 tbsp.	38	90	1	1	24	6	35	.6	106	Tr	.01	.03	.2	0
Molasses(light)	1 tbsp.	20	50	--	--	13	33	9	.9	183	--	.01	.01	Tr	--
Table Blends	1 tbsp.	21	60	0	0	15	9	3	.8	1	0	0	0	0	0
Sugar (White granulated)	1 tbsp.	12	45	0	0	12	0	0	Tr	Tr	0	0	0	0	0
Powdered Sugar	1 cup	100	385	0	0	100	0	0	.1	3	0	0	0	0	0
Vegetable/Vegetable Products															
Asparagus:															
(Frozen Cuts & Tips)	1 cup	180	40	6	Tr	6	40	115	2.2	396	1530	.25	.23	1.8	41
(Frozen Spears)	4	60	15	2	Tr	2	13	40	.7	143	470	.10	.08	.7	16
(Canned Spears)	4	80	15	2	Tr	3	15	42	1.5	133	640	.05	.08	.6	12
Beans:															
Navy	1 cup	190	225	15	1	40	95	281	5.1	790	1	.27	.13	1.3	0
Kidney	1 cup	255	230	15	1	42	74	278	4.6	673	10	.13	.10	1.5	--
Lima	1 cup	190	260	16	1	49	55	293	5.9	1163	--	.25	.11	1.3	--
Snap Green	1 cup	125	30	2	Tr	7	63	46	.8	189	680	.09	.11	.6	15
French Style	1 cup	130	35	2	Tr	8	49	39	1.2	177	690	.08	.10	.4	9
Yellow/Waxed	1 cup	135	35	2	Tr	8	47	42	.9	221	140	.09	.11	.5	8
Bean Sprouts	1 cup	125	35	4	Tr	7	21	60	1.1	195	30	.11	.13	.9	8
Beets															
(Whole)	2	100	30	1	Tr	7	14	23	.5	208	20	.03	.04	.3	6
(Diced/Sliced)	1 cup	170	55	2	Tr	12	24	39	.9	354	30	.05	.07	.5	10
Blackeyed Peas	1 cup	170	220	15	1	40	43	286	4.8	573	290	.68	.19	2.4	15
Broccoli	1 cup	155	40	5	Tr	7	136	96	1.2	414	3880	.14	.31	1.2	140
Brussel Sprouts	1 cup	155	55	7	1	10	50	112	1.7	423	810	.12	.22	1.2	135
Cabbage															
(Raw, shredded)	1 cup	90	20	1	Tr	5	44	26	.4	210	120	.05	.05	.3	42
(Cooked)	1 cup	145	30	2	Tr	6	64	29	.4	236	190	.06	.06	.4	48
Carrots															
(Raw,7x1 in.)	1	72	30	1	Tr	7	27	26	.5	246	7930	.04	.04	.4	6
(Cooked)	1 cup	155	50	1	Tr	11	51	48	.9	344	16280	.08	.08	.8	9
Cauliflower															
(Flowerets-cooked)	1 cup	180	30	3	Tr	6	31	68	.9	373	50	.07	.09	.7	74
(Raw/chopped)	1 cup	115	31	3	Tr	6	29	64	1.3	339	70	.13	.12	.8	90
Celery															
(Raw)	1	40	5	Tr	Tr	2	16	11	.1	136	110	.01	.01	.1	4
Collards															
(Cooked)	1 cup	170	50	5	1	10	299	87	1.7	401	11560	.10	.24	1.0	56

259

	Amount	Grams (g)	Calories	Protein (g)	Fat (g)	Carbohydrates (g)	Calcium (mg)	Phosphorus (mg)	Iron (mg)	Potassium (mg)	Vitamin A (I. Units)	Thiamine (mg)	Riboflavin (mg)	Niacin (mg)	Ascorbic acid (mg)

Vegetable and Vegetable Products, continued

	Amount	Grams	Calories	Protein	Fat	Carb	Calcium	Phosphorus	Iron	Potassium	Vitamin A	Thiamine	Riboflavin	Niacin	Ascorbic acid
Corn															
(Ear-5 in.)	1	229	120	4	1	27	4	121	1.0	291	440	.18	.10	2.1	9
(Kernels)	1 cup	165	130	5	1	31	5	120	1.3	304	580	.15	.10	2.5	8
(Creamed)	1 cup	256	210	5	2	51	8	143	1.5	248	840	.08	.13	2.6	13
Cucumber															
(Slices-large 2 1/8 in.)	6	28	5	Tr	Tr	1	5	5	0.1	45	Tr	0.01	0.01	0.1	3
Lettuce-Iceberg															
(Wedge-1/4 of a head)	1	135	20	1	Tr	4	27	30	.7	236	450	.08	.08	.4	8
(Pieces-shredded)	1cup	55	5	Tr	Tr	2	11	12	.3	96	180	.03	.03	.2	3
Mushrooms, raw	1 cup	70	20	2	Tr	3	4	81	.6	290	Tr	.07	.32	2.9	2
Onions															
(Raw/Chopped)	1 cup	170	65	3	Tr	15	46	61	.9	267	Tr	.05	.07	.3	17
(Sliced)	1 cup	115	45	2	Tr	10	31	41	.6	181	Tr	.03	.05	.2	12
Peas															
(Canned)	1 cup	170	150	8	1	29	44	129	3.2	163	1170	.15	.10	1.4	14
(Frozen-cooked)	1 cup	160	110	8	Tr	19	30	138	3.0	216	960	.43	.14	2.7	21
Potatos:															
Baked	1	156	145	4	Tr	33	14	101	1.1	782	Tr	.15	.07	2.7	31
Boiled	1	137	105	3	Tr	23	10	72	.8	556	Tr	.12	.05	2.0	22
French Fries-Strip)	10	50	135	2	7	18	8	56	.7	427	Tr	.07	.04	1.6	11
Hash browns	1 cup	155	345	3	18	45	28	78	1.9	439	Tr	.11	.03	1.6	12
Mashed(with milk)	1 cup	210	135	4	2	27	50	103	.8	548	40	.17	.11	2.1	21

Miscellaneous Items

	Amount	Grams	Calories	Protein	Fat	Carb	Calcium	Phosphorus	Iron	Potassium	Vitamin A	Thiamine	Riboflavin	Niacin	Ascorbic acid
Barbecue Sauce	1 cup	250	230	4	17	20	53	50	2.0	435	900	.03	.03	.8	13
Beverages, Carbonated:															
Cola	12 oz.	369	145	0	0	37	--	--	--	--	0	0	0	0	0
Fruit-flavored soda	12 oz.	372	170	0	0	45	--	--	--	--	0	0	0	0	0
Ginger ale	12 oz.	366	115	0	0	29	--	--	--	0	0	0	0.	0	0
Root beer	12 oz.	370	150	0	0	39	--	--	--	0	0	0	0	0	0
Gelatin Dessert	1 cup	240	140	4	0	34	--	--	--	--	--	--	--	--	--
Olives:															
Green	4 med.	16	15	Tr	2	Tr	8	2	.2	7	40	--	--	--	--
Ripe Mission	2 lg.	10	15	Tr	2	Tr	9	1	.1	2	10	Tr	Tr	--	--
Pickles:															
Dill	1 med.	65	5	Tr	Tr	1	17	14	.7	130	70	Tr	.01	Tr	4
Sweet-2 1/2 in.	1	15	20	Tr	Tr	5	2	2	.2	--	10	Tr	Tr	Tr	1
Relish	1 tbsp.	15	20	Tr	Tr	5	3	2	.1	--	--	--	--	--	--
Soup:															
(Canned/Condensed with milk)															
Cream of Chicken	1 cup	245	180	7	10	15	172	152	0.5	260	610	0.05	0.27	0.7	2
Cream of Mushroom	1 cup	245	215	7	14	16	191	169	.5	279	250	.05	.34	.7	1
Tomato	1 cup	250	175	7	7	23	168	155	.8	418	1200	.10	.25	1.3	15
(Prepared with water)															
Beef Broth	1 cup	240	30	5	0	3	Tr	31	.5	130	Tr	Tr	.02	1.2	--
Beef Noodle	1 cup	240	65	4	3	7	7	48	1.0	77	50	.05	.07	1.0	Tr
Clam Chowder	1 cup	245	80	2	3	12	34	47	1.0	184	880	.02	.02	1.0	--
Cream of Chicken	1 cup	240	95	3	6	8	24	34	.5	79	410	.02	.05	.5	Tr
Cream of Mushroom	1 cup	240	135	2	10	10	41	50	.5	98	70	.02	.12	.7	Tr
Split Pea	1 cup	245	145	9	3	21	29	149	1.5	270	440	.25	.15	1.5	1
Tomato	1 cup	245	90	2	3	16	15	34	.7	230	1000	.05	.05	1.2	12
Vegetable Beef	1 cup	245	80	5	2	10	12	49	.7	162	2700	.05	.05	1.0	--
Vegetarian	1 cup	245	80	2	2	13	20	39	1.0	172	2940	.05	.05	1.0	--

Caloric Expenditure

Caloric Expenditure Table

Calorie Expenditure per Minute for Various Activities

Activity	Body Weight																					
	90	99	108	117	125	134	143	152	161	170	178	187	196	205	213	222	231	240	249	257	266	275
Archery	3.1	3.4	3.7	4.0	4.5	4.6	4.9	5.2	5.5	5.8	6.1	6.4	6.7	7.0	7.3	7.6	7.9	8.2	8.5	8.8	9.1	9.4
Badminton (recreation)	3.4	3.8	4.1	4.4	4.8	5.1	5.4	5.8	6.1	6.4	6.8	7.1	7.4	7.8	8.1	8.3	8.8	9.1	9.4	9.8	10.1	10.4
Badminton (competition)	5.9	6.4	7.0	7.6	8.1	8.7	9.3	9.9	10.4	11.0	11.6	12.1	12.7	13.3	13.9	14.4	15.0	15.6	16.1	16.7	17.3	17.9
Basebal (player)	2.8	3.1	3.4	3.6	3.9	4.2	4.5	4.7	5.0	5.3	5.5	5.8	6.1	6.4	6.6	6.9	7.2	7.5	7.7	8.0	8.3	8.6
Basebal (pitcher)	3.5	3.9	4.3	4.6	5.0	5.3	5.7	6.0	6.4	6.7	7.1	7.4	7.8	8.1	8.5	8.8	9.2	9.5	9.9	10.2	10.6	10.9
Basketball (half-court)	2.5	3.3	3.5	3.8	4.1	4.4	4.7	4.9	5.3	5.6	5.9	6.2	6.4	6.7	7.0	7.3	7.6	7.6	8.2	8.5	8.8	9.0
Basketball (moderate)	4.2	4.6	5.0	5.5	5.9	6.3	6.7	7.1	7.5	7.9	8.3	8.8	9.2	9.6	10.0	10.4	10.8	11.1	11.6	12.1	12.5	12.9
Basketball (competition)	5.9	6.5	7.1	7.7	8.2	8.8	9.4	10.0	10.6	11.1	11.7	12.3	12.9	13.5	14.0	14.6	15.2	15.8	16.3	16.9	17.5	18.1
Bicycling (level) 5.5 mph	3.0	3.3	3.6	3.9	4.2	4.5	4.8	5.1	5.4	5.6	5.9	6.2	6.5	6.8	7.1	7.4	7.7	8.0	8.3	8.6	8.9	9.2
Bicycling (level) 13 mph	6.4	7.1	7.7	8.3	8.9	9.6	10.2	10.8	11.4	12.1	12.7	13.4	14.0	14.6	15.2	15.9	16.5	17.1	17.8	18.4	19.0	19.6
Bowling (nonstop)	4.0	4.4	4.8	5.2	5.6	5.9	6.3	6.7	7.1	7.5	7.9	8.3	8.7	9.1	9.5	9.8	10.2	10.6	11.0	11.4	11.8	12.2
Boxing (sparring)	3.0	3.3	3.6	3.9	4.2	4.5	4.8	5.1	5.4	5.6	5.9	6.2	6.5	6.8	7.1	7.4	7.7	8.0	8.3	8.6	8.9	9.2
Calisthenics	3.0	3.3	3.6	3.9	4.2	4.5	4.8	5.1	5.4	5.6	5.9	6.2	6.5	6.8	7.1	7.4	7.7	8.0	8.3	8.6	8.9	9.2
Canoeing, 2.5 mph	1.8	1.9	2.0	2.2	2.3	2.5	2.7	3.0	3.2	3.4	3.6	3.7	3.9	4.1	4.3	4.4	4.6	4.8	5.0	5.1	5.3	5.5
Canoeing, 4.0 mph	4.2	4.6	5.0	5.5	5.9	6.3	6.7	7.1	7.5	7.9	8.3	8.7	9.2	9.4	10.0	10.5	10.8	11.2	11.6	12.0	12.4	12.9
Dance, modern (moderate)	2.5	2.8	3.0	3.2	3.5	3.7	4.0	4.2	4.5	4.7	5.0	5.2	5.4	5.7	5.9	6.2	6.4	6.7	6.9	7.2	7.4	7.6
Dance, modern (vigorous)	3.4	3.7	4.1	4.4	4.7	5.1	5.4	5.7	6.1	6.4	6.7	7.1	7.4	7.7	8.1	8.4	8.7	9.1	9.4	9.7	10.1	10.4
Dance, fox-trot	2.7	2.9	3.2	3.4	3.7	4.0	4.2	4.5	4.7	5.0	5.3	5.5	5.8	6.0	6.3	6.6	6.8	7.1	7.3	7.6	7.9	8.1
Dance, rumba	4.2	4.6	5.0	5.4	5.8	6.2	6.6	7.0	7.4	7.8	8.2	8.6	9.0	9.3	9.7	10.2	10.5	11.0	11.5	11.9	12.3	12.6
Dance, square	4.1	4.5	4.9	5.3	5.7	6.1	6.5	6.9	7.3	7.8	8.1	8.5	8.9	9.3	9.7	10.1	10.5	10.9	11.3	11.7	12.1	12.4
Dance, waltz	3.1	3.4	3.7	4.0	4.2	4.6	4.9	5.2	5.5	5.8	6.1	6.4	6.7	7.0	7.3	7.6	7.9	8.2	8.5	8.8	9.1	9.4
Fencing (moderate)	3.0	3.3	3.6	3.9	4.2	4.5	4.8	5.1	5.4	5.6	6.0	6.2	6.5	6.8	7.1	7.4	7.7	8.0	8.3	8.6	8.9	9.2
Fencing (vigorous)	6.2	6.8	7.4	8.0	8.6	9.2	9.8	10.4	11.0	11.6	12.2	12.8	13.4	14.0	14.6	15.2	15.8	16.4	17.0	17.6	18.2	18.8
Football (moderate)	3.0	3.3	3.6	3.9	4.2	4.5	4.8	5.1	5.4	5.7	6.0	6.2	6.5	6.8	7.1	7.4	7.7	8.0	8.3	8.6	8.9	9.2
Football (vigorous)	5.0	5.5	6.0	6.4	6.9	7.4	7.9	8.4	8.9	9.4	9.8	10.3	10.8	11.3	11.8	12.3	12.8	13.2	13.7	14.2	14.7	15.2
Golf, 2-some	3.3	3.6	3.9	4.2	4.5	4.8	5.2	5.5	5.8	6.1	6.4	6.7	7.1	7.4	7.7	8.0	8.3	8.6	9.0	9.3	9.6	10.0
Golf, 4-some	2.4	2.7	2.9	3.2	3.4	3.6	3.9	4.1	4.3	4.6	4.8	5.1	5.3	5.5	5.8	6.0	6.2	6.5	6.7	7.0	7.2	7.4
Handball	5.9	6.4	7.0	7.6	8.1	8.7	9.3	9.9	10.4	11.0	11.6	12.1	12.7	13.3	13.9	14.4	15.0	15.6	16.1	16.7	17.3	17.9
Hiking, 40 lb. pack, 3.0 mph	4.1	4.5	4.9	5.3	5.7	6.1	6.5	6.9	7.3	7.7	8.1	8.5	8.9	9.3	9.7	10.1	10.5	10.9	11.3	11.7	12.1	12.5
Horseback Riding (walk)	2.0	2.3	2.4	2.6	2.8	3.0	3.1	3.3	3.5	3.7	3.9	4.1	4.3	4.5	4.7	4.9	5.1	5.3	5.5	5.7	5.8	6.0
Horseback Riding (trot)	4.1	4.4	4.8	5.2	5.6	6.0	6.4	6.8	7.2	7.6	8.0	8.4	8.8	9.2	9.6	10.0	10.4	10.8	11.2	11.6	12.0	12.4
Horseshoe Pitching	2.1	2.3	2.5	2.7	3.0	3.3	3.4	3.6	3.8	4.0	4.2	4.4	4.6	4.8	5.0	5.2	5.4	5.6	5.8	6.0	6.3	6.5
Judo, Karate	7.7	8.5	9.2	10.0	10.7	11.5	12.2	13.0	13.7	14.5	15.2	16.0	16.7	17.5	18.2	19.0	19.7	20.5	21.2	22.0	22.7	23.5
Mountain Climbing	6.0	6.5	7.2	7.8	8.4	9.0	9.6	10.1	10.7	11.3	11.9	12.5	13.1	13.7	14.4	15.0	15.4	16.0	16.6	17.2	17.8	18.4
Paddleball, Racquetball	5.9	6.4	7.0	7.6	8.1	8.7	9.3	9.9	10.4	11.0	11.6	12.1	12.7	13.3	13.9	14.4	15.0	15.6	16.1	16.7	17.3	17.9
Pool, Billiards	1.1	1.2	1.3	1.4	1.5	1.6	1.7	1.8	1.9	2.0	2.1	2.2	2.4	2.5	2.6	2.7	2.8	2.9	3.0	3.1	3.2	3.3
Push Ups	4.3	4.7	5.1	5.6	6.0	6.4	6.8	7.2	7.7	8.1	8.5	8.9	9.4	9.8	10.2	10.6	11.0	11.5	11.9	12.3	12.7	13.2
Racquetball	6.0	6.6	7.2	7.8	8.3	8.9	9.5	10.1	10.7	11.3	11.9	12.5	13.1	13.7	14.2	14.8	15.4	16.0	16.6	17.2	17.8	18.4

Calorie Expenditure per Minute for Various Activities

	Body Weight																					
	90	99	108	117	125	134	143	152	161	170	178	187	196	205	213	222	231	240	249	257	266	275
Rowing (recreation)	3.0	3.3	3.6	3.9	4.2	4.5	4.8	5.1	5.4	5.6	6.0	6.2	6.5	6.8	7.1	7.5	7.7	8.0	8.3	8.6	8.9	9.2
Rowing (machine)	8.2	9.0	9.8	10.6	11.4	12.2	13.0	13.8	14.6	15.4	16.2	17.0	17.8	18.6	19.4	20.2	21.0	21.8	22.6	23.4	24.2	25.0
Running, 11-min. mile 5.5 mph	6.4	7.1	7.7	8.3	9.0	9.6	10.2	10.8	11.5	12.1	12.7	13.4	14.0	14.6	15.2	15.9	16.5	17.1	17.8	18.4	19.0	19.6
Running, 8.5-min. mile 7 mph	8.4	9.2	10.0	10.8	11.7	12.5	13.3	14.1	14.9	15.7	16.6	17.4	18.2	19.0	19.8	20.7	21.5	22.3	23.1	23.9	24.8	25.6
Running, 7-min. mile 9 mph	9.3	10.2	11.1	12.0	13.1	13.9	14.8	15.7	16.6	17.5	18.9	19.3	20.2	21.1	22.1	23.0	23.9	24.8	25.7	26.6	27.5	28.4
Running, 5-min. mile 12 mph	11.8	13.0	14.1	15.3	16.4	17.6	18.7	19.9	21.0	22.3	23.3	24.5	25.6	26.8	27.9	29.1	30.2	31.4	32.5	33.7	34.9	36.0
Sailing	1.8	2.0	2.1	2.3	2.4	2.7	2.8	3.0	3.2	3.4	3.6	3.8	3.9	4.1	4.3	4.4	4.6	4.8	5.0	5.1	5.3	5.5
Sit ups	4.3	4.7	5.1	5.6	6.0	6.4	6.8	7.2	7.7	8.1	8.5	8.9	9.4	9.8	10.2	10.6	11.0	11.5	11.9	12.4	12.7	13.2
Sprinting	13.8	15.2	16.6	17.9	19.2	20.5	21.9	23.3	24.7	26.1	27.3	28.7	30.0	31.4	32.7	34.0	35.4	36.8	39.2	39.4	40.3	42.2
Skating (moderate)	3.4	3.8	4.1	4.4	4.8	5.1	5.4	5.8	6.1	6.4	6.8	7.1	7.4	7.8	8.1	8.3	8.8	9.1	9.4	9.8	10.1	10.4
Skating (vigorous)	6.2	6.8	7.4	8.0	8.6	9.2	9.8	10.4	11.0	11.6	12.2	12.8	13.4	14.0	14.6	15.2	15.8	16.4	17.0	17.6	18.2	18.8
Skiing (downhill)	5.8	6.4	6.9	7.5	8.1	8.6	9.2	9.8	10.3	10.9	11.4	12.0	12.6	13.1	13.7	14.3	14.8	15.4	16.0	16.5	17.1	17.7
Skiing (level, 5 mph)	7.0	7.7	8.4	9.1	9.8	10.5	11.1	11.8	12.5	13.2	13.9	14.6	15.2	15.9	16.6	17.3	18.0	18.7	19.4	20.0	20.7	21.4
Skiing (racing downhill)	9.9	10.9	11.9	12.9	13.7	14.7	15.7	16.7	17.7	18.7	19.6	20.6	21.6	22.6	23.4	24.4	25.4	26.4	27.4	28.3	29.3	30.2
Snowshoeing (2.3 mph)	3.7	4.1	4.5	4.8	5.2	5.5	5.9	6.3	6.7	7.0	7.4	7.8	8.1	8.5	8.8	9.2	9.6	9.9	10.3	10.6	11.0	11.4
Snowshoeing (2.5 mph)	5.4	5.9	6.5	7.0	7.5	8.0	8.6	9.1	9.7	10.2	10.7	11.2	11.8	12.3	12.8	13.3	13.9	14.4	14.9	15.4	16.0	16.5
Soccer	5.4	5.9	6.4	6.9	7.5	8.0	8.5	9.0	9.6	10.1	10.6	11.1	11.6	12.2	12.7	13.2	13.4	14.3	14.8	15.3	15.9	16.9
Squash	6.2	6.8	7.5	8.1	8.7	9.3	9.9	10.5	11.1	11.7	12.3	12.9	13.5	14.2	14.8	15.4	16.0	16.6	17.2	17.8	18.4	19.0
Stationary Running, 140 counts/min.	14.6	16.1	17.5	18.9	20.4	21.8	23.2	24.6	26.1	27.5	28.9	30.4	31.8	33.2	34.6	36.1	37.5	38.9	40.4	41.8	43.2	44.6
Swimming, pleasure 25 yds./min.	3.6	4.0	4.3	4.7	5.0	5.4	5.7	6.1	6.4	6.8	7.1	7.5	7.8	8.2	8.5	8.9	9.2	9.6	10.0	10.3	10.6	11.0
Swimming, back, 20 yds./min.	2.3	2.6	2.8	3.0	3.2	3.5	3.7	3.9	4.1	4.2	4.6	4.8	5.0	5.3	5.5	5.7	6.0	6.2	6.4	6.6	6.9	7.1
Swimming, back 30 yds./min.	3.2	3.5	3.8	4.1	4.4	4.7	5.1	5.4	5.7	6.0	6.3	6.6	6.9	7.2	7.4	7.9	8.2	8.5	8.8	9.1	9.4	9.7
Swimming, back 40 yds./min.	5.0	5.5	5.8	6.5	7.0	7.5	7.9	8.5	8.9	9.4	9.9	10.4	10.9	11.4	11.9	12.3	12.8	13.3	13.8	14.3	14.8	15.3
Swimming, breast 20 yds./min.	2.9	3.2	3.4	3.8	4.0	4.3	4.6	4.9	5.1	5.4	5.7	6.0	6.3	6.5	6.8	7.1	7.4	7.7	7.9	8.2	8.5	8.8
Swimming, breast 30 yds./min.	4.3	4.8	5.2	5.7	6.0	6.4	6.9	7.3	7.7	8.1	8.6	9.0	9.4	9.9	10.3	10.8	11.1	11.5	11.9	12.4	13.0	13.3
Swimming, breast 40 yds./min.	5.8	6.3	6.9	7.5	8.0	8.6	9.2	9.7	10.3	10.8	11.4	12.0	12.5	13.1	13.7	14.2	14.8	15.4	15.9	16.5	17.0	17.6

Calorie Expenditure per Minute for Various Activities

	Body Weight																					
	90	99	108	117	125	134	143	152	161	170	178	187	196	205	213	222	231	240	249	257	266	275
Swimming, butterfly 50 yds./min.	7.0	7.7	8.4	9.1	9.8	10.5	11.1	11.9	12.5	13.2	13.9	14.6	15.2	15.9	16.6	17.3	18.0	18.7	19.4	20.0	20.7	21.4
Swimming, crawl 20 yds./min.	2.9	3.2	3.4	3.8	4.0	4.3	4.6	4.9	5.1	5.4	5.7	5.8	6.3	6.5	6.8	7.1	7.3	7.7	7.9	8.2	8.5	8.8
Swimming, crawl 45 yds./min.	5.2	5.8	6.3	6.8	7.3	7.8	8.3	8.8	9.3	9.8	10.4	10.9	11.4	11.9	12.4	12.9	13.4	13.9	14.4	15.0	15.5	16.0
Swimming, crawl 50 yds./min.	6.4	7.0	7.6	8.3	8.9	9.5	10.1	10.7	11.4	12.0	12.6	13.2	13.9	14.5	15.1	15.7	16.3	17.0	17.4	17.9	18.8	19.5
Table Tennis	2.3	2.6	2.8	3.0	3.2	3.5	3.7	3.9	4.1	4.2	4.6	4.8	5.0	5.3	5.5	5.7	6.0	6.2	6.4	6.6	6.9	7.1
Tennis (recreation)	4.2	4.6	5.0	5.4	5.8	6.2	6.6	7.0	7.4	7.8	8.2	8.6	9.0	9.4	9.8	10.2	10.6	11.0	11.5	11.9	12.3	12.6
Tennis (competition)	5.9	6.4	7.0	7.6	8.1	8.7	9.3	9.9	10.4	11.0	11.6	12.1	12.7	13.3	13.9	14.4	15.0	15.6	16.1	16.7	17.3	17.9
Timed Calisthenics	8.8	9.6	10.5	11.4	12.2	13.1	13.9	14.8	15.6	16.5	17.4	18.2	19.1	19.9	20.8	21.5	22.5	23.9	24.2	25.1	25.9	26.8
Volleyball (moderate)	3.4	3.8	4.0	4.4	4.8	5.1	5.4	5.8	6.1	6.4	6.8	7.1	7.4	7.8	8.1	8.3	8.8	9.1	9.4	9.8	10.1	10.4
Volleyball (vigorous)	5.9	6.4	7.0	7.6	8.1	8.7	9.3	9.9	10.4	11.0	11.6	12.1	12.7	13.3	13.9	14.4	15.0	15.6	16.1	16.7	17.3	17.9
Walking (2.0 mph)	2.1	2.3	2.5	2.7	2.9	3.1	3.3	3.5	3.7	4.0	4.2	4.4	4.6	4.8	5.0	5.2	5.4	5.6	5.8	6.0	6.2	6.4
Walking (4.5 mph)	4.0	4.4	4.7	5.1	5.5	5.9	6.3	6.7	7.1	7.5	7.8	8.2	8.6	9.0	9.4	9.8	10.1	10.6	10.9	11.3	11.7	12.0
Walking 110-120 steps/min.	3.1	3.4	3.7	4.0	4.3	4.7	5.0	5.3	5.6	5.9	6.2	6.5	6.8	7.1	7.4	7.7	8.0	8.3	8.6	8.9	9.2	9.5
Waterskiing	4.7	5.1	5.6	6.1	6.5	7.0	7.4	7.9	8.3	8.8	9.3	9.7	10.2	10.6	11.1	11.5	12.0	12.5	12.9	13.4	13.8	14.3
Weight Training	4.7	5.1	5.7	6.2	6.7	7.0	7.5	7.9	8.4	8.9	9.4	9.9	10.3	10.8	11.1	11.7	12.2	12.6	13.1	13.5	14.0	14.4
Wrestling	7.7	8.5	9.2	10.0	10.7	11.5	12.2	13.0	13.7	14.5	15.2	16.0	16.7	17.5	18.2	19.0	19.7	20.5	21.2	22.0	22.7	23.5

From Consolazio, Johnson and Pecora, *Physiological Measurements of Metabolic Functions in Man*, McGraw-Hill.

LABORATORY
EXERCISES

Laboratory Exercises

Laboratory		Page
1	Preparticipation Health Survey	269
2	Heart Attack Risk Factors (RISKO)	271
3	Resting Heart Rate	275
4	Blood Pressure	277
5	Target Heart Rate Zone	279
6	1.0 Mile Walk	281
7	12-Minute Run or 1.5 Mile Run	283
8	Step Test Assessment	285
9	Muscular Strength and Endurance	287
10	Optimal Weight	289
11	Fitness Test Record	291
12	Fitness Profile	293
13	Designing Your Exercise Program	295
14	The Exercise Session	297
15	Flexibility Workout	299
16	Aerobics	301
17	Weight Training	303
18	Interval Training	305
19	Recovery Heart Rate	307
20	Blood Pressure Recovery	309
21	Nutrition and Caloric Analysis	311
22	One Day Caloric Analysis	317
23	Calorie Distribution	319
24	Inventory of Eating Habits	321
25	Weight Control	323
26	Blood Cholesterol and Triglyceride Levels	325
27	Lifestyle Modification	327
28	Stresso—A Game To Determine Stress	329
29	Stress Awareness	331
30	Handling Your Stress	333
31	Consumer Awareness	335

LABORATORY EXERCISES

Purpose

The labs which follow focus on assisting you in achieving and maintaining a high level of health and fitness by examining your current lifestyle and health habits.

Your teacher may assign some of the labs as part of your classwork or as an assignment for outside the classroom. You are encouraged to explore other labs on your own.

These lab activities will help you understand more about yourself and will help you select activities for a lifetime program of fitness.

LAB 1. PREPARTICIPATION HEALTH SURVEY

Name _____ Telephone _____

Age _____ Sex _____ Height _____ Weight _____

Emergency contact person _____ Telephone _____

I. Medical History
Please indicate if you currently have or have ever had any of the following conditions (check if yes):

_____	Heart disease/problem	_____	Elevated cholesterol
_____	Asthma	_____	Elevated triglycerides
_____	Respiratory problem	_____	Pregnancy (within last 3 months)
_____	Irregular heart rhythm	_____	Polio
_____	High blood pressure	_____	Epilepsy
_____	Stroke	_____	Allergies
_____	Cancer	_____	Fainting/dizzy spells
_____	Ulcers	_____	Shortness of breath
_____	Liver disease	_____	Severe headaches
_____	Pneumonia	_____	Chest pain
_____	Tuberculosis	_____	Back pain
_____	Diabetes	_____	Arthritis
_____	Kidney Infection	_____	Joint injuries
_____	Anemia	_____	Vision problems
_____	Hepatitis	_____	Hearing problems
_____	Infectious mononucleosis	_____	Other _____

If you answered yes to any of the above conditions, please explain below and include approximate dates.

_____

_____

_____

_____

II. Family Medical History
Please indicate if any close relative has or has had any of the following conditions:

	Yes	No	Relation to you
Heart disease	_____	_____	_____
Stroke	_____	_____	_____
Diabetes	_____	_____	_____
Cancer	_____	_____	_____
Elevated cholesterol	_____	_____	_____

III. Lifestyle

Do you smoke?_____ Number of packs per day _____

Do you drink alcohol?_____ Number of drinks per week _____

How many hours do you usually sleep each night?_____

Do you often feel tired?_____

Do you often feel tense or stressed? _____

Do you handle stress well?_____

How many days per week do you exercise vigorously? _____

   For how many minutes per exercise session? _____

Has your doctor ever advised you to avoid any type of exercise?_____ If yes, please explain.

_____

_____

_____

_____

Do you think you will be able to participate in all activities of this course?_____

If no, please describe any medical limitations which you have and list the activities which may be affected by these limitations.

_____

_____

_____

_____

Signature _____ Date_____

LAB 2. HEART ATTACK RISK FACTORS

Name_____ Section_____ Date_____

Purpose

1. To give you an estimate of your chances of suffering a heart attack.
2. To alert you to certain risk factors in your life which need to be changed if possible.

Procedure

Following the instructions, complete RISKO, A Heart Hazard Appraisal.

Results

1. What is your total score? _____

2. What is your classification?_____

Conclusions and Implications

1. What areas of risk represent your greatest problem?

2. In what areas of risk do you score particularly low?

3. What specific steps can you take to reduce your risk?

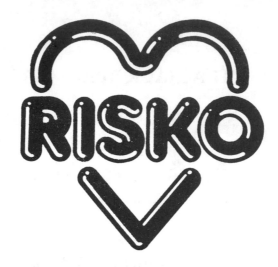

A HEART HAZARD APPRAISAL

RISKO, Copyright 1985 by the American Heart Association, is reproduced with permission.

What Your Score Means

0-4 You have one of the lowest risks of heart disease for your age and sex.

5-9 You have a low to moderate risk of heart disease for your age and sex but there is some room for improvement.

10-14 You have a moderate to high risk of heart disease for your age and sex, with considerable room for improvement on some factors.

15-19 You have a high risk of developing heart disease for your age and sex with a great deal of room for improvement on all factors.

20 & over You have a very high risk of developing heart disease for your age and sex and should take immediate action on all risk factors.

WARNING

* If you have diabetes, gout or a family history of heart disease, your actual risk will be greater than indicated by this appraisal.
* If you do not know your current blood pressure or blood cholesterol level, you should visit your physician or health center to have them measured. Then figure your score again for a more accurate determination of your risk.
* If you are overweight, have high blood pressure or high blood cholesterol, or smoke cigarettes, your long-term risk of heart disease is increased even if your risk in the next several years is low.

How to Reduce Your Risk

* Try to quit smoking permanently. There are many programs available.
* Have your blood pressure checked regularly, preferably every twelve months after age 40. If your blood pressure is high, see your physician. Remember blood pressure medicine is only effective if taken regularly.
* Consider your daily exercise (or lack of it). A half hour of brisk walking, swimming or other enjoyable activity should not be difficult to fit into your day.
* Give some serious thought to your diet. If you are overweight, or eat a lot of foods high in saturated fat or cholesterol (whole milk, cheese, eggs, butter, fatty foods, fried foods) then changes should be made in your diet. Look for the *American Heart Association Cookbook* at your local bookstore.

* Visit or write your local Heart Association for further information and copies of free pamphlets on many related subjects including:
  • Reducing your risk of heart attack.
  • Controlling high blood pressure.
  • Eating to keep your heart healthy.
  • How to stop smoking.
  • Exercising for good health.

Some Words of Caution

* If you have diabetes, gout, or a family history of heart disease, your real risk of developing heart disease will be greater than indicated by your RISKO score. If your score is high and you have one or more of these additional problems, you should give particular attention to reducing your risk.

* If you are a woman under 45 years or a man under 35 years of age, your RISKO score represents an upper limit on your real risk of developing heart disease. In this case, your real risk is probably lower than indicated by your score.
* Using your weight category to estimate your systolic blood pressure or your blood cholesterol level makes your RISKO score less accurate.

* Your score will tend to overestimate your risk if your actual values on these two important factors are average for someone of your height and weight.
* Your score will underestimate your risk if your actual blood pressure or cholesterol level is above average for someone of your height or weight.

WOMEN

Find the column for your age group. Everyone starts with a score of 10 points. Work down the page *adding* points to your score or *subtracting* points from your score.

	54 OR YOUNGER	55 OR OLDER

1. WEIGHT

Locate your weight category in the table below. If you are in . . .

	54 OR YOUNGER	55 OR OLDER
	STARTING SCORE **10**	STARTING SCORE **10**
weight category A	SUBTRACT 2	SUBTRACT 2
weight category B	SUBTRACT 1	SUBTRACT 1
weight category C	ADD 1	ADD 1
weight category D	ADD 2	ADD 1
	EQUALS ☐	EQUALS ☐

2. SYSTOLIC BLOOD PRESSURE

Use the "first" or "higher" number from your most recent blood pressure measurement. If you do not know your blood pressure, estimate it by using the letter for your weight category. If your blood pressure is . . .

		54 OR YOUNGER	55 OR OLDER
A	119 or less	SUBTRACT 2	SUBTRACT 3
B	between 120 and 139	SUBTRACT 1	ADD 0
C	between 140 and 159	ADD 0	ADD 3
D	160 or greater	ADD 1	ADD 6
		EQUALS ☐	EQUALS ☐

3. BLOOD CHOLESTEROL LEVEL

Use the number from your most recent blood cholesterol test. If you do not know your blood cholesterol, estimate it by using the letter for your weight category. If your blood cholesterol is . . .

		54 OR YOUNGER	55 OR OLDER
A	199 or less	SUBTRACT 1	SUBTRACT 3
B	between 200 and 224	ADD 0	SUBTRACT 1
C	between 225 and 249	ADD 0	ADD 1
D	250 or higher	ADD 1	ADD 3
		EQUALS ☐	EQUALS ☐

4. CIGARETTE SMOKING

If you . . .

	54 OR YOUNGER	55 OR OLDER
do not smoke	SUBTRACT 1	SUBTRACT 2
smoke less than a pack a day	ADD 0	SUBTRACT 1
smoke a pack a day	ADD 1	ADD 1
smoke more than a pack a day	ADD 2	ADD 4
	FINAL SCORE EQUALS ☐	FINAL SCORE EQUALS ☐

WEIGHT TABLE FOR WOMEN

Look for your height (without shoes) in the far left column and then read across to find the category into which your weight (in indoor clothing) would fall.

YOUR HEIGHT FT IN	WEIGHT CATEGORY (lbs.) A	B	C	D
4 8	up to 101	102-122	123-143	144 plus
4 9	up to 103	104-125	126-146	147 plus
4 10	up to 106	107-128	129-150	151 plus
4 11	up to 109	110-132	133-154	155 plus
5 0	up to 112	113-136	137-158	159 plus
5 1	up to 115	116-139	140-162	163 plus
5 2	up to 119	120-144	145-168	169 plus
5 3	up to 122	123-148	149-172	173 plus
5 4	up to 127	128-154	155-179	180 plus
5 5	up to 131	132-158	159-185	186 plus
5 6	up to 135	136-163	164-190	191 plus
5 7	up to 139	140-168	169-196	197 plus
5 8	up to 143	144-173	174-202	203 plus
5 9	up to 147	148-178	179-207	208 plus
5 10	up to 151	152-182	183-213	214 plus
5 11	up to 155	156-187	188-218	219 plus
6 0	up to 159	160-191	192-224	225 plus
6 1	up to 163	164-196	197-229	230 plus
ESTIMATE OF SYSTOLIC BLOOD PRESSURE	119 or less	120 to 139	140 to 159	160 or more
ESTIMATE OF BLOOD CHOLESTEROL	199 or less	200 to 224	225 to 249	250 or more

Because both blood pressure and blood cholesterol are related to weight, an estimate of these risk factors for each weight category is printed at the bottom of the table.

MEN

Find the column for your age group. Everyone starts with a score of 10 points. Work down the page *adding* points to your score or *subtracting* points from your score.

		54 OR YOUNGER	55 OR OLDER

1. WEIGHT

Locate your weight category in the table below. If you are in . . .

	54 OR YOUNGER	55 OR OLDER
	STARTING SCORE [10]	STARTING SCORE [10]
weight category A	SUBTRACT 2	SUBTRACT 2
weight category B	SUBTRACT 1	ADD 0
weight category C	ADD 1	ADD 1
weight category D	ADD 2	ADD 3

2. SYSTOLIC BLOOD PRESSURE

Use the "first" or "higher" number from your most recent blood pressure measurement. If you do not know your blood pressure, estimate it by using the letter for your weight category. If your blood pressure is . . .

		54 OR YOUNGER	55 OR OLDER
		EQUALS [ ]	EQUALS [ ]
A	119 or less	SUBTRACT 1	SUBTRACT 5
B	between 120 and 139	ADD 0	SUBTRACT 2
C	between 140 and 159	ADD 0	ADD 1
D	160 or greater	ADD 1	ADD 4

3. BLOOD CHOLESTEROL LEVEL

Use the number from your most recent blood cholesterol test. If you do not know your blood cholesterol, estimate it by using the letter for your weight category. If your blood cholesterol is . . .

		54 OR YOUNGER	55 OR OLDER
		EQUALS [ ]	EQUALS [ ]
A	199 or less	SUBTRACT 2	SUBTRACT 1
B	between 200 and 224	SUBTRACT 1	SUBTRACT 1
C	between 225 and 249	ADD 0	ADD 0
D	250 or higher	ADD 1	ADD 0

4. CIGARETTE SMOKING

If you . . .

(If you smoke a pipe, but not cigarettes, use the same score adjustment as those cigarette smokers who smoke less than a pack a day.)

	54 OR YOUNGER	55 OR OLDER
	EQUALS [ ]	EQUALS [ ]
do not smoke	SUBTRACT 1	SUBTRACT 2
smoke less than a pack a day	ADD 0	SUBTRACT 1
smoke a pack a day	ADD 1	ADD 0
smoke more than a pack a day	ADD 2	ADD 3
	FINAL SCORE EQUALS [ ]	FINAL SCORE EQUALS [ ]

WEIGHT TABLE FOR MEN

Look for your height (without shoes) in the far left column and then read across to find the category into which your weight (in indoor clothing) would fall.

YOUR HEIGHT FT IN	WEIGHT CATEGORY (lbs.) A	B	C	D
5 1	up to 123	124-148	149-173	174 plus
5 2	up to 126	127-152	153-178	179 plus
5 3	up to 129	130-156	157-182	183 plus
5 4	up to 132	133-160	161-186	187 plus
5 5	up to 135	136-163	164-190	191 plus
5 6	up to 139	140-168	169-196	197 plus
5 7	up to 144	145-174	175-203	204 plus
5 8	up to 148	149-179	180-209	210 plus
5 9	up to 152	153-184	185-214	215 plus
5 10	up to 157	158-190	191-221	222 plus
5 11	up to 161	162-194	195-227	228 plus
6 0	up to 165	166-199	200-232	233 plus
6 1	up to 170	171-205	206-239	240 plus
6 2	up to 175	176-211	212-246	247 plus
6 3	up to 180	181-217	218-253	254 plus
6 4	up to 185	186-223	224-260	261 plus
6 5	up to 190	191-229	230-267	268 plus
6 6	up to 195	196-235	236-274	275 plus
ESTIMATE OF SYSTOLIC BLOOD PRESSURE	119 or less	120 to 139	140 to 159	160 or more
ESTIMATE OF BLOOD CHOLESTEROL	199 or less	200 to 224	225 to 249	250 or more

Because both blood pressure and blood cholesterol are related to weight, an estimate of these risk factors for each weight category is printed at the bottom of the table.

LAB 3. RESTING HEART RATE

Name_____ Section_____ Date_____

Purpose
To assist you in establishing your resting heart rate.

Procedure
1. Put a watch or a clock with a second hand next to your bed. Upon awakening the next morning, locate your pulse and count your heartbeats for one minute. Repeat for three days and record your scores below.

2. Find your average resting heart rate by dividing the total for four days by four.

Day 1_____beats per minute

Day 2_____beats per minute

Day 3_____beats per minute

Day 4_____beats per minute

Total for four days _____ = _____
                         4

My average resting heart rate is _____

Conclusions and Implications
1. Why is it desirable to have a low resting heart rate?

2. If there were any great variations in your resting heart rate from one day to the next, what do you think was the cause?

LAB 4. BLOOD PRESSURE

Name_____ Section_____ Date_____

Purpose
To assist you in establishing your usual blood pressure.

Procedure
Have your blood pressure taken for at least four days* and record the results below.

Results

	Date	Time	Blood Pressure	Where Taken
1.	_____	_____	_____/_____	_____
2.	_____	_____	_____/_____	_____
3.	_____	_____	_____/_____	_____
4.	_____	_____	_____/_____	_____
5.	_____	_____	_____/_____	_____

* Check with your instructor as to possible places to have your blood pressure checked, such as school nurse, class labs, or by using a home blood pressure kit.

Conclusions and Implications
1. What was your typical blood pressure?_____/_____.

2. Is your systolic pressure within normal range?_____

   Is your diastolic pressure within normal range?_____

3. If there were any fluctuations or great variations in your blood pressure, what do you think was the reason?

4. List six factors which could affect your blood pressure.

5. What is hypertension?

6. What effect do you think age has on your blood pressure?

LAB 5. TARGET HEART RATE ZONE

Name_____Section_____Date_____

Target heart rate zone identifies for each person the safe and comfortable range in which aerobic exercise should be performed in order to achieve a training effect.

Purpose
1. To assist you in determining your target heart rate zone. (Chapter 3 includes information on target heart rate.)
2. To acquaint you with a method which can be used throughout your life to determine the target zone.

Procedures
1. Determine your maximum heart rate according to your age.
   The formula is: 220 – age = Maximum Heart Rate
   Example: 220 – 18 (age) = 202 (MHR)

Although, under supervised conditions, you could possibly work at this maximum level, it is not a safe situation for you. Therefore, you must identify your **target zone** —the safe upper limit and minimum lower limit necessary for aerobic training to occur. This rate should be based on your **current resting heart rate.**

2. Subtract your resting heart rate from you maximum heart rate, which gives you your heart rate reserve (HRR)
   Example: 202 (MHR) – 65 (RHR) = 137 (HRR)

3. Multiply your heart rate reserve (HRR) by your training percentages. People who have been inactive and/or possess a low level of fitness should use 60% for the lower limit and 75% for the upper limit. People who have an average level of fitness should use 70% and 85% for training percentages. Then add back in your resting heart rate.
   Example: 137 (HRR) x .70 = 99.90 + 65 (RHR) = 161
   137 (HRR) x .85 = 116.45 + 65 (RHR) = 181
   The target heart rate zone in the example is from 161 to 181 beats per minute.

Calculate your target heart rate zone:

Lower Limit		Upper Limit	
220		220	
-____	(age)	-____	(age)
____	(MHR)	____	(MHR)
-____	(RHR)	-____	(RHR)
____	(HRR)	____	(HRR)
x____	(Lower %)	x____	(Upper %)
____		____	
+____	(RHR)	+____	(RHR)
=____	Target Heart Rate	=____	Target Heart Rate

Conclusions and Implications

1. What is your target heart rate training zone?_____

2. Why is age an implication in determining your target heart rate?

3. Why is your resting heart rate taken into consideration?

4. Why is it necessary to elevate your heart rate above the lower limit during exercise?

5. Should you ever exceed the 85% upper limit?

LAB 6. 1.0 MILE WALK TEST

Name_____ Section_____ Date_____

Purpose
1. To assist you in evaluating your cardiovascular fitness level.

2. To acquaint you with a simple, effective method that you can use to periodically assess your cardiovascular fitness level.

Procedure
1. Wear exercise clothing, including walking or jogging shoes.

2. Determine your pre-exercise heart rate.

3. Perform the 1.0 Mile Walk Test, preferably on a school track or a premeasured course.

4. Upon completion, take your post-exercise heart rate.

Results
Pre-exercise heart rate_____

1.0 Mile Walk Test time:_____minutes,_____seconds

Post-exercise heart rate_____

Conclusions and Implications
1. What was the difference in your pre-exercise and post-exercise heart rates?_____

2. Was this a strenuous exercise for you? Why?

3. What is your fitness category? (See Appendix B.)

LAB 7.   12-MINUTE RUN OR 1.5 MILE RUN

Name_____ Section_____ Date_____

Purpose
1. To assist you in evaluating your cardiovascular fitness level by means of a field test.

2. To acquaint you with an effective means of evaluating your cardiovascular fitness through out life.

Procedure
1. Perform the 12-Minute Run Test or the 1.5 Mile Run Test, following the directions in Chapter two. Try to establish a steady pace that you can maintain for the entire run.

Results
1. What distance did you complete in the 12 minutes?_____
                    or
What was your time for the 1.5 Mile Run?_____

2. What is your rating? (See Appendix B-2.)_____

Conclusions and Implications
1. Did you score as well as you thought you would?

2. Were you able to maintain a steady pace throughout the test?

3. Do you feel this test indicates your true cardiovascular fitness level? Why or why not?

4. What implications does the test have for your exercise needs?

LAB 8. STEP TEST ASSESSMENT

Name_____ Section_____ Date_____

Purpose
1. To assist you in evaluating your cardiovascular fitness level by means of a step test.

2. To acquaint you with effective methods of evaluating your cardiovascular fitness throughout life.

Procedure
Perform either the Harvard Step Test and/or the One-Minute Step Test described in Appendix A-3 or A-4.

Results
1. What was your total score for the Harvard Step Test?_____

   What was your fitness classification?_____

   Did you complete 5 minutes of stepping?_____ _____

2. What was your total score for the One-Minute Step Test?_____

   What was your fitness classification?_____ _____

   Did you complete one minute of stepping?_____

Conclusions and Implications
1. How do the results of these tests compare to each other?

2. If there is a difference, what do you think the reason is?

3. How do these tests compare to your other measures of cardiovascular fitness?

4. Which cardiovascular test seemed the most difficult for you to complete?

5. Do you feel a step test is an accurate measure of your cardiovascular fitness level? Why or why not?

LAB 9. MUSCULAR STRENGTH AND ENDURANCE

Name_____ Section_____ Date_____

Purpose
1. To assist you in evaluating your overall level of muscular strength and endurance.

2. To acquaint you with effective methods of evaluating your level of strength and endurance throughout life.

Procedure
Following the instructions and guidelines in Appendix A-8, perform the various tests of strength and endurance.

Results
Record the results of each test below:

	Score	Rating
Back Lift	_____	_____
Leg Lift	_____	_____
Grip: Dominant Hand	_____	_____
Non-Dominant Hand	_____	_____
Pull-Ups (Males)	_____	_____
Inclined Pull-Up (Females)	_____	_____
Dips	_____	_____
Push-Ups	_____	_____
Crunches	_____	_____

Conclusions and Implications
1. Did you score as well as you thought you would on all tests?

   Which ones surprised you?

2. Which areas of your body seem to be the weakest?

   The strongest?

3. What implications do the tests have for your exercise needs?

LAB 10. OPTIMAL WEIGHT

Name_____ Section_____ Date_____

Purpose
1. To assist you in determining the optimal body weight.

2. To acquaint you with a method of determining optimal body weight which can be utilized throughout life.

Procedure
1. Determine your percentage of body fat by following the procedures in Appendix A-6.

2. Determine your current body weight_____and height_____.

3. Compute for optimal weight using the formula below:

   1. Fat Weight = $\dfrac{\text{Weight x \% fat}}{100}$

   2. Fat Free Weight = Weight – Fat Weight

   3. Desired Weight
      Women at 18% Fat = $\dfrac{\text{Fat Free Weight}}{.82}$

      Men at 12% Fat = $\dfrac{\text{Fat Free Weight}}{0.88}$

Results
1. What is your optimal or desired weight according to the formula?

2. How many pounds are you currently over- or underweight?

Conclusions and Implications
1. How does this calculation compare with your desired weight as determined from the height-weight chart in Chapter 6?

2. Do you feel that this calculation reflects a realistic desired weight for you?

3. What implications do these results have for your diet and exercise plans?

LAB 11. FITNESS TEST RECORD

Name_____ Age _____ Sex _____

TEST AREA	PRE-TEST	POST-TEST
Cardiovascular		
Resting heart rate	_____	_____
Resting blood pressure	_____	_____
Post-exercise blood pressure	_____	_____
Bicycle ergometer	_____	_____
Workload	_____	_____
Steady state heart rate	_____	_____
Liters/minute	_____	_____
ml/kg/min	_____	_____
Vital capacity	_____	_____
One mile walk	_____	_____
1.5 mile/12 min. run	_____	_____
Target heart rate	_____	_____
Body composition		
Weight	_____	_____
Height	_____	_____
Skinfold measurements	_____	_____
chest	_____	_____
abdomen	_____	_____
thigh	_____	_____
triceps	_____	_____
iliac	_____	_____
_____	_____	_____
Body fat %	_____	_____
Pounds of fat	_____	_____
Flexibility		
Trunk extension	_____	_____
Shoulder lift	_____	_____
Sit and reach	_____	_____
_____		
Muscular Strength/Endurance		
Grip strength — dominant hand	_____	_____
— non-dominant hand	_____	_____
Crunches	_____	_____
Push-ups	_____	_____
Pull-ups	_____	_____
_____	_____	_____

LAB 12. FITNESS PROFILE

Name_____ Section_____ Date_____

Purpose
To assist you in evaluating your fitness test results.

Procedure
Plot your fitness pre-test results on the chart below. At the end of the semester, record the post test results, using a pen or pencil of a different color.

RESULTS	1.0 Mile Walk	1.5 Mile/ 12 Min.	Sub Max VO2	Vital Capacity	Body Fat %	Sit and Reach	Trunk Ext.	Shoulder Lift	Abd. Endur	Push Ups	Grip Dom	Grip Non Dom.
Excellent												
Good												
Fair												
Poor												
Very Poor												

Conclusions and Implications
1. On which tests did you score the best?

2. Which areas of fitness need the greatest improvement?

3. Were you pleased with your test results? Why?

LAB 13. DESIGNING YOUR EXERCISE PROGRAM

Name_____ Section_____ Date_____

Purpose
To monitor and improve your fitness level through personal assessment and a self-designed exercise program.

Procedure
Fill out the charts below.

WEIGHT_____RESTING HEART RATE_____RESTING BLOOD PRESSURE _____/_____

Fitness Area	Current Level	Activity or Activities	Specific Exercises	Place	No. Days	Time of Day	How Long	Alone or with Others	Cost
Cardio-vascular									
Flexibility									
Muscular Strength & Endurance									

List below any sports or recreational activities which you plan to include in your exercise program. Be certain to include any intramural, varsity, or recreational sports in which you participate.

Sport or Recreational Activity	Your Skill Level	How Often	How Long	Fitness Benefits of Activity

295

LAB 14. THE EXERCISE SESSION

Name_____ Section_____ Date_____

Purpose
1. To determine whether or not you are reaching your target heart rate during the exercise session.
2. To measure the heart rate during the warmup and cool-down periods.
3. To acquaint you with a method of evaluating the effect of the exercise session on the heart rate.

Procedure
1. Select an aerobic exercise of either jogging, cycling, swimming, or aerobic dance and do it for at least 3 days.
2. Measure the pulse before starting to exercise and record it.
3. At least once during warmup (toward end of the warmup) measure pulse and record.
4. During the exercise session measure the pulse 2 or 3 times, if possible, and record it.
5. Measure the pulse immediately upon stopping the exercise.
6. During the cool-down, measure the pulse 2 or 3 times and record it. Continue to measure the pulse until it is back to your original starting pulse (within a few beats). Note the time it takes for the pulse to go below 120 and to reach the starting point.

Results
Fill in the chart on the next page. Using the space provided below, plot a record of your average pulse rate as you went through the various phases of the exercise session. The chart on page 28 may be used as an example.

EXERCISE SELECTED _____   *TARGET HEART RATE* _____

HEART RATE	Resting	Warm-up	Workout	Cool-down	Recovery
185					
180					
170					
160					
150					
140					
130					
120					
110					
100					
90					
80					
70					
60					
50					

297

HEART RATES

	Day 1	Day 2	Day 3	Day 4	Average
Starting pulse (before exercise)					
During warmup					
During exercise					
Post exercise (at conclusion of exercise)					

	Day 1	Day 2	Day 3	Day 4	Average
During cooldown					
Time to reach less than 120					
Time to reach starting pulse					

Conclusions and Implications

1. What do the results of your lab indicate in regard to your exercise session?

2. What changes do you plan to make in future exercise sessions?

LAB 15. FLEXIBILITY WORKOUT

Name_____ Section_____ Date_____

Purpose

1. To give you an opportunity to experience an exercise program specifically designed to develop flexibility.

2. To acquaint you with an exercise program which you might want to consider as a part of your daily activities.

Procedure

Following the instructions and guidelines, perform the flexibility exercises in Chapter 4.

Results

1. Check below as you complete each exercise.

Exercise

_____ Calf Stretches	_____ Quad Stretch
_____ Side Winder	_____ Shin Stretch
_____ Forward Hurdle Stretch	_____ Inner Thigh Stretch
_____ Back Lotus	_____ Hip Stretch
_____ Neck Stretch	_____ Quadriceps Stretch
_____ Upper Leg and Back Stretch	_____ Hip Flexor
_____ Saddle Stretch	_____ Gastrocnemius & Achilles Tendon Stretch
_____ Hamstring Stretch	_____ Hip & Calf Stretch
_____ Shoulder Stretch	_____ Low Lunge Stretch
_____ Back Stretch	_____ Quadriceps Stretch

2. What type of warmup program did you use?

Conclusions and Implications

1. Were any of the exercises difficult for you? If so, which?

2. Which exercises were the easiest?

3. Which areas of your body seem to need the most work? the least?

4. Which additional exercises would you include in your future flexibility workouts?

5. What are your plans in regard to a regular flexibility exercise program?

LAB 16. AEROBICS

Name_____Section_____Date_____

Purpose
1. To give you an opportunity to experience an exercise program specifically designed to develop cardiovascular fitness, i.e., walking, jogging, cycling, rope skipping.

2. To acquaint you with an exercise program which you might want to continue as part of your daily activities.

Procedure
1. Select one of the exercise programs described in Chapter 4 in the section on Aerobics. Become familiar with how the exercise is to be performed and which level is an appropriate starting point for you.

2. Following the recommended guidelines for the exercises, participate for at least 3 days at a level sufficient for an aerobics workout.

Results
1. Which activity did you choose and why?

2. Complete the following immediately after each day's workout.

	1st Day	2nd Day	3rd Day	4th Day	5th Day	6th Day	7th Day
Time (indicate length of time at target heart rate)							
Intensity (indicate exercise heart rates)							
Duration (indicate length of time at target hear rate)							

3. What type of warmup procedure did you use?

4. What type of cool-down program did you use?

Conclusions and Implications

1. Have you ever participated in this type of exercise program before?

2. Do you think you will continue this type of program?

Why or Why not?

LAB 17. WEIGHT TRAINING

Name_____ Section_____ Date_____

Purpose
1. To give you an opportunity to experience a weight training program specifically designed to develop strength.

2. To acquaint you with a weight training program which you might want to continue as a part of your daily activities.

Procedure
Following the guidelines presented in Chapter 4, select and perform a series of weight training exercises for a total body workout.

Results
1. Indicate below the exercises performed:

   Type of Equipment

   _____Universal Gym   _____Nautilus   _____Hydra-gym

   _____Free Weights   _____Other

   Exercises (List type and number of repetitions)

2. What type of warmup procedure did you use?

   What type of cool-down program did you use?

Conclusions and Implications

1. Why did you choose this particular workout program?

2. Which exercises were the most difficult for you?

3. Which were the easiest?

4. Which areas of your body seem to need the most work?

   The least?

5. Have you participated in this type of weight training program before?

6. Do you plan to continue this type of program in the future?

   Why or why not?

LAB 18. INTERVAL TRAINING

Name_____ Section_____ Date_____

Purpose
1. To give you an opportunity to experience an exercise program designed to develop cardiovascular fitness through the use of an interval training program.

2. To acquaint you with an exercise program you can utilize throughout your life.

Procedure
Read Chapter 4, which describes an interval program, and then perform the series of exercises listed below. You will notice the program starts gradually, becomes progressively more difficult, has recovery periods included, reaches a peak, and then slows down again.

1. Walk 2 laps around the area (basketball court, rectangle, or field) at a moderate pace.
2. Fast walk one-half lap and easy jog one-half lap.
3. Perform stretching and flexibility exercises for 3 to 5 minutes.
4. Walk 2 laps.
5. Jog 1 lap slowly.
6. Walk 1/2 lap to recover.
7. Jog 1 lap at a moderate pace.
8. Slide 1 lap.
9. Jog 1 lap at a moderate pace.
10. Skip 1 lap slowly.
11. Jog 2 laps at a moderate pace.
12. Sprint 1 lap, walk 1/2 lap, sprint 1 lap.
13. Jog 3 laps. (Check heart rate immediately after finishing 3rd lap.)
14. Walk 1/2 lap.
15. Run in place, knees high for 15 seconds.

16. 10 curl ups.
17. Run in place—15 seconds.
18. On back, scissor kick for 15 seconds.
19. Run in place—15 seconds.
20. 10 push-ups.
21. Hop on right foot—15 seconds.
22. 10 Squat jumps.
23. Hop on left foot—15 seconds.
24. On stomach, flutter kick for 15 seconds.
25. Hop on both feet—15 seconds.
26. 10 jackknife sit ups.
27. Run in place 15 seconds. (Check heart rate immediately.)
28. Jog 1 lap slowly.
29. Jog 3 laps at a moderate pace—walk 1 lap.
30. Jog 1 lap at a moderate pace—walk 2 laps to recover.
31. Cool down by doing easy stretching exercises standing and seated.

Results

1. Were you able to complete all the exercises in the program?

   If not, which ones were you unable to complete?

2. Did you reach your target heart rate both times?

Conclusions and Implications

1. Do you consider this a good cardiovascular workout program?

   Why or why not?

2. What could you do to make the program more difficult?

3. Would you be likely to include this type of workout in your exercise program?

LAB 19. RECOVERY HEART RATE

Name_____ Section_____ Date_____

Purpose
1. To determine whether you are returning to a normal heart rate after exercising to reach the target heart rate zone.

2. To acquaint you with a method of evaluating your recovery heart rate.

Procedure
1. Assume a resting position for 5 minutes.

2. Measure starting pulse for 1 minute and record.

3. Figure target heart rate at 70% and 85% levels. You may use 60% and 75% if your fitness level is low.

4. Exercise (on the bicycle, jumping rope, running, step testing, etc.) until the 70% target heart rate is achieved.

5. After the workout, immediately check your pulse. This is your **exercise heart rate**. Your exercise heart rate should not be above the 85% level. If it is, then you worked too hard and should slow down during the next workout.

6. Continue to cool down by walking and resting. Five minutes after your exercise ends, get another heart rate reading. This is your recovery heart rate and it should be **120 or lower.** If your recovery rate is higher than 120, it is another indication that you worked too hard and that you must slow down. Enter your recovery rate in the appropriate space.

7. If your recovery heart rate was above 120 after 5 minutes, check your heart rate again after 10 minutes of rest. By this time your heart rate should be below 100. Record this recovery rate in the appropriate space.

Starting Pulse　　　　　　　　_____
70% Target HR　　　　　　　　_____
85% Target HR　　　　　　　　_____
Length of Time Exercising　　_____
Exercise Heart Rate　　　　　 _____
(immediately after exercise)
Recovery Heart Rate　　　　　_____
(5 minutes after exercise)

Conclusions and Implications

1. What do the results of this lab indicate in regard to the intensity of your exercise program?

2. What specific changes might be appropriate?

3. Physically, how did you feel during and after the workout?

LAB 20. BLOOD PRESSURE RECOVERY

Name_____ Section_____ Date_____

Purpose
To determine the effect of exercise on your blood pressure and to see how quickly your blood pressure returns to the starting level.

Procedure
1. Assume a sitting position for 5 minutes. Measure blood pressure and record.

2. Exercise (on the bicycle, jogging, jumping rope, step testing, etc.) until the 70% target heart rate is reached. (You may use 60% if your fitness level is low)

3. Stop exercising and again assume a sitting position. Partner will determine blood pressure immediately following the exercise bout.

4. Partner will continue to take blood pressure and record it until it returns to the starting rate.

Starting Blood Pressure   _____
70% Target Heart Rate   _____
Exercise Blood Pressure   _____
Recovery Blood Pressure   _____
            1 minute   _____
            3 minutes   _____
            5 minutes   _____
            10 minutes   _____

Conclusions and Implications
1. What do the results of the lab indicate in regard to your blood pressure:
before exercise_____

_____

immediately after exercise_____

_____

recovery rate after exercise_____

_____

2. What other factors besides exercise might cause your blood pressure values to change?

3. How does the well-trained individual's blood pressure respond during exercise?

LAB 21. NUTRITION AND CALORIC ANALYSIS

Name_____ Section_____ Date_____

Purpose
1. To evaluate the foods you eat in regard to calories consumed and nutritional qualities.

2. To provide you with a basis for improving your daily diet.

Procedure
1. Record everything you eat or drink for five days on the chart provided at the end of this lab (or your instructor may have a computer analysis program available for your use). Record what was consumed, how much, and when. Eat as normally as you can.

2. Using Appendix C, estimate the number of calories, grams of carbohydrates, protein, fat, etc., consumed for each day.

Steps for Analysis
1. Total all columns for each day and for the five-day period.

2. Total all calories for each meal of each day.

3. Transfer figures to the Diet Recall Summary form.

4. List the total calories for each meal.

5. Determine the average daily intake in all columns by dividing by 5.

6. Determine average calories from fat, protein, and carbohydrates by multiplying daily average by 9, 4, and 4, respectively.

7. Get percent carbohydrates, fat, and protein intake by dividing total calories into daily average in the area and compare with the optimal.

Conclusions and Implications
1. Circle all carbohydrate figures that were "sweet-tasting" foods (ice cream, soft drinks, sugar, cakes, pies, etc.). This will give you an estimate of sucrose intake.

2. On how many days out of the five did you eat the correct number of servings from the basic food groups?

3. Which food group do you tend to omit?

4. In which food group do you tend to overeat?

5. Did you gain, lose, or maintain your weight during this five-day period?

6. List the vitamins and minerals in which you were deficient and the foods you need to include to correct this deficiency. (If you do not have access to the computer analysis program, you may not be able to answer this question.)

7. Based on your nutrition and caloric analysis (i.e., nutrient percentages, calories, fiber, etc.), what specific recommendations do you have regarding your current eating habits?

NUTRITION AND CALORIE ANALYSIS

Food	Amount	Calories	Protein	Unsaturated Fat	Saturated Fat	Carbo-hydrates	Fiber
TOTALS							

DIET RECALL SUMMARY

1. Total Calories for Each Meal

	1	2	3	4	5
Breakfast					
Lunch					
Dinner					
Snacks					
TOTALS					

2. Totals for 5 days

a. Calories _____

b. Grams of protein _____

c. Grams of fat _____

d. Grams of saturated fat _____

e. Grams of unsaturated fat _____

f. Grams of carbohydrates _____

g. Grams of fiber _____

3. Average Per Day

a. Calories _____

b. Grams of protein _____

c. Grams of fat _____

d. Grams of saturated fat _____

e. Grams of unsaturated fat _____

f. Grams of carbohydrates _____

g. Grams of fiber _____

314

4. Average Calories Per Day Per Nutrient

   a. Multiply average grams of protein per day by 4   _____

   b. Multiply average grams of fat by 9   _____

   c. Multiply average grams of saturated fat by 9   _____

   d. Multiply average grams of unsaturated fat by 9   _____

   e. Multiply average grams of carbohydrates by 4   _____

5. Percentage of Calories from Each Nutrient

   a. Divide average calories per day from protein by average total calories per day.

     Total calories
     per day   ) Calories from protein

   b. Divide average calories per day from fat by average total calories per day.

     Total calories
     per day   ) Calories from fat

   c. Divide average calories per day from saturated fat by average total calories per day.

     Total calories
     per day   ) Calories from saturated fat

   d. Divide average calories per day from unsaturated fat by average total calories per day.

     Total calories
     per day   ) Calories from unsaturated fat

   e. Divide average calories per day from carbohydrates by average total calories.

     Total calories
     per day   ) Calories from carbohydrates

315

LAB 22. ONE DAY CALORIC ANALYSIS

Name_____ Section_____ Date_____

Purpose
1. To analyze types of carbohydrates and amounts of carbohydrates consumed in one day.
2. To analyze fat content in food consumed in one day.
3. To analyze types of protein and amount of protein consumed in one day.

Procedure
1. Record everything you eat or drink in one typical day on the chart provided at the end of this lab.
2. Using Appendix C, estimate the number of calories and grams of carbohydrates, fats, and protein consumed in one day.

Conclusions and Implications
1. a. Identify the complex carbohydrates consumed:

   b. Identify the simple carbohydrates consumed:

   c. Identify the carbohydrates high in fiber:

   d. What was your total number of calories from carbohydrates?

   What percentage of your total calories came from carbohydrates?

2. a. List the foods that contributed the most fat. Place an asterisk (*) next to those foods which are high in nutrients.

   b. List the foods high in saturated fats.

   c. What could you substitute for those foods high in saturated fat?

   d. What was your total number of calories from fats?

   What percentage of your total calories came from fats?

3. a. Determine your protein intake in grams_____. Did it exceed the recommended number of grams?_____(Multiply your body weight in pounds x .36 grams (the RDA for protein). If so, what changes could you make in your diet?

   b. List the foods which contained complete proteins.

   c. List the foods which contained incomplete proteins.

   d. What was your total number of calories from proteins?

   What percentage of your total number of calories came from proteins?

NUTRITION AND CALORIE ANALYSIS

Food	Amount	Calories	Protein	Unsaturated Fat	Saturated Fat	Carbo-hydrates	Fiber
TOTALS							

LAB 23. CALORIC DISTRIBUTION
IN FOOD AND FAT PERCENTAGE

Name_____ Section_____ Date_____

Purpose
1. To enable you to evaluate the processed foods you eat with regard to calories of carbohydrates, fats, and proteins.

2. To enable you to calculate the percent of calories from fat in processed foods.

Procedure
1. Use three processed foods that you eat on a regular basis. From the labels, calculate the information below.

2. Food_____Portion Size_____oz. Calories per portion____

    Protein: _____grams x 4 calories = _____calories

    Carbohydrate: _____grams x 4 calories = _____calories

    Fat: _____grams x 9 calories = _____calories

    Total Calories   = _____

Percent of calories from fat = $\dfrac{\text{grams of fat x 9}}{\text{total calories x 100}}$

Percent of calories from fat = _____%

    Food_____Portion Size_____oz. Calories per portion____

    Protein: _____grams x 4 calories = _____calories

    Carbohydrate: _____grams x 4 calories = _____calories

    Fat: _____grams x 9 calories = _____calories

    Total Calories   = _____

Percent of calories from fat = $\dfrac{\text{grams of fat x 9}}{\text{total calories x 100}}$

Percent of calories from fat = _____%

Food_____Portion Size_____oz. Calories per portion____

Protein: _____grams x 4 calories = _____calories

Carbohydrate: _____grams x 4 calories = _____calories

Fat: _____grams x 9 calories = _____calories

Total Calories = _____

Percent of calories from fat = $\dfrac{\text{grams of fat x 9}}{\text{total calories x 100}}$

Percent of calories from fat = _____%

Conclusions and Implications

1. Do these foods provide more fat than is good for you?

2. How often do you eat them?

3. Could you substitute other foods which contain less fat for these foods? List the substitutes.

LAB 24. INVENTORY OF EATING HABITS

Name_____ Section_____ Date_____

Purpose

1. To help you become more aware of your eating habits.

2. To assist you in understanding the part emotions play in your eating.

3. To help you identify your appetite and eating problems.

Procedure

Using the inventory on the next page:

1. Circle the answer that best describes your eating behavior.

2. Total your score and check your classification.

Results

1. What is your total score?_____

2. What is your classification?_____

Conclusions and Implications

1. How would you summarize the major problems in your eating habits, based on this inventory?

2. What steps do you think you can take to improve your eating habits?

3. Do you believe you can really change your eating habits? Why or why not?

INVENTORY OF EATING HABITS

Read each item and circle the number which best describes your eating habits.

	Very Frequently	Often	Occasionally	Seldom	Never
1. Go for long periods without food.	4	3	2	1	0
2. Been unsuccessful in attempts to lose weight permanently by dieting.	4	3	2	1	0
3. Especially susceptible to the smell, sight, or thought of food.	4	3	2	1	0
4. Feel uneasy if I cannot reach for a snack or drink between meals.	4	3	2	1	0
5. Feel tormented by love/hate feelings about eating.	4	3	2	1	0
6. Avoid eating in public and then eat secretly afterwards.	4	3	2	1	0
7. "Don't care" attitude about my weight.	4	3	2	1	0
8. Wish I looked different.	4	3	2	1	0
9. A rushed feeling prevents planning meals.	4	3	2	1	0
10. Abnormal eating periods.	4	3	2	1	0
11. Others easily influence met to eat even when I am not hungry.	4	3	2	1	0
12. Follow a "binge" with induced vomiting or punitive fasting.	4	3	2	1	0
13. Eat excessively when bored or depressed.	4	3	2	1	0
14. Eat foods I know are "bad" for me.	4	3	2	1	0
15. Parents used, made available, or encouraged sweets.	4	3	2	1	0
16. Fear weight gain.	4	3	2	1	0
17. Sneak or hide foods.	4	3	2	1	0
18. Use drugs (tranquilizers, sleeping pills, apetite suppresants, etc.).	4	3	2	1	0
19. Self-conscius of how my body looks.	4	3	2	1	0
20. Feelings of being in the midst of a "struggle" (over diet or weight).	4	3	2	1	0
21. Fatigue or "wiped out" feelings.	4	3	2	1	0
22. Gulp my food.	4	3	2	1	0
23. Uncontrollable hunger urges.	4	3	2	1	0
24. Stuff myself.	4	3	2	1	0
25. Indulge in sweets.	4	3	2	1	0
26. Eat "on the run."	4	3	2	1	0
27. Eat when not hungry.	4	3	2	1	0
28. Cravings for sweets.	4	3	2	1	0
29. Meals or heavy snacks after 7:00 PM.	4	3	2	1	0
30. Eating binges.	4	3	2	1	0

Classification
Total Score:

59 and below	Healthy eating habits
60 - 80	Average eating habits
81 - 95	Moderately unhealthy eating habits; eating based too much on emotional factors.
96 and above	Unhealthy eating habits based excessively on emotional factors.

LAB 25. WEIGHT CONTROL

Name_____ Section_____ Date_____

Purpose
1. To assist you in establishing specific goals for weight control based on calorie intake and expenditure.

2. To acquaint you with a method of weight control you can utilize throughout your life.

Procedure
Complete each of the steps below using information gained from your nutrition and calorie analysis. Then attempt to utilize the information gained for one week.

Results
Weight_____Optimal Weight_____

Calorie Expenditure
1. Exercise preference   _____
2. Calories expended per minute (see Chart in Appendix D).   _____
3. Number of minutes to exercise each day   _____
4. Calories expended per day (line 2 x line 3)   _____
5. Number of days to exercise each week   _____
6. Number of calories expended in exercise each   _____
    week (line 4 x line 5)
7. Average number of calories expended daily in exercise   _____
    (line 6 ÷ 7 days)

Calorie Intake
8. Average calorie intake from Nutrition Analysis Lab   _____
9. Calorie reduction per day to lose two pounds per week.   _____
10. Total daily calorie intake, without exercise to lose two   _____
    pounds a week (line 8 - line 9)
11. Daily calorie intake to lose 2 pounds per week,   _____
    including exercise (line 10 + line 7).

This total should not be below 1200 for women or 1500 for men.

Indicate on the following chart whether you reached your goal for actual calorie expenditure and intake.

Day	Calorie Expenditure Goal Achieved	Calorie Intake Goal Achieved
Monday	_____	_____
Tuesday	_____	_____
Wednesday	_____	_____
Thursday	_____	_____
Friday	_____	_____
Saturday	_____	_____
Sunday	_____	_____

Conclusions and Implications

1. If you were unable to meet your goal in either area, what were the reasons?

2. Did you gain or lose weight? How much?

3. What implications does this have for future exercise and diet plans?

LAB 26. BLOOD CHOLESTEROL AND TRIGLYCERIDE LEVELS

Name_____ Section_____ Date_____

Purpose
1. To help you understand and evaluate the results of blood cholesterol and triglyceride tests.
2. To acquaint you with the relationships between cardiovascular disease and blood cholesterol and triglyceride levels.
3. To acquaint you with methods of controlling levels of blood cholesterol and triglycerides.

Procedure
1. Have a blood cholesterol and triglyceride analysis performed by a reputable lab.
2. Using the information available in Chapters 2, 5, and 7, evaluate your cholesterol and triglyceride levels as they relate to risk of cardiovascular disease.

Results
Place of blood test _____ Date _____

	Level	*Risk*
Total blood cholesterol	_____	_____
LDL cholesterol	_____	_____
HDL cholesterol	_____	_____
Total cholesterol/HDL ratio	_____	_____
Triglycerides	_____	_____

Conclusions and Implications
1. List three methods to reduce blood cholesterol.

_____

_____

_____

2. What is the importance of the levels of high density lipoproteins and low density lipoproteins to your total cholesterol level?

_____

_____

_____

_____

3. List five foods which should be avoided or eaten in moderation in order to help lower your cholesterol intake. Include milligrams of cholesterol in each food.

Food   Mg of cholesterol

_____   _____

_____   _____

_____   _____

_____   _____

_____   _____

4. The recommended dietary intake of cholesterol should be below _____ mg per day.

5. List three things you can do to help control your blood triglyceride level.

_____

_____

_____

LAB 27. LIFESTYLE MODIFICATION

Name_____ Section_____ Date_____

Purpose
To help you establish goals and plans for modifying your lifestyle.

Procedure
1. Begin by setting realistic goals for changes in your lifestyle in the four areas outlined below.
   Suggestions for Goals:
   Exercise: Flexibility exercises, aerobic program, strength training, low back exercises.
   Nutrition: Fresh fruit and vegetables daily, whole grains, low fat protein and dairy products.
   Stress Management: Relaxation technique, patience, less aggressiveness, remaining calm, time control.
   Drug Dependence: Cutting back on excess use of caffeine, alcohol, tobacco, and other drugs and medications.

2. Then attempt to achieve these goals during the week that follows.

3. Make note of your progress in reaching these goals by using the following chart.

Results

	EXERCISE	NUTRITION	STRESS MANAGEMENT	DRUG DEPENDENCY
GOALS				
Monday				
Tuesday				
Wednesday				
Thursday				
Friday				
Saturday				
Sunday				

Conclusions and Implications

1. Which goals were the most difficult for you to achieve? Why?

2. Do you think you will be able to maintain these goals in the future?

3. Which additional goals do you feel should be added to the list?

LAB 28. STRESSO—A GAME TO DETERMINE STRESS

Name_____ Section_____ Date_____

Purpose: To determine your current stress level.

Procedure: Answer the following questions in the spaces provided below.

STRESSO

Answer the following questions by checking the appropriate ( ) with an **X**.

YES	NO	AT TIMES		
( )	( )	( )	1.	Do you frequently drum your fingers on a table or desk top?
( )	( )	( )	2.	When thinking do you frequently pull a lock of hair, your ear, or scratch your scalp?
( )	( )	( )	3.	Do you curl up your toes when sitting?
( )	( )	( )	4.	Do you grip a pencil so tight your fingers become numb?
( )	( )	( )	5.	Do you frequently clasp or unclasp your hands, or twist objects in your hands?
( )	( )	( )	6.	Do you frequently grind your teeth while awake or asleep?
( )	( )	( )	7.	Does your posture and movement appear stiff?
( )	( )	( )	8.	Do you frequently twist your ring, cross or uncross your legs, or wrap your feet around each other?
( )	( )	( )	9.	Do you worry a lot or have tension headaches?
( )	( )	( )	10.	Are you frequently tired, angry, or frustrated?
( )	( )	( )	11.	Are you frequently constipated?
( )	( )	( )	12.	Do you have trouble sleeping?

SCORING: After checking each question give yourself a +1 for every NO answer; a -1 for every YES answer; and a -1/2 for every AT TIMES answer.

+

			–	
8-12	"Far Out Man or Lady"		8-12	"Like a Clock Spring"
5-7	Loose		5-7	Highly Stressed
3-4	Above Average Looseness		3-4	Above Average Stress
1-2	Average Looseness		1-2	Average Stress

329

LAB 29. STRESS AWARENESS

Name_____ Section_____ Date_____

Purpose
To determine your awareness of stress in your life by tell-tale indicators.

Procedure
Read the symptoms below and check the ones that apply to you.

Psychological	Physical	Behavior
___Nervousness	___No energy	___Nervous Laughter
___Excess worry	___Allergic reactions	___Use of drugs
___Boredom	___Increased heart rate	___Withdrawing
___Lack of concentration	___Backaches	___Foot tapper or finger drummer
___Forgetfulness	___Stiff neck, jaw muscles	___Eat too much
___Irritability	___High blood pressure	___Loudness
___Apathy	___Many colds-flu	___Excess alcohol
___Feeling of hopelessness	___Stomach problems	___Can't sleep
___Anxiety	___Headaches	___Listless
___Hostility-Anger	___Dizziness	___Accident Prone
___Other	___Other	___Other

Conclusions and Implications
Which items bother you most?

What can you do to improve your situation?

Which stress item will be the hardest to change?

LAB 30. HANDLING YOUR STRESS

Name_____Section_____Date_____

Purpose
To understand the reasons why you experience stress in hopes of coping better with stressful situations as they occur.

Procedure
Answer the questions below for a better understanding of the causes of stress in your life.

How often do you feel stressed?

_____All the time
_____Frequently
_____Occasionally
_____Seldom

Describe the most common stressful situations you face and the people who are involved.

Do you experience any of the symptoms of stress? (Depression, headache, fatigue, stomach pains, etc.) If so, describe the situation and the symptom.

How do you usually cope with your stress?

Do you feel you are handling your stressful situations well?

What could you do to improve your handling of the situations?

LAB 31. CONSUMER AWARENESS

Name_____ Section_____ Date_____

Procedure
1. Visit a local health spa, exercise center or sports club.
2. Record answers to the questions listed below.
3. Get copies of any brochures of flyers about the program and a membership contract.

Results
1. Name of center_____

2. Manager or Salesperson's name_____

3. Location_____

4. Number of instructors_____

5. Ages of instructors_____

6. Educational background of instructors_____

7. Hours it is open_____

8. Equipment available_____

9. Special programs available (aerobic dance, fitness evaluation, nutrition analysis, etc.)

_____

_____

10. When and how often is instruction and assistance given (in groups, by appointment, at established times)? _____

11. What is the cost for membership?_____

12. Are there extra charges for any activities or programs?_____

13. Are there any restrictions on when certain pieces of exercise equipment or certain facilities are available?_____

14. Are there locker room and shower facilities?_____

Conclusions and Implications

1. Would you recommend joining this center?

   Why or why not?

2. What did you like most about the center?

3. What did you feel was the greatest drawback to the center?

4. Did the people in charge seem knowledgeable and enthusiastic?

5. Would you personally be interested in joining this center?

   Why or why not?

INDEX

Acesulfame K, 83
Achilles tendonitis, 180
Aerobic, defined, 36
Aerobic dance, 190
Aerobic exercise to music, 39
Aerobic metabolism, 147
Agility, 8
Aging, 140-141
    and exercise, 9, 73-74
    and cholesterol, 138
AIDS, 185-186
Alarm phase, 166
Alcohol use/abuse, 2, 77, 140, 182-183, 192
All-or-none principle, 159
Alveoli, 145
Amenorrhea, 192
Amino acids, 86
Anabolic steroids, 183-184, 193
Anaerobic metabolism, 147
Anaerobic threshold, 150, 160
Angina pectoris, 134
Ankle weights, 190-191
Anorexia nervosa, 120
"Apple" shape, 20, 77, 117
Aqua dynamics, 41
    Program, 45-49
Anemia, 108, 129
Arteries, 125-127, 133-134
Arteriosclerosis, 134
Artificial sweeteners, 82-83
Aspartame, 83
Asthma, 154
Atherosclerosis, 133-134

Back exercises, 187-189
Back lift, 224
Back pain, 186-187
Balance, 8
Basal metabolism rate (BMR), 113-115
    Calculation of, 114
Basic food groups. See Food Groups.
Behavior, 3, 4
Behavior modification, 115, 121-122
Bicycle ergometer test, 17, 209, 235
Blisters, 180
Blood, 128-129
Blood types, 129
Blood pressure, 4, 5, 12, 13, 76
    Evaluation of, 227, 230-231
BMR, 113-115
Body composition, 7, 18-20, 29
    Evaluation of, 18-20, 217-219, 242
Body mass index, 19-20
Breast soreness, 191
Bronchiole(i), 145
Brown sugar, 81
Bulimia, 120
Bursitis, 163

Caffeine, 104, 106
Calcium, 101, 102, 107, 184, 189
Calorie, 113
Caloric expenditure, 72, 112, 113-114
Cancer
    and diet, 108
    and fats, 87, 88

and fiber, 85
and sun, 181-182
Capillaries, 127-128
Carbohydrates, 80-85, 115
    Complex, 80
    Simple, 80
Cardiac muscle, 161
Cardiovascular disease, 130-139, 140-141
    See also Heart disease, Heart attack
Cardiovascular endurance, 7, 29
    Testing, 16-18
Cardiovascular fitness programs, 36-49
Cardiovascular risk factors, 4-5, 12, 14, 130
    See also Heart disease, Cardiovascular disease
Cardiovascular system, 125-142
    Effects of training on, 34, 142
Cardiovascular training pattern, 27
Cartilage, 157
Cellulite, 123
Cholesterol, 4, 5, 12, 14-15, 76, 77, 92-94, 95-97, 130,
        136-139, 141, 142
    and caffeine, 104
    and fats, 87-88, 89
    and fiber, 85
    and fish oil supplements, 107
    and obesity, 111
    HDL, 14-15, 88, 92, 136-137
    LDL, 14-15, 92, 136-137
    Recommended levels, 15, 92-93
    Sources, 92, 93
    Testing, 14-15
    Triglycerides, 14-15
    VLDL, 136-137
Cilia, 147
Coffee, 14, 104, 140
    See Also Caffeine.
Cold-related problems, 181
Complete proteins, 86
Components of fitness, 6-8
    Evaluation of, 12-21
Concentric contraction, 73, 161
Congenital heart defect, 134
Consent form, 12
Consumer concerns, 76, 195-198
Continuous passive motion (CPM) tables, 198
Cool-down, 23, 28, 36
Cooper, Kenneth, 10, 17, 142, 167, 171, 172
Coordination, 8
Coronary heart disease, 4, 5, 12
Cramp, muscle, 163, 178
Cross training, 41-42
Crunches, 222
Cycling, 39
    Program, 44

Deep breathing exercises, 173
Designing training program, 30-31
Diabetes, 4, 12, 111, 130
Diaphragm, 145
Diastole, 13, 125
Diet aids, 118
Diet analysis, 122
Diet plans, 119
Dietary goals (U.S.), 76-77
Diets, 115-123

Disaccharides, 81
Distress, 166
Drinks, 104
Drug use, 2, 189, 192

Eating disorders, 120
Eccentric contraction, 73, 161
Education (and fitness), 10
Electrical impedance, 19
Electrolytes, 101, 103-104
Emphysema, 151
Endorphins, 172
Energy production, 160
Environment, 3, 4
Essential amino acids, 86
Essential fatty acids, 87
Equipment, 197-198
Eustress, 166
Evaluation of fitness components, 12 - 21
Exercise, 2, 5-6
   and aging, 9
   and basal metabolic rate, 115
   and disease, 9-10
   and heart disease, 139
   and muscular system, '61
   and respiratory system, 148-150, 154-155
   and smoking, 153
   and stress, 170-172
   and water, 103-104
   and weight control, 112, 113, 115, 117, 122
   Guidelines, 23, 24
Exercise induced asthma, 154
Exercise program sample, 31
Exercise session, 23-24, 28
Exercises for major muscle groups, 56
Exercises, potentially harmful, 69-71
Exhaustion phase, 167

Fad diets, 117-119
Fast Foods, 95-97, 107
Fasting, 118
Fast-twitch muscle fibers, 157, 159-160
Fat-soluble vitamins, 98
Fats, 77, 87-91
   and cancer, 87, 88
   and fast foods, 95
   and heart disease, 88, 134
   Choices, 89-91
   Functions of, 87-88
   Sources, 91
   Substitutes, 90
Fatty acids, 87
   Monounsaturated, 87-89
   Polyunsaturated, 87-89
   Saturated, 87-89, 90
Fiber, 84-85
   Water insoluble, 84
   Water soluble, 84
   Food choices, 85
"Finger-stick" cholesterol test, 15
Fish oil supplements, 207
Fitness clubs, 196-108
Fitness programs, 36-74
Fitness tests, 16-21, 208-247
   Bicycle ergometer, 17, 209, 235
   Body composition, 18-20, 217-219, 242
   Cardiovascular endurance, 16-18

Harvard Step, 18, 213-214
Muscular fitness, 20-21
One-Mile run, 16-17, 236
One-Mile walking, 16-17
One Minute step, 18, 215, 235
Twelve-Minute/1.5 Mile run, 17-18, 237-239
Flexibility, 7, 21, 29, 63
   Exercises, 64-68
   Evaluation of, 21, 220-221, 247
   Program, 63-68
      Guidelines, 64
Food groups, 77-79
Food labels, 104-106
Foot problems/injuries, 179-180
Framingham Heart Epidemiology Study, 5, 15
Fraud, 195196
Frequency (of exercise), 25, 36
Fructose, 81, 83

Gender, 4
General Adaptation Syndrome, 166-167
Glucose, 81, 104
Glucose-electrolyte replacement solutions (GES), 104
Glycogen, 81, 83
Goals, 2
Grip (test), 226, 243
Guidelines for training, 29, 30

Hand weights, 190-191
Harmful exercises, 69-71
Harvard Step Test, 18, 213-214
HDL cholesterol, 14-15, 92, 132, 136-138, 142
Health. *See* Wellness.
Health questionnaire, 12
Health-related fitness, 3, 6-7
   Tests, 16-21
Health screening tests, 13-16
Hemoglobin, 129
Heart, 125-126
Heart attacks, 5
Heart disease. *See also* Cardiovascular disease.
   and fats, 88
   and fish oil supplements, 107
   and obesity, 111
Heat
   and water intake, 103
   problems related to, 180-181
Heat exhaustion, 181
Heat stroke, 181, 191
Heel pain, 179
Heredity, 3, 4, 130, 134
High blood pressure, 4, 5, 130, 140
   and obesity, 111
   and teenagers, 140
High-density lipoprotein. *See* HDL cholesterol.
High-fructose corn syrup, 82, 83
HIV/AIDS, 185-186
Home exercise program, 58-62
Homeostasis, 166
Honey, 81, 82, 83
Hydrogenation, 87, 88
Hypertension, 13, 101, 134, 135-136
   See Also High blood pressure.
Hypoglycemia, 81, 82
Hypokinetic disease, 7

Imagery, 173
Inactivity, 3

Incomplete proteins, 86
Injuries, 176-180
    Prevention of, 176-177
    Treatment of, 177-178
Insomnia, 170
Institute for Aerobics Research, 5
Intensity (of exercise), 25, 27, 30
Interval training, 38-39
    Program, 44
Iron, 108
Isokinetic, 49, 51
Isometric, 49, 52-53
Isotonic, 49-51

Jogging, 37-38, 72, 74, 191, 192
    Program, 43
    Risks, 74
Junk Food, 95

Knee problems/pain, 179

Labels (food), 104-106
    Terms, 105-106
Laboratory exercises, 267-336
Lactic acid, 160
Lactose, 82
LDL cholesterol, 14-15, 92, 137-139, 142
Leg lift, 225
Leg problems/injuries, 179-180
Lifestyle, 2, 112, 122
Ligaments, 157
Low impact aerobics, 39
Low-density lipoprotein. *See* LDL cholesterol.
Lung capacity, 16, 232-234
Lungs. *See* Respiratory system.

Marijuana smoking, 151-152
Massage, 198
Maximum oxygen uptake, 147, 154
Medical examination, 12
Meditation, 172-173
Menstrual cramps, 192
Mental health, 6
METS, 113
Minerals, 101-103
    Macrominerals, 101, 102
    Trace, 101, 102
Minimum Daily Requirement (MDR), 101
Mitochondria, 157
Molasses, 81
Monosaccharides, 80-81
Monounsaturated fat, 87-89, 91
Motor unit, 159
Muscle
    Balance, 42
    Contractions, 161-162
    Cramps, 178
    Fibers, 159-160
    Pulls, 178
    Resistance methods, 53
    Soreness, 33, 178
    Structure, 157-160
    Toning, 23, 24
Muscles of the body, 54-55
    effects of training on, 162-163
    types of, 160-162
    problems (injuries), 178
Muscular endurance, 7, 20, 29
    Evaluation of, 20, 222-226, 243-247

    Program for, 49-62
Muscular fitness, 20
Muscular strength, 7, 20, 29
    Evaluation of, 20
    Program for, 49-62
Muscular system, 157-164
Myofibrils, 157
Myoglobin, 157

New American Eating Guide, 78-79
Nutrients, 80-104
Nutrition, 2, 3, 75-109
    Advice, 109
    Labels, 104-106
Nutritive value of foods, 250-259

Obesity, 4, 6, 111-112
One-Mile Run Test, 16-17, 236
One-Mile Walking Test, 16-17
One Minute Step Test, 18, 215, 235
Osteoporosis, 184, 189
Overload, 24, 25, 27, 30
Overweight, 111-112
Oxygen capacity continuum, 149
Oxygen consumption, 147-148
Oxygen debt, 147
Oxygen deficit, 36, 147

Passive smoke, 154
"Pear" shape, 20, 77, 117, 123
Peripheral vascular disease, 134
Physical fitness, defined, 6-8
Plantar fasciitis, 179
Plasma (blood), 129
Platelets (blood), 129
Polysaccharides, 81
Polyunsaturated fat, 87-89, 91
Posture, 20
Power, 8
Pregnancy
    and caffeine, 104
    and exercise, 189
    and obesity, 111
    and smoking, 153-154
Premature death, 4, 6
Premenstrual Syndrome (PMS), 104
Principles of training, 24-26
Program, selection of, 35-74
Progression, 24, 25, 27, 30
Progressive muscle relaxation, 172, 173
Prone trunk extension test, 220-221, 247
Proprioceptive Neuromuscular Facilitation (PNF), 63-64
Protein(s), 86-87, 107-108, 115
    Complete, 86
    Incomplete, 86
    Sources, 86
Pull-ups, 223-224, 244
Pulse, 13-14, 72, 128
Push-ups, 222-223, 245-246

Quacks, Quackery, 195-198

Reaction time, 8
Recommended Dietary Allowance (RDA), 99-100, 101, 102, 104, 105
Recovery heart rate, 27, 28
Recreational activity, 2
Red blood cells, 128-129
Resistance phase, 167

Respiratory system, 145-155
Response rates (to training), 26
Rest, 2
Resting heart rate, 13-14, 26-27
    Evaluation of, 232
Retrogression, 26
RICE (treatment), 178
Risk factors. *See* Cardiovascular Risk Factors.
Rockport Walking Institute/Walking Test, 16, 17, 208, 240-241
Rope jumping, 40-41
    Program, 45
Rubberized suits, 190
Running, 37-38, 43, 142, 191

Saccharin, 83
Safety in exercise, 33, 51
Salt, 77, 101, 103
    Substitutes, 103
Sarcolemma, 157
Sarcoplasm, 157
Saturated fat, 77, 87-89, 90, 91
Second wind, 33
Selecting fitness program, 35-74
Set point, 123
Shin splints, 179
Shoulder lift test, 221, 247
Sit and reach test, 220, 245
Skeletal muscle, 164
Skill, 26
Skill-related fitness, 8
Skinfold calipers, 18-19, 217
Sleep, 2, 169-170
Sleeping pills, 174
Slow-twitch muscle fibers, 157, 159-160
Smoking, 2, 4, 5, 14, 130, 139, 151-154
Smoking cessation, 152
Smooth muscle, 161
Sodium, 77, 101, 103
Sorbitol, 82, 83
Sore muscles, 163, 178
Spas, 196-197
Specificity, 24, 25-26
Speed, 8
Sphygmomanometer, 13
Spirometer, 6
Spot reducing, 123
Sprains, 179-180
Static contraction, 162
Steady state, 147-148
Step aerobics, 40
Steroids. *See* anabolic steroids.
"Stitch in the side," 190
Stress, 2, 130, 165-174
    Sources of, 168-169
    Warning signs, 167
Stress management, 3, 165-174
Stressor, 166
Striated muscle, 161
Stroke, 134
Sucrose. *See* Sugar.
Sugar, 77, 81-83
    Content of foods, 250
    Substitutes, 82-83
Suicide, 6
Sun
    and cancer, 181-182

    and eyes, 193
Sun screens, 182
Sunglasses, 193
Supplements, 98, 107
Sweating, 33
Systole, 13, 125

Tanning salons, 198
Target fat rate, 88
Target heart rate, 26-28, 36
Tendons, 157
Time (duration) of exercise, 24, 27
Total fitness, 2, 3, 6
Trachea, 145
Training, 23
    Principles of, 24-26
Training Program, 23-32
    Guidelines, 29, 30
Tranquilizers, 174
Triglycerides, 14-15, 87, 136
Twelve-Minute Run/1.5 Mile Test, 17-18237-239
Type A personality, 174

Varicose veins, 128, 191
Vascular problems, 133-135
Vegetarian diet, 108-109
Veins, 127-128
Very low density lipoprotein (VLDL), 136, 137
Vital lung capacity, 16, 147, 216
Vitamins, 98-101
    Fat-soluble, 98
    MDR, 101
    RDA, 101
    Sources, 98, 99-100
    Supplements, 98
    Water-soluble, 98

Walking, 36-37, 74
    Program, 43
    Test (Rockport), 208, 240-241
Warm-up, 23, 28, 36, 159
Warning signals, 2
Water, 103-104
    and exercise, 103-104
    Bottled, 109
Water workout, 72
Water-soluble vitamins, 98
Weight, healthy, 76-77, 112
Weight control, 2,3, 111-123, 136
    Guidelines, 115-117
Weight gain, 121
Weight loss, 115-119
Weight training, 49-51, 73, 74
    Safety precautions, 51
Wellness, 2
    Components of, 2
    Physical (physiological), 2, 3
    Psychological, 2, 3
    Social, 2, 3
Wellness continuum, 2
White blood cells, 129
Women
    and alcohol, 140, 192
    and iron intake, 108
    and maximum oxygen intake
    and physical activity, 33
    and weight training, 50-51, 73
Workout, 23-24, 28